More Than Meets the Eye

More Than Meets the Eye

WHAT BLINDNESS BRINGS TO ART

Georgina Kleege

OXFORD
UNIVERSITY PRESS

OXFORD
UNIVERSITY PRESS

Oxford University Press is a department of the University of Oxford. It furthers the University's objective of excellence in research, scholarship, and education by publishing worldwide. Oxford is a registered trade mark of Oxford University Press in the UK and certain other countries.

Published in the United States of America by Oxford University Press
198 Madison Avenue, New York, NY 10016, United States of America.

CIP data is on file at the Library of Congress
ISBN 978-0-19-060436-3 (pbk.)
ISBN 978-0-19-060435-6 (hbk.)

For Arien

The blindness in this story isn't a metaphor.

—ANNE FINGER, "*THE BLIND MARKSMAN*"

{ CONTENTS }

{ ACKNOWLEDGMENTS }

Portions of this book have appeared in *Disability Studies Quarterly, Journal of Literary and Cultural Disability Studies, Representations, Social Research*, and *The Journal of Visual Culture*. I am grateful to all the editors for their support of this project.

In 2002, Fiona Candlin and Caro Howell invited me to speak at a symposium called "Challenging Occularcentricity in Museum Practice," at the Tate Modern in London, which set this project in motion. I am also grateful to Martin Jay for inviting me to the "Show and Tell" conference at Berkeley in 2004, where my investigation of the Hypothetical Blind Man began. Katherine Sherwood and Elizabeth Dungan curated the "Blind at the Museum" exhibit in 2005, which introduced me to several of the artists featured in the book. The "Blind Creations" conference at Royal Holloway, University of London in 2015, organized by Hannah Thompson and Vanessa Warren introduced me to several others. I am also thankful to David Feeney and Daniel Thornton for inviting me to participate in a panel called "More Than Meets the Eye" at the Edinburgh International Film festival in 2013, which gave the book its title.

Time and again I have turned to artists Suzanne Lacke and Katherine Sherwood to describe images, explain painting and drawing techniques, and generally share their knowledge and expertise.

Gabriella Wyatt helped select images and obtain the permissions to reproduce them.

I am indebted to the following people for their advice, suggestions, friendship, and description of images, without which this book would not have happened: Elizabeth Abel, Patrick Anderson, Devon Bella, Brenda Jo Brueggemann, Anastasia Howe Bukowski, Will Butler, Amanda Cachia, Catherine Cole, Michael Davidson, Piet Devos, Nadia Ellis, Anne Finger, Lakshmi Fjord, Maria Flamich, Ann Fox, Rosemarie Garland-Thomson, Florian Grond, Gili Hammer, Leon Hilton, Rita Hoffman, Catherine J, Kudlick, Petra Kuppers, Nina Levent, Victoria Lewis, Heather Love, Victoria Marks, Darrin Martin, Josh Miele, Mara Mills, Karen Nakamura, Corbett O'Toole, Joan Muyskens Pursley, Babette Schmidt, Susan M. Schweik, C. Namwali Serpell, Jennifer Sutton, Scott Wallin, Zina Weygand.

At Oxford University Press I am grateful to Brendan O'Neill for his faith in this project and to Sarah Pirovitz for her ongoing support. Abigail Johnson has been endlessly helpful. India Gray has been a vigilant copyeditor and Rajakumari Ganessin has managed the many phases of the production with efficiency and grace.

{ A NOTE ON CAPTIONS AND IMAGES }

I have tried to describe all the images in the body of the text, while the captions simply provide the titles, artist, and the necessary copyright information. I hope that this will be less intrusive for people who read aurally and tactually.

More Than Meets the Eye

Introduction

The topic for this book came to me almost by accident. In 2002, I was invited to speak at a symposium at the Tate Modern in London, on the topic of access to the visual arts for people who are blind and visually impaired. The symposium organizers had read my book, *Sight Unseen*, where I describe, among other things, growing up as the legally blind daughter of two visual artists. Due to this family background, and the personal inclination that grew out of it, I have always spent a lot of time in art museums. I have been known to travel some distances to attend exhibits of favorite artists and would generally classify myself as an art lover. At the time, however, I had never looked into access programs because I was accustomed to providing my own access, in the person(s) of friends and family members who went with me to look at art. Typically, they would read me the labels and enhance whatever impressions my impaired perceptions allowed me to form through their opinions and insights. I knew that with the passage of antidiscrimination legislation like the Americans with Disabilities Act, art museums, like other public institutions, were tasked with making their facilities and collections accessible to people with disabilities. I had observed the addition of ramps and automatic doors to many museums I visited at home and abroad but had never really thought much about what access to visual art would mean for blind people.

When I began to research access programming that was already in place at institutions around the world, I was at first heartened by what I discovered. There was a lot going on. With a little effort or advance warning, it was possible to find some sort of program nearly everywhere. But as I looked deeper, what I discovered was somewhat disturbing. The vast majority of these programs seemed aimed at one of two overlapping groups. The first target audience was blind children. I have no problem with this. In fact, with the general decline of arts education in the public schools, it seems admirable and desirable that museums should take over this task, for the benefit of both blind and sighted children. But the other target audience was a bit at odds with reality. Programs seemed aimed at totally and congenitally blind adults who not only had no prior experience of art or art history but also little or no knowledge of visual terminology. This seemed to me to defy logic and demographics, when one considers that the vast majority of blind and visually impaired people in the industrialized world are adults who were formerly sighted. Furthermore, it seemed logical that the average blind adult likely to seek out these services, born that way or not, would have some prior knowledge of visual art, art history, and visual terms and concepts. This then was my starting point. Is there a way to provide access to the visual arts for blind people that does not demean those who are supposed to benefit?

When I tell people that I'm working on a book about blindness and visual art, I have come to expect a particular response. To put the words *blindness* and *visual art* in the same sentence may seem like the punchline to a tasteless joke or part of a simile denoting futility, as in, "that makes about as much sense as a blind person in an art museum." In my defense, I'd point out that I'm not the first person to pair blindness with visual art. Indeed, the history of speculation on visual art, and human vision in general, is haunted by ideas about blindness. For example, Denis Diderot's essay, "Notes on Painting" (1765) begins with a description of a blind woman. Of all the many subjects and styles of painting he could use to launch his discussion, why choose an image of blindness? Since then, when theorists imagine a spectrum of human visual experience they place the blind man at one end, standing for the complete absence of vision. The other endpoint is occupied not by a person with merely average vision, but by the artist, someone understood to possess extra special vision. The artist is depicted as a sort of superman of seeing, able to see more or better than ordinary people, and to show, not just what he sees but also how best to look at it. Consider this example where the critic, Leo Steinberg imagines a dialogue about art between a blind man and Jasper Johns:

> It is part of the fascination of Johns's work that many of his inventions are interpretable as meditations on the nature of painting, pursued as if in dialogue with a questioner of ideal innocence and congenital blindness.
>
> *A picture, you see, is a piece of cotton duck nailed to a stretcher.*
>
> *Like this?* says the blindman, holding it up with its face to the wall. Then Johns makes a picture of that kind of picture to see whether it will make a picture (Johns, *The Canvas*, 1956).[1]

There are also many instances of the familiar cliché about the paradoxical "blindness" of visual artists, which seem to crop up in many depictions of the artistic process. It's a distinctively romantic notion of the artist as so utterly possessed by his muse that he produces the artwork without deliberate effort or even conscious awareness. For example, at the beginning of Henri-Georges Clouzot's documentary *The Mystery of Picasso*, the voiceover intones:

> The painter stands like a blind man in the darkness of the white canvas. The light that slowly appears is paradoxically created by the painter who draws one black curve after another. For the first time, the daily, private drama by the blind genius will be experienced publicly.[2]

Similarly, in *The Object Stares Back*, James Elkins suggests that all drawing has something to do with blindness. Elkins asserts that the visual artist relies on touch at least as much as on sight and that this reliance simulates an experience of blindness.

He also represents blindness as the polar opposite of vision, as a complete void, a force to struggle against and overcome:

> A drawing also begins in blindness, with a pure white sheet. At the moment when the artist sets pencil to paper there is nothing to see, and the first mark is made in isolation and framed by emptiness. As the pencil travels along the page, it always moves into blindness, leaving behind a narrow path of vision. Unless the entire page is covered with marks (and in the history of drawing, it is rare to find an image that is principally marks, where the marks have won out against the blank page), the drawing exists mostly in blindness. A small fraction of the sheet will be marked out, like paths through a wilderness, and the remainder will be a trackless surface. A drawing is an expression of a dialogue with blindness, and the most beautiful drawings are beautiful because they show it is sometimes possible to win that battle and produce a form out of nothing. [3]

Here, blindness is initially the purity of the blank sheet of paper, but it rapidly morphs into a trackless wilderness. Then the dialogue with blindness becomes less a mutual exchange than a life and death battle that must be won. Beauty in art only occurs when the artist is victorious in this mortal combat.

I am interested in these metaphorical depictions of blind people and artists, as well as the many stories, novels, films, and other cultural texts that extend these metaphors into narratives. I am also intrigued, and at times horrified, by how much early philosophical speculation and contemporary cognitive science use blind people, both imaginary and real, to theorize how human beings understand pictorial representation. An additional concern, however, is more practical and personal. As a potential consumer of access programs now available at museums, I'm interested in exploring how well they work and how they might work better. While I am gratified by the proliferation of access programs, I feel compelled to scrutinize ideas about blindness that shape the image of the intended audience for these services.

This might prompt the comment, "When you say blind access to visual art, you mean people like you, people who are only partially blind, people who remember being sighted, not people who are really blind, blind since birth, totally blind."

My use of the word "blind" to encompass the widest possible range of visual impairments has a long history. For instance, the National Federation of the Blind, founded in 1940, has long held that calibrating distinctions between the totally, congenitally blind, the adventitiously blind, the visually impaired, the partially sighted and so forth, actually dilutes the political impact of a group of admittedly diverse individuals who nevertheless have common social, educational, and vocational goals. For instance, the editor of *The Braille Monitor*, the Federation's newsletter, introducing an article on a tactile museum in Athens, Greece, noted that in her original text the author

> was scrupulous about always referring to both blind and visually impaired people. Since we recognize everyone with a significant visual impairment as legally or functionally blind, I have simplified these references. Those who are not used to grouping people with significant vision loss into a single category should understand that all people who experience difficulty in seeing museum displays are included in this discussion.[4]

There are many purists who prefer to reserve the word *blind* to designate only those individuals who were born with no visual experience at all. Total congenital blindness, however, is a rare occurrence in the industrialized world today. Only about 3 newborns out of 10,000 births have no visual perception. Furthermore, blind adults who might be consumers of access programs are self-selecting. It's safe to assume that a recently blinded person who is still traumatized by the loss of sight, whether total or partial, is probably unlikely to seek out these programs. So statistically speaking, the typical consumer of these services is, in fact, someone like me.

A little autobiographical information may be necessary here. I was not born blind, but became blind at about the age of eleven. I am not totally blind. The technical designation for someone like me is legally blind with some usable sight. Legality comes into it in that my vision impairment is significant enough to make me legally eligible for certain federal and state educational and rehabilitation programs. It's worth noting the definition of legal blindness that came into being in the 1930s turns on two specific facets of visual functioning—visual acuity and peripheral vision. In effect, blindness is determined according to the person's inability to perform two culturally significant visual activities—reading print and maneuvering unaided through space. The eyes of the law are not concerned with the person's ability to perceive color, light, or form, visual skills that might have more to do with looking at art.

The "some usable sight" aspect of my vision impairment is a bit murkier. I do see something. For instance, I can tell light from darkness, can identify most colors, and can perceive motion with some degree of accuracy. I cannot perceive fine detail such as print on a page or features on a face. Forms appear amorphous with unstable outlines that seem constantly on the verge of merging into their surroundings. The degree to which I actively use this visual experience varies widely. I can make sense of the wavering forms and blurry blobs before my eyes mainly because I have a good sense of what's out there.

People tell me that I don't look blind. Much of the time I think this is because I don't have the blank zombie stare and tentative, groping movements that most sighted actors assume when portraying a blind character on stage or screen. When people talk to me, I turn my face in their direction, and my eyes may line up more or less with theirs. Apparently this looks like eye contact, even though it feels like nothing for me. But I think that people also assume that when I do things I must be using my residual vision, when in fact I may be employing no visual discernment. Once, a neighbor commented that my house looked very clean. I said that I'd just vacuumed. She at first expressed surprise that I could vacuum by myself but then amended, "Oh, but you can see something." While it's true that I can generally make out the forms of the furniture, I know where it is because I put it there. But I cannot see the dust on the floor. Isn't that why anyone uses a vacuum cleaner—to clean up the dirt they cannot see?

If others assume that I use my eyes more than I actually do, I too am sometimes prone to give my eyes more credit than they deserve. Sometimes I engage in what I call "wishful seeing." By this I mean that I sometimes actively attempt to interpret the impaired images my eyes give me in a way that anticipates a desired outcome. When I am waiting for the bus, I train my gaze down the street and attend to every change in the visual array. The vehicles moving toward me, light reflected off their surfaces or filtering through leaves overhead all combine to give the illusion that the bus is there, only a block away. But every time, I hear the bus's telltale wheezing transmission long before it's anywhere near where I might be able to identify it visually. On a couple of occasions when the jack hammers of some nearby street work drowned out all the regular sounds, the bus actually surprised me as it pulled up at the stop even though I was looking for it.

While these particularities of my impairment are not unusual, there are some aspects to my blind identity that make me perhaps atypical. The first is that I know a lot about the visual arts. Because both my parents were visual artists, I grew up surrounded by their work, their materials, and tools. Even more significantly, I grew up surrounded by their talk about visual art and visual matters. I spent a lot of time in artists' studios, art galleries and museums, and heard a lot of talk about what artists see in one another's work and in the world in general. Still the knowledge I claim to have about art is mostly based on hearsay—what I have heard said or read about it. In fact, much of what I know about many of the artists in my parents' circle is in the order of gossip about their love affairs and drunken misbehavior. My firsthand knowledge of art is limited, except of course for those works I have been allowed to touch. Incidentally, it has been my experience that artists are a lot less squeamish about letting people touch their work then are art conservators. Without name-dropping, I admit here that my fingerprints are all over any number of mid-twentieth-century art on display in museums and private collections around the world.

On top of what I claim to know about visual art, I know a good deal about vision. Having written extensively about blindness, I have studied human visual perception. I can name all the parts of the eyeball, describe all the conditions that impair sight, identify regions of the brain related to different aspects of vision, and refer to major research studies.

Another complicating factor in my blind identity, however, is that while I know a lot about vision and visual art, or at least can speak with some semblance of knowledge on these subjects, my vision is not at the forefront of my consciousness. In my book, *Sight Unseen*, I tried to create a detailed phenomenology of my impaired vision. I did this because ophthalmology and perception texts I consulted did what I considered an inadequate job. Those descriptions were written from the perspective of someone looking at flawed eyes from the outside, while extrapolating what the visible imperfections there would do to what an undamaged eye would see. In other words, authors of those texts took an image then erased the parts they understood to be affected by a particular impairment. They rarely consulted anyone looking at the world through that impairment. At best, they could come up with a list of symptoms that an eye-care specialist should expect to hear from a patient experiencing some new vision loss. More importantly, these medical descriptions did not consider how the experience of lost vision might change over time. A facet of vision loss that is seldom contemplated is that, over time, one loses faith in vision that has ceased to be faithful to reality.

As I was finishing *Sight Unseen*, one night I was washing potatoes for dinner. Because of the book, I was practicing putting my visual experiences into words. Every activity, no matter how mundane, provided additional opportunities. On this occasion, I was trying to find words to express the look of the running water and the sheen of the chrome faucet. I was having trouble separating what I was seeing from what I was feeling—the slightly fizzy stream of warm water—and what I was hearing—the shush of the water over the faint gurgle of the drain. I could tell that the sounds were influencing the image. The vibration that is always at the center of my visual field was somehow in synch with the sound.

And then I told myself to let it go. I had already written enough examples. This one was at once too complex and too silly. Instantly everything changed. The image did not go blank or black. It simply receded from the taut center of my attention. I relaxed into the sensations coming from my hand as my fingers rubbed the skin of the potato where the few last remnants of dirt flaked off and dissolved in the running water.

Since I have lived with impaired vision for over forty years, blindness is normal for me. In everyday situations, at home, at work, traveling to and fro,

I rarely make use of my residual vision. The residual vision that I have is so unreliable and inadequate that it would be foolish and unsafe to attempt to use it in these contexts. In fact, the only occasion when I regularly make use of the vision I have is when I visit an art museum. Saying this can give the mistaken impression that I can turn my vision on and off, as if it were a binary system. People might wonder why, if I can use my vision to look at a painting, why can't I use it to read the print on my computer screen? The answer is that my synthesized-voice screen reader allows me to perform that task more efficiently and painlessly than my eyes ever will. As yet, there is no analogous technology for looking at art, which is why I am interested in access programs that can enhance my impaired perceptions.

Note that in defining my blind identity, the degree of sight loss is only one of many factors. It is equally significant to consider age of onset and what we might call visual interest or literacy. The simple binary—blindness versus sightedness—is not adequate here. There are people, both sighted and blind, who simply are not all that interested in visual art or visual matters. But I assume that none of them will read this book. And in any case, all this is probably more information than my concerned interlocutor—who was only making polite inquiries about the subject of my new book—wants to know about me. Perhaps I should simply respond that when I talk about blind access to visual art of course I'm not talking about those blind people, the totally, congenitally blind people, the truly blind, the pure blind. I'm talking about people like me: the adventitiously blind, the visually impaired with some usable sight and some prior knowledge of visual art, the legally blind who admit to the illegal touching of valuable works of art.

But what if I am talking about *those* blind people? What, if anything, does that change? After all, I know totally congenitally blind people who might be interested in visual art if given the opportunity. And there is a danger in subscribing to a hierarchy of impairment, pitting those who can be accommodated with minimal effort and expense against others for whom accommodation requires more ingenuity. I prefer to start from the premise that a totally blind person, even one who has never had any visual perception at all, can nevertheless conceptualize features of visual experience. I believe that even *those* blind people have some understanding of such things because they live in the same visual culture as the rest of us. They grew up, attended school, and work among sighted people. They read books; listen to radio, TV, and movies; and inhabit architecture, created by and for sighted people. In fact, I would argue that the average totally, congenitally blind person knows infinitely more about what it means to be sighted than the average sighted person knows about what it means to be blind.

Let's zero in on one of these features of visual experience—color. Is it possible to talk about color to someone who has never seen it? It would be next to impossible for a totally, congenitally blind child to avoid encountering the names of colors in story books, school lessons, and conversation. Parents and teachers must employ a good deal of imagination to explain the meaning of these words, but fortunately there is an abundance of color-related idioms to provide accessible associations. The child may learn that grass is green and that it is greener on the other side of the fence. But she will also learn that there are other shades of the color associated with other objects, such as limes, acid, olives, and bottles. Later, in science class, the child may learn why grass, and other plants are green, and what it means when it turns another color such as yellow or brown. She will also learn that greenness in a fruit may denote unripeness while in a vegetable it can indicate freshness and vitamin content. She may also learn that while Martians are supposed to be green, Earthlings do not come in this color, though they may be said to be green when seasick or envious. Indeed, according to Shakespeare, envy is a green-eyed monster. The blind child will learn that green paint can be made from equal parts of blue and yellow, and that green light has a measurable wavelength a bit shorter than blue light and a bit longer than red. While most of this blind child's knowledge of green requires rote memorization, the same can be said for a sighted child who can physically perceive the color but acquires the other associations from sources outside her own perception. And it is these associations that should allow us to talk about the effect of a particular shade of green used by whatever artist we are considering.

But even if we talk about a blind person who has led an unusually isolated life, what would be so terrible about explaining visual phenomena and concepts relevant to art. How, for instance, does linear perspective work? What effect does it have on the viewer? What values do people ascribe to different colors? Why do we talk about warm or cool colors, when to the touch the pigments would have the same temperature? What do we mean when we say that a portrait is a good likeness? How does a good likeness differ from caricature? What about abstraction? What about conceptual art, when the point is more about the idea than the technical execution. And then there are more general questions about why looking at art is pleasurable, and why it matters. But the risk is that the blind museum visitor is cast in the role of Leo Steinberg's blind man, posing naïve questions to the sighted service provider, which are edifying to the general public, but do nothing in particular for the blind person.

Leaving aside the prickly aesthetic questions about the value and pleasure of looking at art, there are practical considerations. Does access to the visual arts for blind people need to occur at the museum or gallery? Blind people interested in art can already acquire a good deal of information without visiting the museum. They can read books, articles, reviews. They can find detailed descriptions of particular works, styles or periods in art history, and find biographies of artists. If they have some of the right kind of vision, they can use assistive technology to enlarge images of works of art available on museum websites and other virtual venues. All this can be done from the comfort of their own homes. So why go to a crowded, noisy museum?

Historically, the blind and people with other disabilities have been asked this type of question too many times. Society still sends the message, especially to newly disabled people, that the correct response is a smiling acceptance of one's limitations and a cheerful abandonment of old interests and activities. The underlying advice is to stay at home, out of sight and out of mind. The disability rights movement has challenged the "just stay home" messages. In some sense, when blind people show up at an art museum, we assert that we have a place in this society and a right to public institutions.

In raising the issue of civil rights however, I invite the objection that my topic is trivial when we take into account that the vast majority of blind Americans, including those with residual sight, are undereducated and unemployed. Only about 45 percent of students with severe visual impairments or blindness graduate high school compared with 80 percent of their sighted peers.[5] Unemployment among working-age blind Americans still hovers around 70 percent.[6] I am not arguing that access to the visual arts will improve these disturbing statistics, but I believe that social change needs to happen on many fronts at once. If we as a society can enlarge our understanding of what blind people can do, we can perhaps raise the low expectations among the people who educate and rehabilitate the blind. Scrutiny of one cultural issue—access to arts institutions—and one subset of the disabled population—blind people—can have larger, more general implications.

Apart from the abstract value of a more inclusive society though, is there a benefit in encouraging blind people to come to the museum?

To answer this question, we need to consider the many ways museums function in society. Museums are more than repositories to preserve culturally valued artifacts. They are also educational institutions, providing information and inspiration both to the general public, and to future artists. Long before there were art academies, or MFA programs, aspiring artists visited museums to gain a sense of their artistic heritage and to pick up technical tips. If we provide museum access to blind people, some fraction of that population might become artists in the future. If the visual arts represent a pinnacle of human self-expression, than the blind too, given the right cultural opportunities, have selves worthy of expression. This is true despite the fact that blindness is usually spoken of as something that takes away from or even destroys identity. We speak of losing sight, never of gaining blindness except in terms of the supernatural, extrasensory compensatory powers blind people are supposed to have. I am suggesting rather that there is more to the experience of blindness that might find expression in art.

Again, this prompts the question: "When you talk about blind artists, you're not talking about real blind people, are you? You're talking about artists who used to be sighted, and still have partial sight. Surely, a totally, congenitally blind person, even aided by knowledge derived from the sorts of access programs now becoming available, still could not produce art, real art, art that was anything more than a novelty, or some kind of misguided therapy. After all, how could they judge what they were doing? At best, they'd have to rely on a sighted assistant to tell them what they'd produced, and then, wouldn't the resulting art work really be the product of the sighted person? Shouldn't the blind person seek to satisfy her artistic impulses in the time-honored media already accessible to blind people—literature and music? And if she had to produce something in the visual arena, wouldn't she more naturally gravitate toward sculpture?"

It's true that the vast majority of blind artists working today and exhibiting in a growing number of shows around the world are people who were formally sighted or else retain some residual vision. So again, statistically speaking, when I refer to blind artists I'm talking about adventitiously visually impaired artists with some usable sight and/or visual memory and/or a prior history of art practice. But what if I'm imagining a future for real blind people creating real art? What would that art look like? Or would the look of it be the most relevant aspect. If for instance, the blind artist I'm imagining was making sculpture meant to be experienced tactually, as she experienced it, what materials would she have to use. How should it be displayed? Should the museum hand out blindfolds for sighted visitors? Would we need to enlarge our vocabulary to describe this new aesthetic experience? And how would these new, previously unstudied tactile aesthetics expand outward from the realm of the fine arts to influence other aspects of the culture?

The Plan of the Book

I will begin this study with four chapters about traditional representations of blindness. Chapter 1 surveys the figure I call the Hypothetical Blind Man in philosophical thought. In his *Optics*, Descartes compared the human visual system to the way a blind man uses a stick to move through space. Later, William Molyneux posed his famous question to John Locke: If a man, born blind, who has learned to recognize geometrical figures such as a sphere and a cube through touch, then has his sight restored by some hypothetical operation, will he be able to recognize the same figures through sight alone? Both these instances rely on an over-determined analogy relating touch in the blind to sight in the sighted. I will argue that these theories fail to take into account the presence of other senses or the ability of blind people to draw analogies from nonvisual experience to develop concepts about visual phenomena. Touch in the blind is not necessarily more sensitive than touch in the sighted. The difference is that experienced blind people learn to interpret their tactile perceptions with a higher degree of conscious awareness, as many have described in their autobiographical accounts. Yet, the Hypothetical Blind Man continues to reside in the imaginations of many researchers in cognitive science, perception, and visual studies, as I will show in chapter 2. Chapter 3 will argue that the use of Braille in public sites and works of contemporary art often serve merely as signifiers of blindness rather than as a true access tool. In chapter 4, I will describe my experience of touch tours at art museums around the world. I argue that these programs risk failure when they are based on a limited definition of touch perception and a rudimentary notion of aesthetic pleasure. Too often, programmers assume that the point of tactile exploration is to recognize forms through tracing their outlines, as if viewing a work of art were merely a matter of identifying the objects depicted. I have found that the most rewarding touch tours engage the full spectrum of touch sensation—texture, temperature, resiliency, as well as form—and draw attention to features that are not apparent to the naked eye. I go on to suggest that since the majority of art lovers are denied the opportunity to touch the art, museum educators would do well to collect the observations of the privileged few who enjoy this exceptional access. Thus touch tours would cease to be random acts of charity and become a way to enlarge cultural understanding of art.

The next four chapters will shift focus from the tactile to the verbal. In chapter 5, I will return briefly to Denis Diderot. His *Letter on the Blind* (1749) builds on and also diverges from other philosophical treatments. Ideas about blindness engaged him throughout his life even when he was writing on other topics. I will argue that this preoccupation contributed to the ways he wrote about art. In his Salon criticism, he employed a remarkable range of techniques to describe art works for readers who were not present to view them for themselves and had no access to reliable reproductions. He combined detailed descriptions, invented narratives and mocking rebukes of the artists to express his opinions and to recreate his viewing experiences. In a quite literal way, Diderot was writing for readers who were blind to the art he described. His criticism not only gives us models for verbal description of art but also proclaims that the experience of art is inextricably tied to language and thus is not entirely dependent on vision. His criticism offers a powerful warrant for bringing the specter of blindness out of the shadows and into the foreground of visual experience.

Chapter 6 surveys literary depictions that pair blindness with visual art. While these representations still follow the contours of the Hypothetical Blind Man, they also allow authors to extol the power of language to perform even the most difficult tasks, such as describing visual experience to the blind. In chapters 7 and 8, I combine these observations to critique the theory and practice of audio description for the blind. Originally invented to provide blind people access to live theater, film, and television, audio description would seem the ideal choice to give blind people access to works of art that cannot be touched. However, while a picture may be worth a thousand words, the assumption seems to be that those thousand words—or even a million words—will not do justice to the picture. This holds even though ekphrasis, or poetry that describes visual art, has been around at least since Homer. Guidelines for audio description seem founded on the most reductive notion of what blind people can conceptualize. While I critique the current practices, I call for innovations that could elevate audio description to the status of a new literary and interpretative genre that can serve all audiences of visual culture.

I conclude the book with a discussion of artists with impaired sight, specifically their self-portraits. When celebrated artists such as Monet and Degas lose sight late in life, biographers tend to represent it as a tragic irony and call for predictable responses of pity and admiration. But a careful reading of these artists' accounts of the experience presents a more complex picture. After a lifetime of coordinating their eyes, hands, and minds to create images, their adaptation to diminished sight involved a heightened reliance on tactile and cognitive skills. But here I am mainly concerned with artists who also make blindness a theme of their work and speculate on how acceptance of the idea of blind artists and blind art lovers can change future museum practices and aesthetic values.

When I began this project more than a decade ago, I thought I could write about all the blind artists then practicing in the world. Now, even my imperfect research finds so many that I have to choose only a very small sample whose work seeks to remake the image of blindness. I don't know if this is due to the fact that I was ignorant back then. Or if there has been a proliferation of the number of artists with impaired vision. Has the rise, however incremental in awareness and accessibility for blind people, encouraged artists who lose their sight to continue their practice and encouraged other blind people to consider art as a pastime or career?

It is fitting that I end this book with the words, ideas, and art work of blind people. Indeed, throughout the book I seek to put blind people in dialogue with the philosophers, scientists, and educators who study blindness and speak on behalf of the blind. It's not that I think that artists who become blind and find ways to continue their art practice deserve extra recognition beyond what may have been accorded them before. From writing a book about Helen Keller, I recognize that when a disabled individual is put on a pedestal and praised as exceptional and inspirational, it is just another form of exclusion. My point is rather that artists who continue working even after sight loss seem in the best position to advise the museum art educators designing programs for blind visitors. Sometimes, arts institutions gesture in this direction. At conferences about access for museum professionals, a few blind or visually impaired artists may be mentioned or invited to speak about their work. Many museums offer art-making classes for blind children and adults. Frequently the work of professional artists and amateur novices is conflated. Museum professionals do not always reckon with what the artists are doing beyond formulaic admiration for their fortitude. The fact that they may be invited into the museum to comment on access programming does not necessarily inspire museums to commission or acquire their work. This has a great deal to do with the hierarchies within arts institutions where art educators and collection curators exist in very different realms, remote from each other. Still, art educators seem more engaged with cognitive scientists who investigate what blind people can and cannot conceptualize, when surely the work and testimony of blind artists can enlarge and enliven general cultural understanding.

This book is not a how-to manual for museum professionals. In fact, I've observed in the rise of books, conferences, and websites devoted to arts access that the reification of rules can be counterproductive. Moreover, as will be apparent to scholars in these fields, I am not a philosopher, scientist, or art historian, but I hope this collection of observations suggests new avenues of research. Furthermore, I hope others can extrapolate from this example of blind people and visual art to examine other cases of cultural marginalization.

In the quarter-century since the Americans with Disabilities Act, blind and other disabled people have become minimally more visible, though as the statistics cited earlier indicate this visibility has not necessarily resulted in higher levels of education or employment. The general public is aware that the law requires wheelchair ramps, Braille signage in elevators, and closed captioning on television, but apart from an abstract notion that this is more humane than sequestering disabled people in institutions, there has been little articulation of the larger benefits of these accommodations. True access needs to be understood as something more than a one-sided act of generosity or charity. The presence of those formerly excluded people must be understood to invite a wholesale scrutiny of what the culture takes for granted about itself. So the ultimate goal is not merely to explain visual art to blind people in the hope that this cultural access will compensate for the loss of sight. Rather, the hope is that blind people can bring a perspective that has not been articulated before. If we can abandon the notion that blindness can only diminish, damage or destroy identity, and adopt instead the idea that the experience of blindness, in all its varieties, can in fact shape and inform other facets of personality and personal history, we will move toward a more genuinely inclusive society. The integration of blind perceptions and experiences will change the foundational assumptions of the culture; change how the human condition is defined. And I believe this is the goal worth working toward.

{1}

The Tenacious Life of the Hypothetical Blind Man

When I claim to know something about visual art, I collide with a long philosophical tradition that conflates seeing and knowing. According to this tradition, because I am blind, my knowledge of art is merely hearsay and secondhand. So before I can address the question of art access for blind people, I need to reckon with traditional understandings of blindness. The Man Born Blind, as he is often called, or the Hypothetical Blind Man,[1] is one of the stock characters of the Western philosophical tradition. The Hypothetical Blind Man—or the Hypothetical as I will call him for the sake of brevity—has long played a useful, though thankless, role as a prop for theories of consciousness. He is the patient subject of endless thought experiments where the experience of the world through four senses can be compared to the experience of the world through five. He is asked to describe his understanding of specific visual phenomena—perspective, reflection, refraction, color, form recognition—as well as visual aids and enhancements—mirrors, lenses, telescopes, microscopes. He is understood to lead a hermit-like existence, so far at the margins of his society that he has never discussed this visual terminology before the philosophers inquired. Like the blind man that Leo Steinberg invented to converse with Jasper Johns, the Hypothetical is "a questioner of ideal innocence and congenital blindness." Part of the emotional baggage he hauls around with him comes from other cultural representations of blindness, such as Oedipus and the many Biblical figures whose sight is withdrawn by the wrathful God of the Old Testament or restored by the redeemer of the New. Sometimes he follows the tradition of the Blind Seer, like Tiresias, or the Blind Poet, like Homer, who deliver unexpected insights from the perpetual darkness they are assumed to inhabit. But his primary function is to highlight the importance of sight and to elicit a frisson of awe and pity which promotes gratitude among the sighted theorists for the vision they possess.

I will not attempt to survey every depiction of the Hypothetical throughout the history of philosophy.[2] It is enough to cite a few of his more memorable appearances, and then to suggest what happens when he is brought face-to-face with actual blind people through their firsthand accounts.

Let us begin then, with Rene Descartes. In his *La Dioptrique* (1637) Descartes invites his reader to imagine using a stick to find his way in darkness:

> It has sometimes doubtless happened to you, while walking in the night without a light through places which are a little difficult, that it became necessary to use a stick in order to guide yourself; and you may then have been able to notice that you felt, through the medium of this stick, the diverse objects placed around you, and that you could even tell whether there were trees, or stones, or sand, or water, or grass, or mud, or any other such thing. True, this kind of sensation is somewhat confused and obscure in those who do not have long practice with it; but consider it in those born blind, who have made use of it all their lives: with them, you will find it is so perfect and so exact, that one might almost say that they see with their hands, or that their stick is the organ of some sixth sense given to them in place of sight.[3]

Descartes' introduction of the Hypothetical here is remarkable in that he posits an advantage to congenital blindness in this situation. While the sighted man's perceptions are confused and obscure, the Hypothetical's discernment is imagined to be so precise and exact as to constitute a new sixth sense. Descartes reinforces the traditional view that blind people's tactile sensations are in excess of a sighted person's. He at once explains it as a supernatural power given in compensation for the absent sight, while at the same time emphasizing that it develops over a lifetime of practice. I will be churlish and point out that by labeling it as a sixth sense, he gets the math wrong; since the Hypothetical is without sight, this extra-special stick-wielding touch sensation would therefore only count as his fifth. It would only count as a sixth sense for the sighted man who already has the regular, daylight, stick-less form of touch plus his four other senses.

I also have to comment that the sighted man Descartes addresses seems inordinately helpless here. Does one really need a stick to tell water from sand or mud? Wouldn't the foot be the better organ of perception in this instance? I note too that the scene Descartes imagines is unnaturally silent. In the real world, trees emit sounds even on a still night. The poor sighted man is so busy tapping around in the mud that he seems oblivious to this and other sensory features of the landscape. For instance, it might help him to observe that vegetation and soil exhale telltale scents, and that the temperature changes as he leaves a wooded area or approaches water.

In other words, Descartes' description reflects a basic misunderstanding. He imagines that the blind man uses the stick to construct a mental image of his surroundings, mapping the location of specifically identified objects, while his other senses, not to mention memory and cognition, remain inactive. In fact, then as now, a stick or white cane is a poor tool for this kind of mental imaging. Speaking from my experience, the cane is more of an obstacle detector than a tool to map the environment. The cane's tip proceeds me as I move through space, alerting me to objects I need to step over or around. It merely announces the presence of an obstacle, without distinguishing between a rock or a tree root. If I need to make this distinction, it will usually come from a sound cue—a tap versus a thud—rather than a tactile assessment of the objects' forms or relative densities. Although, many blind people are adept at interpreting echoes of the cane's taps to judge the environment around them. Canadian social practice artist Carmen Papalia draws attention to aural rather than tactile navigation in his project, "Mobility Device" (Fig. 1.1). He abandoned his white cane and substituted a high school marching band. The band spontaneously improvises a vocabulary of sounds to alert him to obstacles and help guide him from place to place. Together, they navigate city streets, enter sandwich shops, board buses, and so forth. Here, the artist appears in the midst of his band, wearing the standard costume for his performances—a tailored vest and a fedora. His arms are at his sides and his head is lowered slightly as he attends to the sounds around him. The band, in their vaguely military uniforms, surround him. Sunlight glints off the bells of the tubas. The band director, his arms raised, conducts from the left side. Behind them passers-by in ordinary dress look on and follow along as they move across the street.

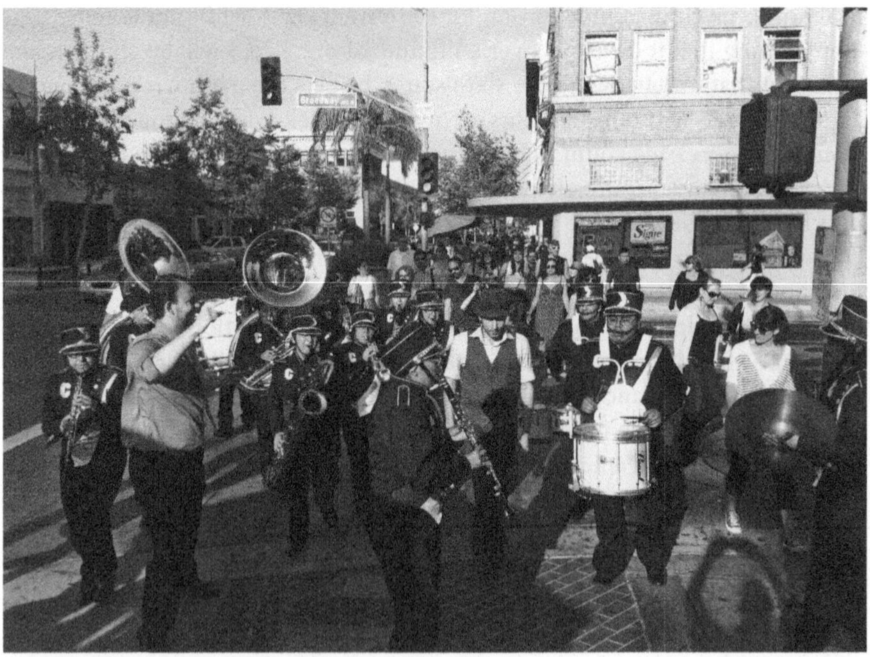

FIGURE 1.1 *Carmen Papalia,* Mobility Device *(2013).*
Courtesy of the Grand Central Arts Center.

I'm speaking anachronistically of course. White canes today are made of space age materials, carbon fiber with a metal tip, and were designed to be used in a paved environment. The Hypothetical's stick—or those used by his real-world brethren—was probably fashioned from a tree branch, and the terrain underfoot would be uneven and unpaved, so the auditory effects would have been different. But the point remains that Descartes utterly ignores the role hearing, smell, or other aspects of touch sensation might play in the blind man's navigation. And in any case, Descartes is making an analogy here. He's trying to describe the way light connects the eye to distant objects in the same way that the blind man's stick touches objects that are out of reach of his hand. In a later discussion of binocular depth perception, Descartes performs a thought experiment, giving the Hypothetical a second stick that he could use to judge the distance between two objects by calculating the angle formed when he touches each object with one of the sticks. Descartes explains that the Hypothetical performs this calculation through some "natural geometry," [4] which is perhaps another, seventh sense. But he does not explain how he can avoid running into things while doing so. I doubt that Descartes actually believed that any blind person ever used two sticks in this way. In fact, the illustration that accompanies this discussion shows the Hypothetical, in rather ragged robes, handling the two sticks somewhat awkwardly. Alphabet letters appear to suggest the geometrical calculations he may be performing in his mind. Meanwhile his dog, attached by a leash to the Hypothetical's belt (since his hands are full), is curled up and sound asleep on the ground, indicating that the Hypothetical is going nowhere (Fig. 1.2). But what is significant for future depictions of blindness, is the way that Descartes' desire to describe vision as an extension of, or hypersensitive form of touch, makes him recreate the blind man in his own image, where the eye must correspond directly to the hand extended by one or perhaps two sticks.

Thus it is established that if the sighted theorist is all eyes, the Hypothetical Blind Man is all hands. In all subsequent treatments of the Hypothetical the focus is riveted on his tactile perception to the complete exclusion of all his other senses. For example, in 1693, William Molyneux wrote his famous letter to John Locke where he proposed the following thought experiment, summarized here by Locke:

> Suppose a man born blind, and now adult, and taught by his touch to distinguish between a cube and a sphere of the same metal, and nighly of the same bigness, so as to tell, when he felt one and the other, which is the cube, which the sphere. Suppose then the cube and sphere placed on a table, and the blind man to be made to see; quaere, Whether by his sight, before he touched them, he could now distinguish and tell which is the globe, which the cube? To which the acute and judicious proposer answers: Not. For

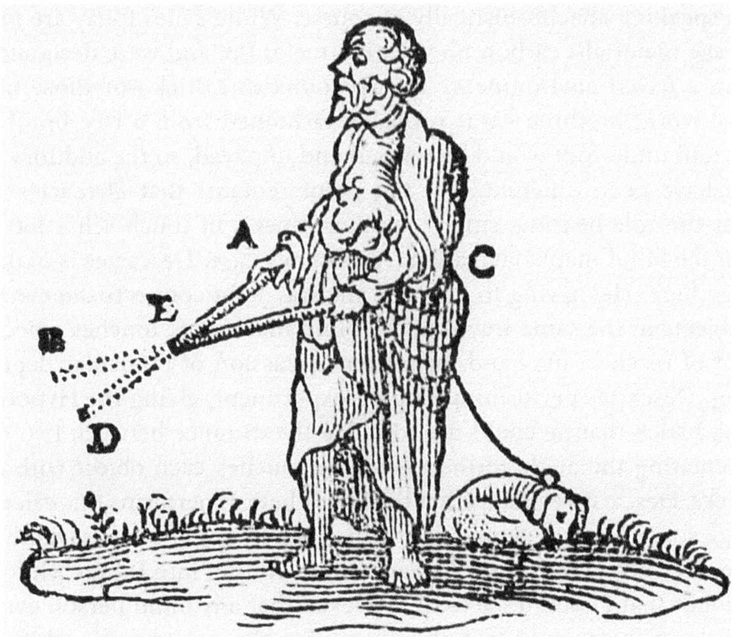

FIGURE 1.2 *From Rene Descartes.* La Dioptrique *(1637).*
Image reproduced with the permission of the Bibliothèque nationael de France.

> though he has obtained the experience of how a globe, how a cube, affects his touch; yet he has not yet obtained the experience, that what affects his touch so or so, must affect his sight so or so; or that a protuberant angle in the cube, that pressed his hand unequally, shall appear to his eye as it does in the cube.[5]

Locke and Molyneux are careful to construct their experiment according to a scientific method with controlled conditions. The globe and the cube are not only made of the same material and close to the same size, but they also emit no sound or scent. And the newly sighted Hypothetical is not only at a prescribed distance but also unable to move nearer to or around the objects. The philosophers took the Hypothetical's failure at this task as confirmation of the theory that there are no innate ideas common to human beings. Ideas come from experience, and the Hypothetical's touch experience would not automatically translate into sight experience after the operation. Interestingly neither Locke nor Molyneux doubted that the Hypothetical would see something. They imagined that the operation would act on the blind man like the lifting of a blindfold from the eyes of a sighted man. This facet of the Molyneux question was immediately debated by other theorists who predicted that it would take some time before the Hypothetical would be able to see the sphere and cube, much less name them.

Apparently, Molyneux was married to a blind woman, which has always led me to wonder why he did not pose his hypothetical question about her. Perhaps he knew that others would object that marriage to a philosopher might contaminate the experimental data. There would be a risk that the philosopher might prime her answers or otherwise rig the results. More significantly to the experiment, she was not born blind so there was a chance she might retain some memory of spheres and cubes.

Certainly in commentary on actual cases of restored sight, there is always a good deal of quibbling about the date of onset and degree of blindness. For example, in 1728, William Cheselden published a case study entitled, "An account of some observations made by a young gentleman, who was born blind, or lost his sight so early, that he had no remembrance of ever having seen, and was couch'd between 13 and 14 years of age." Cheselden seems on the defensive against devotees of the Hypothetical as he attempts to quantify the young gentleman's visual experience prior to the operation. Like many people with congenital cataracts, the young man was able to distinguish light from darkness, and even to identify some colors, though he reported that his color perception was vastly improved after the operation. Cheselden did not try the cube versus sphere experiment; it's unclear whether he was familiar with the Molyneux question. But the young gentleman was unable to tell the dog from the cat, until he touched them. Cheselden records that he scooped up the cat, looked at it attentively for a while and then said, "So Puss! I shall know you another time."[6] In so doing, he was breaking the rules of the Molyneux problem. Simultaneously touching and looking at the cat, gave him an opportunity to make a connection between his previous tactile recognition and his new visual experience. And I half suspect that in addressing the cat, he may have been inviting it to give him an aural cue next time as well.

Cheselden's account of this real-life case of restored sight made it plain to philosophers that the Hypothetical needed a makeover to accommodate for the messiness of reality. For example, the Abbé de Condillac replaced the Hypothetical with a statue to which he could add and subtract various sensations and capacities. Since the statue had no previous experience, no memory, it made a tidier subject for contemplation. On the other hand, Denis Diderot focused his speculation on real rather than hypothetical blind men. His 1749 *Letter on the Blind for the Use of Those Who See* deals with two men, one identified only as the blind man from Puiseaux, the other, Nicholas Saunderson, the English mathematician. As he introduces the blind man of Puiseaux, Diderot is at pains to supply details of his family history and early life to persuade his reader that this is a real person. His father taught philosophy at the university in Paris, and he knew a bit about chemistry and botany. He made a modest living through the sale of a liqueur he distilled himself. Significantly the man from Puiseaux is first encountered helping his young son with his studies, demonstrating both that he is a loving family man and capable of intellectual activity. Still, the questions Diderot poses generally fall under the prevue of the Hypothetical. Certainly, many of his remarks help support Descartes' one-to-one correspondence between the sighted man's eyes and the blind man's hands. For instance:

> I asked him what he meant by *a* mirror: "an instrument," answered he, "which sets things in relief at a distance from themselves, when properly placed with regard to it. It is like my hand, which, to feel an object, I must not reach to one side of it."
>
> Had Descartes been born blind, he might, I think, have hugged himself for such a definition.[7]

It is almost too perfect. The blind man even repeats Descartes' analogy saying that the light is to the sighted man's eyes as his stick is to his hand. It leads me to wonder if the blind man's philosopher father read him Descartes. Diderot and his company go on to describe other visual aids:

> One of our company thought to ask our blind man if he would like to have eyes. "If it were not for curiosity," he replied, "I would just as soon have long arms: it seems to me my hands would tell me more of what goes on in the moon than your eyes or your telescopes."[8]

As the interview progresses, I sense a growing irritation in the blind man's tone. Perhaps I am only projecting, but it is as if he recognizes that the questions are reshaping him to conform to the pattern of the Hypothetical. Or perhaps it is the way Diderot suddenly digresses into musings on how dangerous the blind man would be if he had a rock or gun in his hand. And why shouldn't the blind man be irritable? Who are all these philosophers anyway? Will any of them even spring for a bottle of liqueur?

While Diderot praises the blind man's ability to make philosophical surmises about vision, he shifts rapidly from pondering the blind man's literal touch sensation to speculation on moral issues—the blind man's presumed lack of fellow feeling for others:

> As of all the external signs which raise our pity and ideas of pain the blind are affected only by cries, I have in general no high thought of their humanity. What difference is there to a blind man between a man making water and one bleeding in silence?[9]

This is a rare instance where a philosopher considers the blind man's hearing rather than touch sensation. And the phrasing of the question here suggests an afterthought. I imagine Diderot, at his table, conjuring up two men, one pissing, one bleeding. While his visual imagination is practiced in making these sorts of mental images, he is less adept at tuning his mind's ear. He recognizes that for the blood to be spilt at a rate sufficient to create the same sound as flowing urine, the bleeding man would normally cry out in pain. So he imagines, in effect, a bleeding mute. But he fails to take into account the relative viscosity, not to mention the different odors, of the two fluids.

While it's easy to make fun of Diderot's bleeding mute, it is not as if his low opinion of the Hypothetical's ability to empathize with others' pain has no correlation to contemporary attitudes about blindness. Consider this anecdote from recent history. Some weeks after September 11, 2001, the blind musician Ray Charles was interviewed about his rendition of "America the Beautiful," which received a good deal of air time during the period of heightened patriotism that followed that event. The interviewer, Jim Gray, commented that Charles should consider himself lucky that his blindness prevented him from viewing the images of the World Trade Center's collapse, and the Pentagon in flames: "Was this maybe one time in your life where not having the ability to see was a relief?"[10] Like Diderot, the interviewer assumed that true horror can only be evinced through the eyes. Many eyewitness accounts of the event, however, were strikingly nonvisual. Many people who were in the vicinity of Ground Zero during and soon after the disaster found it hard to put what they saw into words, in part because visibility in the area was obscured by smoke and ash, and in part because what they were seeing did not correspond to any visual experience for which they had language. People described instead the sound of falling bodies hitting the ground, the smell of the burning jet fuel, and the particular texture of the ankle-deep dust that filled the streets. But for the majority of television viewers, eyewitnesses from a distance, those events are recalled as images, indelible, powerful, and eloquent. To many, like the reporter interviewing Ray Charles, it is the images rather than the fact of the events that produce the emotional response. The assumption seems to be that because the blind are immune to images they must also be immune to the significance of the events, and therefore must be somehow detached from or indifferent to the nation's collective horror and grief.

But let us return to Diderot. In speculating on the blind man's morality, Diderot is laying the ground work for his discussion of Nicholas Saunderson, the English blind mathematician. His account, however, is based on hearsay, as the two men never met. And in fact, it was Diderot's creation of Saunderson's fictional deathbed conversation with a priest that got him in so much trouble. He put blasphemous words in the blind man's mouth. When the priest describes the visible wonders of the world, Diderot has Saunderson say:

> Don't talk to me of this magnificent spectacle, which it has never been my lot to enjoy. I have been condemned to spend my life in darkness, and you cite wonders quite out of my understanding, and which are only evidence for you and for those who see as you do. If you want to make me believe in God you must make me touch Him.[11]

The authorities were not duped by Diderot's fiction, and he had to spend some time in jail.

While Diderot's contemporary critics may have seen *Letter on the Blind* as merely a vehicle for him to veil his more radical ideas, his treatment of blindness was at once far more complex and far more compassionate than that of other philosophers. For instance, in his discussion of the Molyneux question, he not only refutes the assumption that the Hypothetical would be able to see immediately after the operation, but he also proposes that the newly sighted man's response would depend on his background. He allows for the possibility that he might have been a blind geometer like Saunderson, or even a blind, or deaf-blind philosopher:

> If ever a philosopher, blind and deaf from his birth, were to construct a man after the fashion of Descartes, I can assure you, madam, that he would put the seat of the soul at the fingers' ends, for it is from these that the greater part of the sensations and all his knowledge are derived.[12]

The more enlightened view of blind people's potential that Diderot exemplified can be said to have led to a rise in educational opportunities. Valentin Haüy, who founded the first blind school in the world in Paris in 1785, cited Diderot as an inspiration. Schools elsewhere in Europe and America opened in the following decades. With the rise in literacy among blind people, autobiographical texts by actual blind people began to appear in the late eighteenth and early nineteenth centuries. And these often directly confront the Hypothetical's characteristics and values. One such account is a text written in 1825, by a twenty-two-year-old blind French woman named Thérèse-Adèle Husson. Born in Nancy into a petit bourgeois household, Husson became blind at nine months following a bout of smallpox. Her case attracted the attention of the local gentry, who sponsored a convent education for her and encouraged her to cultivate her interests in literature and music. At the age of twenty she left home for Paris where she hoped to pursue a literary career. Her first text, "Reflections on the Moral and Physical Condition of the Blind" seems to have been written as a part of her petition for aid from the Hospice des Quinze-Vingts, an institution that provided shelter and financial support to the indigent blind of Paris. For the most part, her text follows the example of comportment and educational manuals of the time, offering advice to parents and caretakers on the correct way to raise a blind child, and to young blind people themselves on their role in society. It is by turns formulaically obsequious and radically assertive, since she writes from the premise—revolutionary for the time—that her firsthand experience of blindness gives her a level of expertise that equals or surpasses that of the institution's sighted administrators. While it is unlikely that Husson's convent education would have exposed her to the work of Descartes or Diderot, she considers some of the same questions previously posed to the Hypothetical. It is possible that the provincial aristocrats, who took up her education, may have engaged in amateurish philosophizing in her presence. For instance, like Diderot's blind man of Puiseaux, she prefers her sense of touch to the sight she lacks. She recounts how, at the time of her first communion, her mother promised her a dress made of chiffon, then, either as a joke or in an attempt to economize, purchased cheaper percale instead. When the young Husson easily detected the difference through touch, her mother persisted in her deception, and even brought in neighbor women to corroborate. Whether playing along with the joke, or as a genuine rebuke of her mother's attempt to deceive her, Husson retorted:

> I prefer my touch to your eyes, because it allows me to appreciate things for what they really are, whereas it seems to me that your sight fools you now and then, for this is percale and not chiffon.[13]

In a later discussion of her ability to recognize household objects through touch, her impatience seems out of proportion, unless we imagine that she frequently found herself the object of philosophical speculation by literal-minded practitioners:

> We know full well that a chest of drawers is square, but more long than tall. Again I hear my readers ask what is a square object! I am accommodating enough to satisfy all their questions. Therefore, I would say to them that it is easy enough to know the difference between objects by touching them, for not all of them have the same shape. For example, a dinner plate, a dish, a glass can't begin to be compared with a chest of drawers, for the first two are round, while the other is hollow; but people will probably point out that it is only after having heard the names of the articles that I designate that it became possible for me to acquire the certainty that they were hollow, round, square. I will admit that they are right, but tell me, you with the eyes of Argus, if you had never heard objects described, would you be in any better position to speak of them than I?[14]

Her emphasis on square versus round objects as well as her tone and her taunt, "You with the eyes of Argus," suggests an irritation that may come from hearing the Molyneux question one too many times. She is also arguing against the notion that such words as "square" and "round" designate solely visual phenomena, to which the blind have no access and therefore no right to use these words.

Almost a century later, Helen Keller gives vent to a similar irritation at literal-minded readers. In her 1908 book, *The World I Live In*, she gives a detailed phenomenological account of her daily experience of deaf-blindness. Early on, she footnotes her use of the verb "see" in the phrase, "I was taken to see a woman":

> The excellent proof-reader has put a query to my use of the word "see." If I had said "visit," he would have asked no questions, yet what does "visit" mean but "see" (*visitare*)? Later I will try to defend myself for using as much of the English language as I have succeeded in learning.[15]

Keller makes good use of her Radcliffe education to show that the more one knows about language, the harder it is to find vocabulary that does not have some root in sighted or hearing experience. But, she argues, to deny her the use of seeing-hearing vocabulary would be to deny her the ability to communicate at all. She goes on to engage directly with theorists of the Hypothetical:

> Critics delight to tell us what we cannot do. They assume that blindness and deafness sever us completely from the things which the seeing and the hearing enjoy, and hence they assert we have no moral right to talk about beauty, the skies, mountains, the song of birds, and colors. They declare that the very sensations we have from the sense of touch are "vicarious," as though our friends felt the sun for us. They deny *a priori* what they have not seen and I have felt. Some brave doubters have gone so far even as to deny my existence. In order, therefore, that I may know that I exist, I resort to Descartes's method: "I think, therefore I am." Thus I am metaphysically established, and I throw upon the doubters the burden of proving my non-existence.[16]

Keller's reference to critics who denigrate her experience as merely vicarious is a direct response to the one negative review of her first book *The Story of My Life* (1903). The critic in question took her to task for describing various events and scenes using visual terminology. But here she extends her resentment to any commentator who assumes that the experience of deaf-blindness is partial or secondhand. Writing from what she calls the "borderland of experience," she describes the ways she uses her sense of smell, which she identifies as the fallen angel of the senses. She contradicts the general definition of smell as a proximal sense and describes using it to map her environment:

> Sometimes, when there is no wind, the odors are so grouped that I know the character of the country, and can place a hayfield, a country store, a garden, a barn, a grove of pines, a farm-house with the windows open.[17]

More significantly, in describing her touch sensation, she does not limit herself to the process of mental mapping and form recognition that Descartes imagines. She points out that the hand is only one of many organs of touch perception and enumerates at least three different aspects of touch sensation that she finds meaningful—texture, temperature, and vibration. In fact, she understands sound as vibrations that the hearing feel in their ears while the deaf can feel them through other parts of their bodies. Thus she could feel thunder by pressing the palm of her hand against a windowpane, or someone's footsteps by pressing the soles of her feet against floorboards. In several instances, she offers detailed, play-by-play accounts of her everyday sensory experience:

> The other day I went to walk toward a familiar wood. Suddenly a disturbing odor made me pause in dismay. Then followed a peculiar, measured jar, followed by dull, heavy thunder. I understood the odor and the jar only too

> well. The trees were being cut down . . . to-day an unfamiliar rush of air and an unwonted outburst of sun told me that my tree friends were gone. The place was empty, like a deserted dwelling. I stretched out my hand. Where once stood the steadfast pines, great, beautiful, sweet, my hand touched raw, moist stumps.[18]

Keller is struck first by an odor and then by two different vibrations. She feels an unfamiliar airy openness where she expects to feel the shade and shelter of the trees. From this combination of sensation she draws her initial conclusion, which she confirms through touching the fresh stumps. What's most significant here is how she presents the way her tactual and olfactory perceptions work sequentially and in concert. Though this book of Keller's is sometimes quoted by philosophers, for instance William James with whom she corresponded, she failed to achieve the status of deaf-blind philosopher that Diderot imagined. Her gender, as well as her disability, held her back. And the general public was happier to restrict her to the status of inspirational icon.

It took almost another century for a blind philosopher to enter this discussion. In their 1995 book, *On Blindness*, two philosophers, one sighted and one blind, conduct an epistolary debate that might seem to put to rest all the old hypothetical questions. Unfortunately, Martin Milligan, the blind philosopher, died before the discussion was fully underway. If he had lived, we can assume not only that he and his sighted colleague, Bryan Magee, would have gotten further with their debate, but also that they would have edited some testy quibbles about which terms to use and which translation of Aristotle is more accurate. Milligan, who worked primarily in moral and political philosophy, and was an activist in blind causes in the United Kingdom, forthrightly keeps the discussion from straying far from the practical and social conditions that affect the lives of real blind people. For instance, he cites an incident from his early life, before he found an academic post, when he was turned down for a job as a telephone typist on a newspaper because the employer assumed that he would not be able to negotiate the stairs in the building. He identifies this as one of thousands of examples of the exaggerated value sighted people place on vision. Any thinking person has to recognize that sight is not required to climb or descend stairs. He asserts that the value of sight would be that it would allow him to move around unfamiliar places with greater ease. He concedes that vision might afford him some aesthetic pleasure while viewing a landscape or painting but insists that he can know what he wants to know about the visible world from verbal descriptions, and that this knowledge is adequate for his needs, and only minimally different from the knowledge of sighted people. He accuses Magee of voicing "visionist" attitudes that the differences between the sighted and the blind must be almost incomprehensibly vast, and that vision is a fundamental aspect of human existence. Milligan says that these statements seem

> to express the passion, the zeal of a missionary preaching to the heathen in outer darkness. Only, of course, your "gospel" isn't "good" news to us heathens, for the message seems to be that ours is a "darkness" from which we can never come in—not the darkness of course that sighted people can know, but the darkness of never being able to know *that* darkness, or of bridging the vast gulf that separates us from those who do.[19]

This prompts Magee to cite his own early work on race and homosexuality, as proof of his credentials as a liberal humanist. He also speculates, somewhat sulkily, about whether the first eighteen months of Milligan's life when his vision was presumed to be normal, might disqualify him as a spokesman for the blind, since he might retain some vestige of a visual memory from that period. Later, Magee consults with a neurologist who assures him that the loss of sight at such an early age would make Milligan's brain indistinguishable from that of a person born blind. And so the discussion continues.

Along the way, Magee makes some claims about sight that seem to me to be far from universal. For instance, he states:

> By the sighted, seeing is felt as a *need*. And it is the feeding of this almost ungovernable craving that constitutes the ongoing pleasure of sight. It is as if we were desperately hungry all the time, in such a way that only if we were eating all the time could we be content—so we eat all the time.[20]

After I read this passage for the first time, I was riding to work on the bus. While blind people are frequently found on public transportation, I assumed that on this day the vast majority of my fellow passengers, plus the driver, were all sighted. I started to wonder if they were experiencing this ravenous and insatiable visual hunger that Magee describes. I found the thought so disturbing that I got off the bus two stops early.

Magee also asserts that when sighted people are obliged to keep their eyes closed even for a short time, it induces a kind of panic. To illustrate his point, he notes that a common method of mistreating prisoners is to keep them blindfolded, and this mistreatment can lead them to feel anxious and disoriented. I suspect that his example is influenced by traditional metaphors that equate blindness with a tomb-like imprisonment. Surely a blind prisoner, accustomed to the privation of sight, might still have similar feelings of anxiety and disorientation, due to the threat, whether stated or implied, of pending bodily harm.

Milligan exhibits laudable patience with all of this and offers his own phenomenology. Like Keller, he refutes the notion that the hand is the only organ of touch. In addition, as a hearing person, he specifies that his ability to map his environment has more to do with aural apprehension:

> Silent objects such as lamp-posts and parked cars with their engines off can be heard by me as I approach them and pass them as atmosphere-thickening

> occupants of space, almost certainly because of the way they absorb and/or echo back the sounds of my footsteps and other small sounds in their vicinity. It isn't usually necessary to make sounds oneself to have this awareness, though it helps. Objects of head height probably slightly affect the air currents reaching my face, which helps towards my awareness of them—which is why some blind people refer to this kind of sense-awareness as their "facial" sense. Since an overwhelming amount of noise, and also profound deafness, seem to obliterate this sense, I agree with what seems to be the opinion of the majority of blind people who have it that this sense—usually well developed in born-blind people, less so in people who have lost their sight late in life—is primarily mediated through the ears, and should be thought of as primarily a kind of "hearing."[21]

Remarkably, Magee identifies with this blind sense and describes his experience of the phenomenon when he was a child attempting to navigate an unfamiliar room in the dark:

> I had a vivid non-visual awareness of the nearness of material objects. I would walk confidently along a pitch black corridor in a strange house and stop dead a few inches short of a closed door, and then put out my hand to grope for the knob. If I woke up in the dark in a strange bedroom and wanted to get to a light-switch on the opposite side of the room I could usually circumnavigate the furniture in between, because I could "feel" where the larger objects in the room were. I might knock small things over, but would almost invariably "feel" the big ones. I say "feel" because the sensation, which I can clearly recall, was as of a feeling-in-the-air with my whole bodily self. Your phrase "atmosphere-thickening occupants of space" describes the apprehension exactly. I suddenly "felt" a certain thickness in the air at a certain point relative to myself in the blackness surrounding me . . . This illustrates your point that the blind develop potentialities that the sighted have also been endowed with but do not develop because they have less need of them.[22]

While Milligan identifies this sense as primarily a function of hearing, Magee recalls it as a matter of feeling. Perhaps Magee finds it hard to shake the one-to-one analogy of the sighted man's eyes to the blind man's hands. However it is significant that Magee puts the emphasis on potentialities that the blind develop, while the sighted child has them initially but loses them as he grows up and becomes more and more dependent on sight alone. Is this then the sixth sense that Descartes described in his first image of the Hypothetical moving across the dark landscape? The two twentieth-century philosophers strive to define a form of perception that partakes of hearing and touch simultaneously, and is experienced kinesthetically and by the body as a whole.

What Milligan, Keller, Husson, and other blind authors have in common is an urgent desire to represent their experiences of blindness as something besides the absence of sight. Unlike the Hypothetical, they do not feel themselves to be deficient or partial—sighted people minus sight—but whole human beings who have learned to attend to their nonvisual senses in different ways. But as we will see in the next chapter, the Hypothetical Blind Man is still alive and well in the minds of many.

{2}

Touching on Science

Of all the hypothetical questions posed about blindness, it is the Molyneux problem that continues to fascinate philosophers and scientists. What if a man who was born blind but had learned to recognize via touch certain geometrical forms, such as a sphere and a cube, were to have his sight restored by an operation, would he then be able to recognize these forms through sight alone? It is estimated that there have only been about twenty such cases in the past thousand years. Twenty cases in a thousand years may seem a statistically insignificant number. But reading the literature, where cases are documented, debated, disputed, analyzed and reanalyzed by subsequent generations of philosophers and scientists, makes it feel like many more.

Moreover, the case studies follow a predictable pattern. Typically, the patients are initially excited and overwhelmed by the visible world. Researchers give them tests and tasks. The newly sighted patients often fail these tests. After a while the newly sighted become disillusioned with the whole business. The visible world is not all rainbows and sunsets. Loved ones turn out not to resemble movie stars. And there are limits to the utility of the restored sight. It is seldom strong enough to read print or recognize people's faces. Depth and distance perception may be impaired, which can hinder free movement through space. When the patients opt for the familiar methods of white cane and Braille, researchers express disappointment. They talk of this choice in terms of relapse, as if the skills of blindness were a bad habit or addiction. Researchers operate in a simple blindness versus sight binary where some sight, no matter how impaired or inadequate, is assumed to be better than none. They are not interested in the murkier phenomenology of such contemporary conditions as "legal blindness with some usable sight" that I touched on in my introduction. They claim to be restoring sight, when in fact they provide their patients a new visual impairment with little or no guidance about how to manage it. Not surprisingly, the formerly blind people become depressed. And this depression may contribute to health problems even early death.

Elsewhere I have speculated that the failures and depression of the formerly blind people may be a function of the researchers' and patients' inflated expectations. For the purposes of this book, I am less concerned with the emotional issues in these studies and more interested to observe how often the newly sighted person is required to look at pictures. It would seem that looking at pictures would be well down the list of visual activities a newly sighted person should wish to master. Of course, a person with some previous visual experience might be eager to become reacquainted with favorite works of art when sight is restored. John Howard Griffin (who would later write *Black Like Me*) was blind for ten years following a head injury sustained during World War II. When his sight suddenly and inexplicably returned, he was happy to see his wife and children for the first time, but soon isolated himself in a monastic retreat where he spent time every day looking at reproductions of Vermeer.[1] His returning sight was fragmented and erratic, so he sought solace in works of art he found peaceful and beautiful.

But for scientists studying people who were blind since birth, the pictures serve another function. From the earliest recorded cases, researchers measure how long it takes the patients to learn to interpret pictorial representations. It's almost as if they believe pictures and reality are the same thing or that humans are born knowing how to understand them. While infants show a preference for pictorial representations of faces over images of other things, face recognition neurons respond even to a smiley face or a similarly simple configuration; show a picture of anything else to a newborn, and she will make nothing of it. Even months later she may respond to it tactually or kinesthetically, crumpling and shredding the page then putting it in her mouth. Adults who read to her will point to and trace elements of the illustrations, naming the objects depicted. Over time, the child will learn to associate certain patterns on the pages with objects in the real world and the words used to name them. But the formerly blind are expected to pick this up much quicker. For instance, in 1728 William Cheselden reported that his young patient had trouble with pictures:

> We thought he soon knew what pictures represented, which were shew'd to him, but we found afterwards we were mistaken; for about two months after he was couch'd, he discovered at once, they represented solid bodies; when to that time he consider'd them only as party-colour'd planes, or surfaces diversified with variety of paint; but even then he was no less surpriz'd, expecting the pictures would feel like the things they represented, and was amaz'd when he found those parts, which by their light and shadow appear'd now round and uneven, felt only flat like the rest; and asked which was the lying sense, feeling, or seeing?[2]

From an art historical perspective, the young gentleman showed remarkable prescience. Initially, he saw the pictures for what they were—painted surfaces. In effect, he expressed a distinctly twentieth-century observation: "Paint is paint, canvas is canvas." It took him another two months to learn to interpret the pictures as two-dimensional projections of three-dimensional space. When he was shown a miniature portrait of his father, he

> acknowledged a likeness, but was vastly surpriz'd; asking, how it could be, that a large face could be express'd in so little room, saying, it should have seem'd as impossible to him, as to put a bushel of anything into a pint.[3]

Here again, the young gentleman's comments seem to anticipate statements by critics and artists in later centuries. For instance, there's a famous, possibly apocryphal, anecdote about Pablo Picasso once being accosted by a stranger who asked why his paintings did not depict reality. When Picasso asked the man what he considered a picture of reality, he produced a photograph of his wife. Picasso scrutinized the photo for a while, then said, "She's very small. And flat." This story reveres Picasso for a profound statement about representation. But for Cheselden, the formerly blind young gentleman's comments are merely silly—a measure of what he had yet to learn. His question about which is the lying sense is dismissed unanswered, since apparently everyone knows that the eyes never lie.

In 1776, almost fifty years after Cheselden's case study, Franz Anton Mesmer, known later as the father of hypnotism, claimed that he had cured blindness through his techniques of animal magnetism. His patient was Maria Theresia von Paradis, an eighteen-year-old pianist and protégée of the Austrian empress for whom she was named.[4] The case, like many of Mesmer's claims, was controversial at the time and continues to rouse skepticism today. Was the cure an early instance of transcranial magnetic stimulation, or was it the result of hypnotic suggestion? Or were the two in cahoots hoping to boost their respective careers with this dramatic story? Certainly accounts are more melodramatic than scientific. Her parents interfered with the doctor's treatment. Mesmer believed it was because they feared she would lose the pension the empress had bestowed on her that supported the whole family. Others said it was because they believed he had seduced the girl. In a scandalous confrontation at Mesmer's home, the mother banged the girl's head against the wall and she lost her sight again. Mesmer restored it briefly, but eventually she returned to her parents and became blind for good. The family left Vienna for Paris where she continued her career as blind pianist, composer, and teacher.

But before all this upheaval, Mesmer attempted to record his patient's progress with something like scientific precision. And Like Cheselden, Mesmer devoted a good deal of time showing Paradis pictures. When she was shown portraits of her uncles she touched them and was troubled to discover their surfaces were flat. She distinguished colors but forgot their names. She could tell black from white because she found the white more painful to look at. This must have been particularly problematic for a pianist, and she found that she could not play while sighted. Fortunately for her future livelihood, she did not stay sighted for long.

Cases from the nineteenth and the twentieth centuries feature more clinically controlled methods. In 1963 R. L. Gregory and J. G. Wallace published their case study of Sidney Bradford, known only by his initials, SB, whose sight had been restored a few years earlier. Initially he showed a knack for transferring his prior tactile knowledge to his new visual experience. For instance, he quickly learned to tell time visually because he had been accustomed to read the angle of the clock's hands by touching his Braille watch. He also was able to identify capital letters that he had been trained to know by touch. He never made much of lowercase letters and never became proficient in reading. He could guess the title of a magazine from the initial letters but did not make much of the photo on the cover. He drew pictures, but his pictures tended to emphasize tactile elements of objects. For instance, when asked to draw a bus, he made the wheels like cart wheels, since these were the kind of wheels he had handled previously.

Oliver Sacks account of the formerly blind Virgil published in 1995 follows Gregory's case study with religious fidelity.[5] He arrived at Virgil's home with the same set of tests and optical illusions. He was surprised that Virgil could identify alphabet letters but could not instantly read. Why should this be surprising? Reading is not a matter of identifying letters in a word, nor is it a matter of scanning along a line. To read with any fluency, the eye must jump from cluster of letters to cluster of letters in regular intervals. This takes some time to master, and it involves a good deal of coordination of motor and cognitive skills. Virgil had similar trouble with pictures, and although he had always enjoyed listening to television, he had trouble making sense of the moving images. At the zoo, he could not perceive the animals as whole entities. It was only once he was allowed to touch a sculpture of a gorilla while he was simultaneously looking at a living animal that he was able to point to and name its parts and features. Like Paradis, he found that sight added nothing to his profession as masseur. In fact, he was troubled by seeing his clients for the first time. Then significant health problems intervened causing him to lose his job and then his house. His restored vision faltered. He went back to being blind. Sacks decamped for more interesting neurological cases elsewhere.

The Molyneux cases follow such a predictable pattern that it is no wonder that they should provide plots for literature and film. Brian Friel's *Molly Sweeney* was inspired by Sacks's account. Though female, Molly is middle-aged, has been blind since infancy, and works as a massage therapist. Like Virgil, the impetus for the surgery comes initially from her spouse rather than from her own desire. Like the historical accounts, Molly is initially elated but soon becomes frustrated, both by her perceived failure and from the constant scrutiny of those around her. Rice, her surgeon, monitors her progress. Frank, her husband, conducts nightly coaching sessions to help her learn to visually identify household objects that she previously knew by touch alone. And the O'Connors, a couple of neuroscientists, study her responses to photographs and optical illusions. Molly complains:

> Tests-tests-tests-tests-tests! Between Mr. Rice and Jean O'Connor and George O'Connor and indeed Frank himself I must have spent months and months being analyzed and answering questions and identifying drawings and making sketches. And, God, those damned tests with photographs and lights and objects—those endless tricks and illusions and distortions—the Zollner illusion, the Ames distorting room, the Staircase illusion, the Miiller-Lyer illusion. And they never told you if you had passed or failed so you always assumed you failed. Such peace—such peace when they were all finished.[6]

Molly's peace is only temporary. At the end of the play she is alone in a psychiatric hospital, suffering from hallucinations. Frank has decamped, and Rice, who had hoped to revive his career with success in Molly's case, now concedes that her failure to adapt to vision only confirms the familiar pattern established by the twenty previous cases and retires from medicine.

The 1999 film *At First Sight* is also inspired by Sacks's account, though it has a happier ending than Friel's play. Here, the emphasis is on the love story between Virgil (Val Kilmer) and Amy (Mira Sorvino). Amy is initially attracted to Virgil because she finds his blindness exotic and interesting. But soon after they become a couple, she urges him to have a sight-restoring operation. His surgeon is perplexed by Virgil's postoperative difficulties and sends him to Phil (Nathen Lane), a "visual therapist." This character might seem to be a stand-in for Oliver Sacks, but he is actually a counselor at a blind school, training newly blind children to adapt to blindness. He takes on the reverse process with Virgil, training him to adapt to his newly acquired sight. His method does not include the battery of tests that Molly Sweeney complained of; it is more improvisational than scientific. For example, in one scene he takes Virgil to a strip club. But as in the real-life cases, there's some emphasis on looking at two-dimensional images. In their first meeting, Phil shows Virgil an apple and then a picture of an apple. Virgil is able to make the connection instantly, though he is surprised when he touches the image and finds it flat, rephrasing the question Cheselden's patient asked, "You mean my eyes can lie?" Amy takes Virgil to look at art. He is perplexed by an installation by Dubuffet, but pleased by some graffiti, and Amy feels compelled to correct his aesthetic judgments. But as in Sacks's account, Virgil does not progress beyond a minimal level of visual proficiency. Eventually he loses his sight again, but here it is due to a different eye disease. He and Amy split up but are reunited in the final scene when she recognizes she had been wrong in wanting to change him. Thus, Hollywood love triumphs even over blindness!

It may be that this happy ending was suggested by a much earlier fictional account of restored sight. Wilkie Collins's 1872 novel, *Poor Miss Finch*, draws on eighteenth- and nineteenth-century speculation on blindness. The plot of this novel defies summary, but the central narrative is about how Licilla, the poor Miss Finch of the title, regains and later loses her sight. Prior to meeting the eye surgeon who will perform the operation, Lucilla is a well-adapted blind person. She paraphrases Diderot's blind man of Puiseaux when she disparages sight as inferior to touch, saying that she would rather have longer arms than working eyes: "I could find out better what was going on at a distance with my hands, than you could with your eyes and your telescopes."[7] She only agrees to go through with the operation because she wants to be able to see her fiancé. The doctor tests her new sight with household objects, asking her to distinguish between a square sheet of paper and a round saucer, not having a cube and sphere as Molyneux prescribes. But he does not show her pictures. Lucilla has the same trouble distinguishing between the cat and the dog that Cheselden's patient had. When her sight eventually fails, it is as much a psychological as a physiological problem. She ignores her surgeons advice to remain calm and becomes so agitated by the melodrama of her love life (her fiancé's twin brother attempts to deceive her into eloping with him) and her blindness returns. Even once she is married to the right twin, she refuses the offer of another surgery and repudiates her former desire to see him. While scientists, who study these cases in the real world, are puzzled by their patients relapse into blindness, Collins's blind Lucilla proclaims her happiness to be restored to her original state: "I look back in horror at what I suffered when I had my sight—my one effort is to forget that miserable time."[8] She recovers from the trauma of temporary sightedness and lives happily ever after.

These fictional narratives make a metaphor of the sight-restoration cases to tell a cautionary tale about the dangers of trying to change something fundamental in another person. The outcome of the real-life Molyneux cases is so dire it is a wonder that any blind person would submit to have the operation. In 2000, Mike May, a California entrepreneur and skiing enthusiast, regained partial sight after forty-three-years of total blindness. He benefited from new stem-cell procedures and anti-rejection drugs that aided his body's acceptance of a corneal transplant. He deliberately did not read the accounts of other sight-restoration cases, and once he did, after the fact, he says he was glad he didn't. They might have discouraged him from agreeing to the surgery. His case has not received the scientific attention of other restored-sight cases, because he lost his sight at age three, which is generally held to be too late to count. Nevertheless, the blog he kept following his operation makes for refreshing reading after the accounts of restored-sight cases done by professionals. This is due, in part, to the fact that here, the patient speaks for himself. He directs his newly restored vision to features in the world which interest him, rather than the time-honored tests devised by researchers. So he is delighted by his first glimpse of clouds from an airplane window and dancing dust motes in sunlight. His restored sight in the right eye is about 20/1000, well below the level of legal blindness. In terms of the utility of this impaired vision, he records that he appreciates how it makes it easier for him to follow people standing on a line and moving through a crowd. But in many other instances, he finds the vision distracting and tends to close his eyes. He continues to use a service dog and Braille. He also uses GPS devices his company developed. Nowhere in his own account is this depicted as a relapse into blindness. The doctors and researchers who work with him do not make him feel guilty for retaining the blind way of doing most things, and so he does not experience the depression of patients like SB and Virgil. He seems to have been immune to the inflated promises about how much his life would improve with vision. A year after the operation he reports that there's nothing he could do with sight that he couldn't do before:

> If I didn't see another day, I have a year of fascinating experiences I can be extremely grateful for. I can't say my life has changed radically because of having vision; it is as crazy and fun filled as ever. Besides seeing my loved friends and family, the highlights of the past year are: Seeing Mont Blanc from Fiona's chalet in Switzerland, seeing and skiing for the first time, seeing the stars, people watching and watching our boys play soccer. Seeing their baby video was pretty emotional for me.
>
> One of the most functional benefits of this limited vision has been being able to catch a ball in the air and to follow people in a line or when walking through crowds. I saw my first mosquito today. Is this a good thing? It is if I can swat it. For the most part, there is nothing I can do today that I couldn't do a year and a day ago without vision. It is a revelation to realize that as well as to savor the mysteries of vision, which I have explored and may continue to explore.[9]

May finds his new visual experience interesting and entertaining but does not feel transformed into a sighted person. May does not report much about looking at pictures per se. The first time he went to the movies with his children, he could not make sense of the moving images. And when he watched football on TV, he had trouble with the cross-cutting between different perspectives. In other words, the conventions of cinematic narrative and television sportscasting made his viewing difficult.

But as I say, researchers interested in the Molyneux problem would disregard Mike May's account because he was not born blind. While the rate of total congenital blindness in the industrialized world is about 3 births in 10,000, in the developing world it is higher; in India, for example, there are about 8 births per 10,000. And blind children in developing countries will typically have fewer educational opportunities and may live in isolation from their peers. They would therefore make better subjects for this kind of research. In 2003 Pawan Sinha, a neuroscientist at MIT, launched Project Prakash, a humanitarian and scientific enterprise to identify, treat, and study blind children in India.[10] The researchers actively seek congenitally blind children in rural areas where there is typically little access to medical care. Those with congenital cataracts are brought to Delhi where the cataracts are removed and synthetic lenses are implanted. Those who wish to volunteer then participate in studies. What separates the Project Prakash research from the studies of the twenty other cases of restored sight over the past thousand years is that the Prakash researchers have the luxury of a comparatively large pool of subjects, and so can focus their inquiries into singular visual tasks rather than wearing out their subjects with a plethora of tests. A recent study employed a pool of eight recently sighted children to test their susceptibility to optical illusions two days after their surgery.[11] Other studies focus on object recognition tasks: How does the brain learn to distinguish an object from its surroundings? It has been discovered that motion is key. The newly sighted people learn to parse out objects from their surroundings when there is some motion involved. It makes sense; infants living in the real world are likely to observe the world in motion around them. This helps explain while earlier patients had so much trouble with static pictures.

But the researchers test the patients using pictures rather than visual arrays in three-dimensional space. The newly sighted patients are asked to trace the outlines of images on a computer screen with their fingertips. Initially they trace both the object and peripheral elements such as shadows. But once the picture is animated, they do better. For example, a researcher may show the patient an image of a square and a circle. Note that the square and the circle replace the cube and sphere of Molineux's problem. At first, the patient will trace the outlines of the square and circle but also identify the shape formed by the overlap of the two forms as a separate object. Once the square and circle are made to move around the computer screen, the patients are then able to perceive and correct their initial error.[12]

While Project Prakash offers new answers to the old Molyneux question, there is a good deal of other research in neuroscience and perceptual psychology that employs blind subjects. Much of this research with blind people is about mapping the brain and speculating on neural plasticity. Brain-imaging technology allows scientists to compare the brains of congenitally blind people with those of congenitally sighted people to determine to what extent the brain rewires itself to compensate for a lack of one kind of sensory stimuli. It has been observed, for instance, that when a totally congenitally blind person who is a fluent Braille reader reads a Braille text while in a MRI machine, areas of the brain typically associated with vision will be activated. But these images of brains of blind people do not, of course, recreate the subjects' experience of their mental images. Is it possible to devise objective representations of blind mental imaging? Does the mind's hand of the blind function the same way as the mind's eye of the sighted?

There is a whole field of research preoccupied by this issue, seeking to determine whether blind people can make sense of images when they are rendered in tactile form. Technologies now exist that allow a blind person to make a drawing with semi-permanent raised lines. With a raised-line drawing kit someone can draw a line with a pointed stylus on a sheet of plastic stretched over a board coated with a rubbery surface. This surface will press back against the pressure of the stylus and will make the plastic pucker to create a tangible line. The drawings produced with this device are extremely simple, with the lines depicting the outlines of objects. It is impossible to depict shading of any kind, and all the lines tend to be of a uniform thickness. Numerous studies observe blind people examining the simple line drawings made with the device, while others observe the blind subjects making drawings of their own. In addition to indicating the age of onset and degree of sight loss, the researchers specify that the subjects have no prior experience with tactile pictures. It seems likely, however, that even someone who has been blind since birth will have some experience of ideas about pictures. As a child, she will learn that story books include illustrations, that television includes images with the sounds. It is also likely that she will handle toys and models that will convey some sense of the stylization required to translate a natural object into a representation, such as a simple contour line drawing. Later, she might learn that people go to art museums to look at pictures, and may ask to have visual terms defined, such as vantage point, perspective, foreshortening, and so forth. Researchers who wish to study how a blind person conceptualizes visual phenomena such as color, or conventions of pictorial representation such as perspective, may consider that the findings are contaminated if the blind person had these concepts explained at some point by parents or teachers.

Perhaps to bypass some of these complications, one researcher did a series of studies at a blind school in Haiti. As far as he could ascertain from the somewhat incomplete medical records, he collected a group of children who had been blind from an acceptably early age. In most cases, the cause of their blindness was severe malnutrition. These children certainly had no prior experience with tactile pictures. Indeed, they had little experience with many commonplaces of North American life. Also, as the researcher discovered, malnutrition in infants affects other systems and processes as well. Nevertheless, the researchers persevered, with somewhat mixed results. For instance one subject tended to laugh "rather than respond directly to questions."[13] It remains unclear whether this was a sign of some cognitive impairment due to infantile malnutrition or a commentary on the tasks she was being asked to perform.

Leaving aside ethical questions about whether the money that funded these studies in Haiti might have been better spent, there is an abundance of other research to consider. Typically researchers begin by showing tactile images to the subjects and recording their interpretations and comments. For example, the blind subjects may be instructed to examine a tactile drawing of a fork, a familiar everyday object that they are accustomed to handling. When they identify it as an animal's paw or a candle, the response is marked as "a near miss,"[14] rather than a complete error, because it makes sense visually. But the researchers fail to acknowledge that the response makes sense tactually as well. The blind subjects seem to be interpreting the tines of the fork as tactile features of another object, in this case features that denote some danger—the pointy claws of the animal, or the singeing heat of the flame. Were there other unrecorded responses that might have made no sense visually, but reveal an interpretation of the tactile patterns as representing tactile features?

Researchers record blind subjects' comments about the inadequacy of two-dimensional representations of three-dimensional objects. For instance, blind subjects point out that a face drawn in profile is inaccurate because it only shows one eye and one ear when in tactile reality there would be two. But the researchers fail to anticipate that exposure to these drawing practices may shape the way these same subjects later respond to certain drawing problems. If asked to draw a table, blind subjects often draw a rectangle to represent its top, and then four lines or other configurations to represent the legs, which might or might not be attached to the top. The rectangular top is certainly an accurate rendering of what a table top feels like. The right angles of the corners are constant no matter where the person is located in relation to it. Researchers may prompt the subjects to revise their original drawing or do additional drawings to show how the parts of the table fit together. The researchers judge the drawing as satisfactory only if there is some attempt to represent perspective, for example, if the drawing shows two legs rather than four to indicate the table is being viewed from the side. It seems that the researchers' prompts communicate a subtle message: the point of drawing is to record visual rather than tactile perception.

Some researchers have sought to understand how blind people conceptualize space and map their environment. Perhaps this research was inspired by Descartes' image of the Hypothetical Blind Man moving effortlessly over the nighttime landscape, while his sighted brother flailed and floundered in the mud. But the research required the subjects to draw maps to show how they understood their movement through space. In one instance, blind children were required to follow a path by holding onto a rope that marked it. At each turning point there was some sort of prize. Afterward, they were asked to draw a line showing the route and indicating the sequence of the prizes.[15] One child drew a more or less straight line, indicating that the first prize was the teddy bear, the second, the toy car, and so forth. The researcher prompted the child to revise the map to indicate the turns in the path, in effect to represent a bird's eye view of the route taken. While it seems to me that the child responded to the researcher's instructions in a perfectly adequate manner, the line representing the temporal sequence of the experience was not how the sighted researcher conceptualized space. The researcher might have benefited from reviewing pilgrimage maps of the Middle Ages, which were written as a list of instructions directing the pilgrims from one location to the next, without any effort to depict the twists and turns of the actual road. The road might go over rivers and through woods, but these details were peripheral to the people making or using these maps.[16] Bird's-eye views and Ariel maps are relatively recent innovations. With the popularity of GPS systems that give drivers turn-by-turn instructions, I wonder how notions of normal mental mapping will change. Since GPS systems are also popular with blind people, their conceptualization of space and way-finding might now become normative.

Among other things, researchers have found that with instruction, blind subjects can learn the principles of linear perspective: making parallel lines converge at a vanishing point, adjusting the scale of objects to indicate their distance from the viewer, and developing some system to indicate how near objects occlude portions of those that are farther away. I can remember learning to draw in perspective. This was in second or third grade when my eyesight was close to average. I remember learning that to draw a road going off into the distance, one should draw not parallel lines but lines that converge at the horizon. I also learned how to draw a rectilinear form, such as a house, in perspective, with an adjustment of the angles to indicate distance from the viewer. Did I believe I was drawing something that resembled reality, or was I simply learning conventional drawing techniques? The houses I drew that featured shuttered windows and chimneys emitting curly-cues of smoke in no way resembled the apartment buildings where I actually lived. I suspect I was simply imitating the images in story books. For me, drawing at school was an academic exercise with rules, right and wrong answers. Left to my own devices, I was far more likely to produce highly colored abstract images similar to the art work at home and at the galleries and studios I visited with my parents.

I was once a subject of a research study involving raised-line drawings. I was at a conference where there happened to be a significant number of blind people present. The researcher approached me during a break and asked if I would like to participate in her project. I agreed, and we sat down on a bench in a corridor where a coffee break was in progress. She asked the usual questions about my age, educational background, degree of vision impairment, and age of sight loss. Although totally congenitally blind people are the prize quarry for such research, studies often include imperfectly blind people such as myself for comparison, and often blindfolded sighted people, usually university undergraduates.

The researcher had small models of geometrical forms—the sphere and cube I would have predicted—and a cone, which was a refreshing innovation. She arranged these on the flat surface of the bench between us, and then showed me raised line drawings and asked me to pick the one that best represented the arrangement. The drawing represented the view looking down from above. The cube was therefore represented by a square, the sphere by a circle, and the cone by a circle with a single dot at its center.

I found this particularly ingenious. I should point out that though I have residual vision, the white on white pattern of a raised-line drawing is invisible to me. I explained this to the researcher. I even offered to wear a blindfold so there would be no question about whether I was performing the task visually. I also knew that there's evidence that being able to see the motion of ones hands can aid tactile discernment. But she didn't seem to care about these issues. She had a stopwatch and recorded how long it took me to identify the correct drawing.

After several different arrangements and sets of drawings, we moved on. Now the drawings were meant to represent a straight-on view. I was meant to imagine that I was viewing the arrangement of objects as if my chin were on the edge of the bench and the objects were all at eye level. I began to quibble; the notion of eye level is somewhat alien, even for me, but I knew what she was up to. She wanted to test if I could understand a drawing in perspective where portions of the forms closer to the viewer would occlude the objects farther back in space. The task was made somewhat easier in that the sphere was still represented by a circle since raised-line drawings do not use shading to indicate curved volumes. The cube was drawn in perspective according to rules that I knew. The cone was a triangle with a curved base. I commented on all this. She did not write it down. When the forms were widely spaced across the table top, the task was relatively easy because I knew that the object that was smallest was meant to show that it was farthest from the viewer. When the objects were closely grouped and the drawing had overlapping outlines, it became trickier. I made educated guesses based on whether I was touching a straight or curved line.

She did not give me my score, but I suspect I did OK: perhaps slower in my judgments than a sighted person looking at similar drawings but perhaps quicker than a young blind child without much experience of raised-line drawing who never had the conventions of drawing explained to her.

I do not know what became of this researcher. She was a graduate student from another country. I do not know if the study I participated in helped her gain an advanced degree. If it did, I'm happy for her. I admire the many blind people, children and adults, who have contributed to understanding human cognition. But the ultimate goal of so much of the modern research on blind subjects seems to have very little practical applications to education or cultural enrichment. Certainly it is useful for a blind person to know how to interpret and produce raised-line diagrams, maps, and drawings.

But beyond this, the researchers seem to be conflating two very different capacities. The research shows that blind subjects can learn the drawing techniques that have evolved for the convenience and enjoyment of sighted people. But does this prove the existence of some sort of universal, innate capacity related to picture making? Are the blind subjects really producing representations of their own perceptions?

This research is frequently cited by arts institutions seeking to develop access programs for people with impaired vision. The art educators extract the message that blind people have the cognitive wherewithal to understand concepts related to art. It is disheartening that this message needs to be reiterated at this late date in human history. I recognize that arts organizations seeking funding for programming for the blind can cite some of this research as scientific proof that the enterprise is not utterly futile. But the focus on total congenital blindness perpetuates a stereotype about blindness as a monolithic experience. And the researchers' obsession with linear perspective fails to take any account of other innovations in pictorial representation over the centuries. A raised-line rendering might help a blind person appreciate the bold drawing and skewed perspective of an artist like Henri Matisse, but it would seem an inadequate reproduction of work by Mark Rothko or Jackson Pollack.

Here's another thought experiment. If we imagine, after the fashion of H. G. Wells's short story, "The Country of the Blind," a culture where everyone was born without sight, would there develop a tradition of tactile picture making? Would the idea of two-dimensional projection of three-dimensional space occur to anyone as a meaningful representational system? Wouldn't it be more likely that these blind people would devise a system of symbols to record tactile features of objects beyond their contours such as texture, temperature, volume, and weight? What would those pictures look like? And would those pictures be recognizable or comprehensible to a sighted viewer?

The point needs to be made that while human beings throughout history and across cultures have an inclination to make pictures, there are conventions of picture making that artists have innovated and that cultures accept. One of my nephews was asked to draw a picture of himself one day at school. In his picture there was a circle. To the right of the circle there were two feet, and to the right of these there was a hand with all five fingers extended with a circle, smaller than the first, right above it. When asked, my nephew explained that it was a picture of him running to catch a ball. It was a picture intended to be read in a sequence, from left to right. It may have been influenced by comic books or maybe television cartoons, where fragments of a whole object are pictured in close up, as it were, then juxtaposed to represent a sequence of events. Or it may have been an example of what are known as "list" drawings, where a series of scribbles and squiggles are made then named by the child to represent different parts of a whole.

My nephew's teacher, however, considered him to be too old to be making drawings in this way. She was concerned that the picture reflected some defect or delay. The right way to draw a picture of oneself, according to the teacher's training, was some elaboration of a full frontal stick figure, with a head and an appropriate number of limbs symmetrically arranged on either side of a vertical axis, representing the upright spine. Also, the figure should be motionless, as if posing for a snapshot.

My father, an artist who had taught drawing for many years and indeed believed he could teach anyone to draw, was outraged. To him, his grandson's drawing reflected an original response to the assigned task. Why should he not represent himself in this way? He was an active boy; stasis was not a natural state for him. Why not draw himself in motion? And he was proud of himself for making the running catch—a feat of eye-hand coordination and motor skills well in advance of his age. But to the teacher drawing was not about art, not about self-expression, or even about making an original response to an assignment. It was about recognizing and employing the conventions of symbolic representation, where certain marks on paper are to be universally understood to mean one thing and one thing only. The teacher was not asking my nephew to be original or to tell a story with images. She meant to assess something about his cognitive capacities from his drawing.

This anecdote illustrates a fundamental disconnect between scientists and the educators who are influenced by their research, and artists. Scientists are using pictures as an indication of cognitive capacities and conceptualization skills. Artists, and their ilk, think of pictures as techniques of representing three-dimensional reality on a two-dimensional plane, with a history and an array of conventions. While it is nice that science has shown that blind people can learn to interpret some standard conventions of drawing, I'm not sure it proves that the drawings they learn to interpret or to make are necessarily an unmediated representation of their own concepts about reality. They may learn to follow the rules of sighted drawing, but when they use the tools to make something to satisfy their own concepts, the results are dismissed as incorrect. We should not forget that all this research, whether with formerly or currently blind people, is not designed to improve the lives or opportunities of blind people. These research subjects replace the Hypothetical Blind Man of philosophical inquiry, to build new theories about human consciousness in general. Educators and rehabilitation specialists might be able to glean some ideas about using tactile diagrams or maps to aid blind people in the study of geometry or way-finding. Some of the research might make art educators less likely to talk down to blind people about art. But I am not convinced that any of this research using blind people brings us closer to understanding the cognitive processes involved in art appreciation or art making.

{3}

Visible Braille, Invisible Blindness

The long-lived analogy linking the Hypothetical Blind Man's hands to the sighted man's eyes has had one major benefit for actual blind people—the Braille reading and writing system. As I noted in chapter 1, Valentin Haüy, the founder of the first school for the blind, was well versed in the philosophy of the Hypothetical and was convinced that blind people could learn to read using their fingers. Even before Haüy founded his school, there were affluent or well-connected blind people whose family and friends sought to devise tactile reading and writing systems, as well as tactile maps and diagrams. Diderot and others commented on Nicholas Saunderson's tactile apparatus to do mathematical calculations. And Haüy consulted with Theresia von Paridis to learn techniques she used for reading and writing music. When he founded his school, Haüy used embossing techniques that were already available to create a library of texts featuring enlarged, raised Roman letters that blind students read by tracing each letter with the fingertip. These texts were readily legible by sighted people, and so teachers of the blind required no special training to use them. But tracing embossed Roman letters with the fingers is a slow and imprecise process. Haüy and others used various methods for blind students to write the Roman alphabet, by, for instance, tracing forms underneath the writing paper, but, of course, the blind students could not read the texts they produced.

In 1824, a fifteen-year-old blind student at the school Haüy founded proposed a reading system that solved the problems of all the previous methods. Louis Braille used patterns of raised dots, each representing but not resembling a letter in the Roman alphabet, and taking up only as much space as the tip of a finger. This meant that the reader did not need to trace around the individual letters. Rather the blind reader moves the finger quickly across the line. The system meant that books could be produced more rapidly and cheaply. Most significantly, Braille's code could be produced and read by blind readers themselves. It was perhaps this feature of the system that made educators of the blind initially reluctant to adopt Braille as an official teaching method.

Teachers needed to learn a new system, and blind students could communicate independently with each other, without the intervention and possible censorship of a sighted amanuensis. The school in Paris did not recognize Braille officially until 1854, two years after its inventor's death. During the late nineteenth and into the twentieth century, there were competing systems in use in Europe and North America. Braille was only adopted by American blind schools in 1916, and it took until 1932 for Braille to replace other systems. Today, Braille has been adapted for all the world's alphabets and languages, and it has been in use for the better part of a century. Still, it remains something of a mystery to sighted people, a secret code that sets blind people apart.

I encounter this attitude whenever I read Braille in public. People often ask to see the Braille text, never having handled one before, and I sometimes find myself conducting an introductory Braille reading lesson. People even make comments about how reading as I do must make me feel closer to the text, as if the physical contact with the Braille must somehow amplify my emotional or intellectual response. The conflation of tactile sensation with the emotions leads to a kind of mystification. If my Braille reading prompts comment, then it is evidence that the blind, like other disabled people, are still invisible in mainstream American life. Our habits and paraphernalia remain unfamiliar and exotic. Blind people continue to be excluded from the educational and employment opportunities that would provide them access to the sort of academic and literary venues where they would be required to read in public. Only about 45 percent of students with severe visual impairments or blindness graduate high school compared with 80 percent of their sighted peers.[1] Unemployment among working-age blind Americans still hovers around 70 percent.[2] In addition to the educational and economic disadvantages that keep blind people out of the public eye, the rate of Braille usage in America has declined significantly since the second half of the twentieth century. From 1963 to 1993 the percentage of legally blind children who used Braille declined from 51 to 9 percent.[3] The decline began with the introduction of magnification devices and recorded books, and then later text-to-speech computer technology. Special education experts determined that these modern innovations made Braille obsolete. More recent research shows, however, that blind people who use Braille achieve higher levels of education and employment,[4] and many states have adopted legislation ensuring that blind children can obtain Braille instruction through the public schools if they wish. So the trend away from Braille may be reversing. But rehabilitation specialists still dissuade people who become blind as adults from learning Braille, claiming it is too hard to master.

Speaking from my experience, I can unequivocally assert that this is a myth. I belong to the first generation of American Braille illiterates—a fact that does not make me proud. I grew up during the period when Braille instruction was actively discouraged in favor of the new low vision technologies. I did not learn Braille until I was over thirty, when I taught it to myself. Like anything worth knowing, learning Braille takes effort and practice. I do not read it as fluently as I would if I had learned it when I first went blind as a child. But it's a useful tool and I'm glad I learned it. Despite the general decline in Braille literacy, the passage of the Americans with Disabilities Act in 1990 meant that Braille began to appear in public places such as the signs on the doors of public restrooms and in government offices, especially those serving blind people, and most prominently, in elevators. The message of these signs is uncontroversial: blind people use public spaces and have a right to the same information available to their sighted peers. But in some instances, the designers of these signs did not think about access all the way through.

Perform the following thought experiment. If you do not happen to be blind already, imagine that you are. You board an elevator in a high-rise office building in a large American city. You wish to go to the twenty-second floor and scan the panel of Braille labels to find the correct button. You can do this even if you don't read Braille since the panel also includes raised Arabic numerals you can trace with your fingers. Acknowledging that not all blind people read Braille, tactile signage typically includes large raised print for non-Braille readers. By whatever means, you find and press the button for the twenty-second floor. Meanwhile other passengers board the elevator and press buttons. The doors close. You go up. The doors open and someone gets off. Again the doors close and you go up. The doors open and two people get off and one gets on. The doors close. You go up. After another interval, the doors open. What floor are you on?

Answer? You do not have enough information to answer. You must resort to the method blind people used prior to the introduction of Braille buttons: you ask your fellow passengers. In fact, you may find it easier to ask them to press the button for you back on the ground floor, since it may be more convenient and polite than to reach around them to scan the panel for the right button.

This is not to say that Braille elevator buttons are not a welcome accommodation. After all, there may not always be other passengers to lend assistance. Braille buttons also send a visual message to anyone using the elevator to allow for the possibility that there are blind people in the world who might end up in the elevator. But they do not solve the whole problem. Some buildings install tactile labels on the exterior frame of the elevator door on each floor, though it often takes a good deal of groping to lay one's hands on these, not to mention the need to always station oneself near the door. Some elevators feature a recorded voice to announce the floor as the doors open, though this solution is often rejected as annoying to seeing-hearing passengers by contributing to the ambient din of noise-polluted public environments. But without some sort of signal indicating each floor, Braille elevator buttons seem to perform a different function altogether. They are a visible sign proving that the building is in compliance with the ADA, whether or not other facets of that code are being observed.

Perhaps the rise in Braille used in public spaces has contributed to the phenomenon of Braille jewelry. Typically, there is a pendant or bracelet charm that features a single word or short phrase in Braille, sometimes paired with the word in Roman print, sometimes not. Often these trinkets are sold to benefit blind schools or other organizations, but it is possible to find examples sold without any reference to blind people. Recently, I was walking in my neighborhood when a woman on a bicycle stopped me. At first I thought she was going to ask directions. Contrary to stereotypes, if you want good directions, always ask a blind person. We are less likely to rely on vague gestures and imprecise phrases such as "over there" or "you can't miss it." But in this instance she asked me if I could read Braille. When I told her that I could, she rummaged in her backpack and produced a ceramic pendent she'd bought at a spiritual retreat's craft fair. It was a circular disk with a shiny teal glaze. The front had a bumpy texture and the back had a few Braille dots. The Braille was slightly undersized and the spacing of the characters was irregular. Initially, I read one of the *e*'s as *ch*. But eventually I made out that it said "peace." In fact, there was almost no need to read it. These things usually feature one of two words: peace or love. It's as if these are the only two words one needs to communicate to blind people. It reminds me of the fact that most Americans know how to say "I love you" in American Sign Language even if they know no other sign. What is the message here? Are blind and deaf people so alien and potentially hostile that they need to be placated in this way? On the street corner I was more struck by the possibility that the Braille might have been mistranscribed to say peach rather than peace, similar to the way tattoo artists often miswrite Chinese or Sanskrit characters. But the woman with the ceramic pendant did not seem interested in these ironies. She produced the card of the artist, and then decided that she wanted "to gift me" with the pendant. I declined. I didn't want to deprive her. But she insisted and then pedaled off to her meditation class. Now that the thing is in my possession, I note that the bumps on the front may represent grapes on a vine. Are the grapes meant to suggest the Braille dots on the back? Are grapes suggestive of peace? Maybe it's just an abstract pattern.

Other uses of braille in public also seem intended to send some sort of message to sighted people rather than to aid the blind. Consider the Alabama state quarter (Fig. 3.1). In 1999, the US Mint began releasing twenty-five cent coins with different designs on the reverse to commemorate each of the fifty states. The Alabama quarter features a portrait of Helen Keller, who was born in the state in 1880. She is pictured seated with a large book in her lap. The slogan "Spirit of Courage" appears in a banner at her feet. Her name is in both Roman letters and a reduced-sized Braille, which is printed to one side. When the coin was issued in 2003, the US Mint made much of the fact that it is the first circulating coin in America to feature Braille, but no one mentioned that the miniscule size of the Braille makes it impossible to read with a fingertip. For that matter, it is nearly impossible to read visually without magnification.

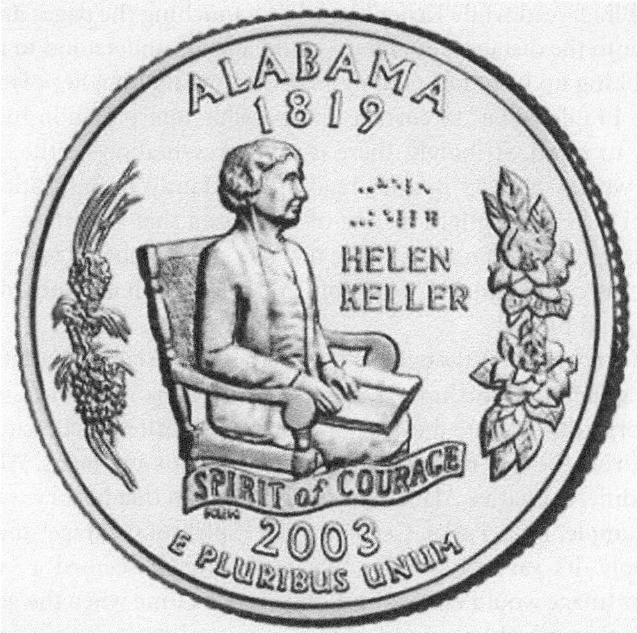

FIGURE 3.1 *The Alabama state quarter featuring Helen Keller reading Braille.*

Even if it were large enough to be read by finger, what is it there to communicate? The words "Helen Keller" do not indicate the value of the coin. And if the braille was there to indicate the denomination, it would be an unnecessary accommodation. Most blind people learn to distinguish between different coins through such tactile features as variations in size and shape, thickness or thinness, milled and smooth edges. Blind people have always had this skill. Indeed, Valentin Haüy initially became convinced that blind children were educable when he observed how easily a blind beggar could recognize the different coins tossed in his bowl.

Since the Braille on the Helen Keller quarter does not denote the coin's value, it seems to be there rather as a visible signifier of her blindness, and to signal that it was her overcoming of her blindness that earns her the "Spirit of Courage" motto. Many Americans, particularly younger Americans may not know who Helen Keller was and why she deserves to be commemorated in this way. It is difficult to represent blindness in a portrait, especially a portrait of such small size. In the reduced scale of a coin image, the blindfolds and dark glasses that are the typical attributes of blindness in painting, photography, and film might be understood as a medical intervention or fashion statement. People in the know may recognize the large format of the book in Keller's lap as characteristic of Braille pages, which are generally about twelve inches square. But it is equally possible that the book is simply a large one, perhaps a Bible. And while Keller's hands are touching the pages and her eyes are aimed into the distance, the image could also be understood to represent a woman looking up from her reading in reflection, holding her place with her finger. The Braille serves to correct this possible interpretation before it can even come to mind. Strikingly, there is no representation on the coin of any other noteworthy activity besides reading—certainly no indication that the book Keller is reading might be one of the dozen that she wrote. Rather the whole message of the coin seems to be that she is remembered for reading, and for having the commendable "Spirit of Courage," which is assumed necessary to learn to read Braille.

It's worth noting that though Keller was born in Alabama, after about age ten she resided in the Northeast—Massachusetts, New York, and Connecticut. Many Americans associate the state of Alabama as a site of activism and racial violence during the civil rights movement of the 1950s and 1960s. We can wonder why a different native Alabaman associated with that history was not chosen, for example, Rosa Parks. Certainly, the "Spirit of Courage" motto would equally apply. It's easy to surmise that Helen Keller seemed a safer choice because her image would not evoke memories of a time when the government of that state was culpable.

Perhaps in response to the criticism of the undersized Braille on the Helen Keller quarter, in 2009 the US Mint issued a noncirculating silver dollar coin commemorating the bicentenary of Louis Braille's birth. This coin has an image of Louis Braille on the face and on the back, the standard sized Braille characters BRL, which is the contracted form for his name. Again, the Braille is not used to identify the denomination of the coin, but at least it is the correct size to be legible. The US Mint seems to have no plans to incorporate Braille or any sort of tactile markings on other coins, or paper currency, where it would be truly helpful.

If the Braille on the Helen Keller quarter helps viewers interpret an otherwise ambiguous image, the Braille on the Franklin D. Roosevelt Memorial in Washington, DC presents a different array of problems. When the memorial opened in 1997, many disabled activists protested that there was no image of Roosevelt in a wheelchair. A massive fundraising campaign was launched and 1.65 million dollars were collected to commission an additional statue of Roosevelt, eventually dedicated in 2001.

At the same time, there was a side controversy about the use of Braille in the monument. A series of bronze bas relief plaques by sculptor Robert Graham depicted social programs Roosevelt instituted during the Depression, through a montage of many figures and faces expressing the anguish and hope of the era. The plaques also include Braille characters spelling out the program names: WPA, CCC, and so forth. The dots in these inscriptions are four to five times the standard size—closer to the size of a bottle cap than to a pin head—and the spacing of the dots is so irregular it makes the inscriptions almost impossible to decipher. A third of the plaques are displayed about eight feet off the ground, putting them well out of the reach of visitors.

At the time of the memorial's opening, Robert Graham said, "My concept of that piece was to have Braille as a kind of invitation to touch, more than anything . . . Braille is not much different than touching a face or anything else . . . That was kind of the graphic idea, the layering of many faces coming out and the layering of the Braille and the layering of several tactile surfaces."[5]

In the artist's mind, the Braille was meant as "an invitation to touch," but to whom? The memorial as a whole is a work of environmental art where touching is understood to be a part of a multisensory, kinesthetic experience. But the many quotations from Roosevelt's speeches on display around the memorial do not include Braille transcriptions, so there does not seem to have been any intention to make the memorial especially blind-friendly. And while the Braille on the Helen Keller quarter is there to indicate Keller's blindness, the faces in Graham's designs are not necessarily those of blind people. Blindness does not seem to have been on the artist's mind. Rather, Graham was using Braille as a decorative motif, an interesting texture, not as an aid to blind visitors. Furthermore, I would have to argue, reading Braille is not at all analogous to touching a face. Braille reading is done with the fingertips; face touching involves all parts of the fingers and palms, since the point of face touching is to grasp the whole form rather than to take in the meaning of the expression.

Graham's mention of face touching refers to the faces in his bas-reliefs, but it suggests that he subscribes to the popular belief that blind people regularly touch others' faces, even those of strangers. This is held to be a way for blind people to learn what others look like, and thus to gain, through the extrasensory perception we are supposed to possess, tactile insight into their characters. Helen Keller is the only blind person I've ever heard of who made a regular practice of this. Or at least she was frequently photographed with her hands on others' faces. Sometimes she was performing "tadoma," a method of tactile lipreading, where an experienced practitioner can interpret another's speech from the movements of the lips, and the vibrations from the throat. But in other images, Keller's hands are all over the other's face, as if trying to blot them out of the picture. On the date of Keller's death in 1968, the *New York Times* printed a photograph of Keller touching Eleanor Roosevelt's face in this way. The 1954 documentary *The Unconquered* features some footage of Keller doing this to President Eisenhower. He visibly stiffens at her touch, while she grins broadly as she prods and palpates a glint in her prosthetic eyes. Given her leftist politics, one senses that the contrived photo op gave her a particularly subversive kick.

Responding to the protests that the Braille was too large to be meaningful to blind people Graham said, "Nothing is life-size in the piece, so you very much have to adjust yourself to the scale."[6] But scale is not the only problem. It is not simply that the Braille dots are oversized; it's that the spacing between the dots is irregular. The dots in Braille elevator buttons are also larger than those in a paper document, but they are legible because the spaces between dots within a single character and the spaces between characters are all standard. Graham's reference to scale mistakenly makes an analogy to oversized print letters as in a giant billboard. But the problem with the Braille in his sculpture is actually analogous to oversized print where letters overlap each other in such a way to make it difficult to determine where one letter ends and the next begins.

All this reflects a basic misunderstanding about how Braille works. Braille readers do not read dot by dot, or even character by character. Braille must be read serially, with the reading finger sliding unencumbered straight across the line. There is no tracing movement involved, no attempt to connect the dots to make them form a Roman letter. Also, Braille depends on active rather than passive touch. Even experienced readers have a hard time identifying Braille characters that are pressed onto the immobile fingertip. Fluent Braille readers do not pause on each cluster of dots but feel a rhythm of rising and falling dots as the finger moves.[7]

The over-sized and irregularly spaced braille at the FDR Memorial can only be deciphered by touching each dot and trying to assemble the pattern by making a mental picture of their arrangement. It is a sighted conception of how Braille must work. The Braille is almost an abstraction, referring to language without actually meaning anything. And while this may have an intellectual appeal, to many blind people who are still seldom imagined as visitors to such public places, this use of Braille as a decorative motif, rather than a meaningful communication, is both frustrating and insulting.

But Graham's use of Braille seems to have more than merely an aesthetic function in the piece. He was relying on sighted viewers to draw on a range of figurative associations about blindness, to suggest the spiritual darkness of the Depression, a period when Americans were "blind" to their economic future. Significantly, the Braille refers to Roosevelt's new deal policies, often disparaged by his critics as "alphabet soup"—a seemingly random collection of acronyms whose coherence was difficult to decipher.

The sculptor Ann Hamilton used Braille in a similar manner in her installation at the American Pavilion of the 1999 Venice Biennale. The installation included a mechanism that sifted a vivid magenta powder over a wall coated in Braille. The powder moved in response to air currents created by passing viewers, and so clung, to then fell from, dots of braille, making portions of it appear highlighted then disappear. The Braille text was taken from two volumes of poetry by Charles Reznikoff titled *Testimony: The United States 1885–1915 Recitative*, based on turn-of-the-century legal documents giving graphic descriptions of acts of violence. Speakers in the gallery played a recording of the artist reading Lincoln's Second Inaugural Address in international phonetic code. Hamilton described her concept as follows: "Both of the references to language, in Braille and phonetic code, are veiled in such a way that language doesn't become the vehicle through which you arrive at a certain set of information."[8]

Of course, Braille is only veiled to someone who doesn't know how to read it. It is unclear whether visitors were allowed to touch the Braille on the wall; perhaps there were concerns about possible allergic reactions to the magenta powder. But it does not seem that Hamilton ever imagined blind people would visit the installation. She could have used writing in another alphabet, Cyrillic or Arabic, even a dead language and alphabet, such as hieroglyphs, but there would always be a chance that a native speaker or scholar might show up, for whom the transcription would have been transparent. There are, of course, sighted people who can read Braille visually—Braille teachers and transcribers. But I suspect these were not the intended audience any more than were blind people.

In an interview occasioned by the Biennale work, Hamilton said that rendering Reznikoff's poems "in braille in some sense mirrors the way this kind of violence is difficult to absorb into the democratic ideal."[9] As in the FDR Memorial, Braille is used to suggest a coded meaning, something difficult to understand or absorb. In the same interview, Hamilton responded to a question about her artistic process: "sometimes you're blind to your own interests. On one level you do this intellectualized research and you think you're really onto something—but it's almost as if you're keeping yourself busy because you're blind to deeper issues."[10] Hamilton is far from alone in her use of the word "blind" to mean ignorant or oblivious. Still, her use of Braille in this piece suggests additional ideas about blindness as something mysterious, mournful, and tragic, an emblem of loss, and for a visual artist, presumably the worst loss imaginable.

The point is not that Hamilton's piece is culturally insensitive or politically incorrect. The metaphor equating blindness with ignorance and prejudice is such a cliché that it is hard to summon the indignation to be offended. What is truly troubling is the way Braille is used to efface actual blind people. Hamilton's piece only works if we assume that the writing on the wall is meaningful only to people who are absent, invisible, people who are never assumed to be visitors to art installations.

Braille functions in a similar way in *Les Mains Pour Voir* (*Hands for Seeing*), a book of fine art photographs by Yoshiko Murakami.[11] The first half of the book is a series of photographs Murakami took over the course of several years when she volunteered as a sighted guide on nature walks organized by a prominent blind agency in Paris. A few lines of Braille appear on each image, usually somewhere near the center of the page. These are lines from three poems, two by Evelyne Commer, and one by the photographer herself. The Braille is a bit less raised than is standard, but is still legible with effort. Sighted people I consulted are struck by the look of the Braille embedded as it is within the images. For instance, the first image shows a branch with dew droplets on its leaves, making the Braille appear to mirror the forms in the image. My sighted informants were, however, equally intrigued by the reverse page where the Braille dots are indentations rather than raised. The Braille does not describe or even comment on the images particularly. For instance, an image of a flat boulder with the branches of a flowering bush stretched across it has the final lines of Murakami's poem: "I saw, reflected in your eyes, / a glint of birds on the wing." Other images feature the blind people with their white canes or service dogs, their hands fondling tree bark and pine cones, or their faces raised skyward, as if listening. The second half of the book has images of the members of a blind theater troop. The photographer met one of the members on one of the nature walks. She is identified only as Isabel. These blind people are shown in more everyday situations: on public transportation, at the beach, playing chess, reading Braille. The service dogs are lovingly pictured. There is no Braille on these images. The book as a whole could be read as the chronicle of an evolution in the photographers understanding of the blind. The early images, which are all framed by black, have a heightened sense of mystery, emphasizing the blind people's other worldliness and super-sensitive touch. The Braille visually reinforces these qualities. The later images, framed by white, suggest greater integration and more quotidian qualities. But even while depicting some progress from the exotic toward equality, it is clear that blind people are not the intended audience for this book.

Mexican photographer, Gerardo Nigenda (1967–2010), who became blind at age twenty-five, inscribed his images with Braille. The Braille text is sometimes descriptive of the image, sometimes a figurative evocation of a mood he hoped to capture, and sometimes a narrative referencing something about how he made the image. The Braille is usually distributed all around the image, in atypical arrangements that require ingenuity to decipher. *Multi-Looks in Corporal Ascension* (2007) (Fig. 3.2) is a black-and-white photograph of a softly lit pair of legs. The top leg is bent at the knee, covering most of the lower leg, except for the upturned sole of the foot. A hand reaches from the left of the image to grasp or stroke the calf. Two fingers of another hand are touching the thigh near the top right of the image. The Braille appears in a horizontal line at the top of the image, in a vertical line along the calf, and whimsically distributed on the fingers and toes. Unlike the use of Braille by Murikami or Hamilton, where the Braille references blindness without necessarily serving a purpose for blind people, Nigenda's work invites a collaborative effort between a sighted viewer and a blind interlocutor. The full meaning of the photographs is only activated when both the visual and tactile elements are set in dialogue with each other.

In addition to these examples from the fine arts, there are a growing number of books created to educate blind children and adults about art that features Braille, raised-line images, and other tactile elements. For instance, the Metropolitan Museum of Art has published a book, *Art and the*

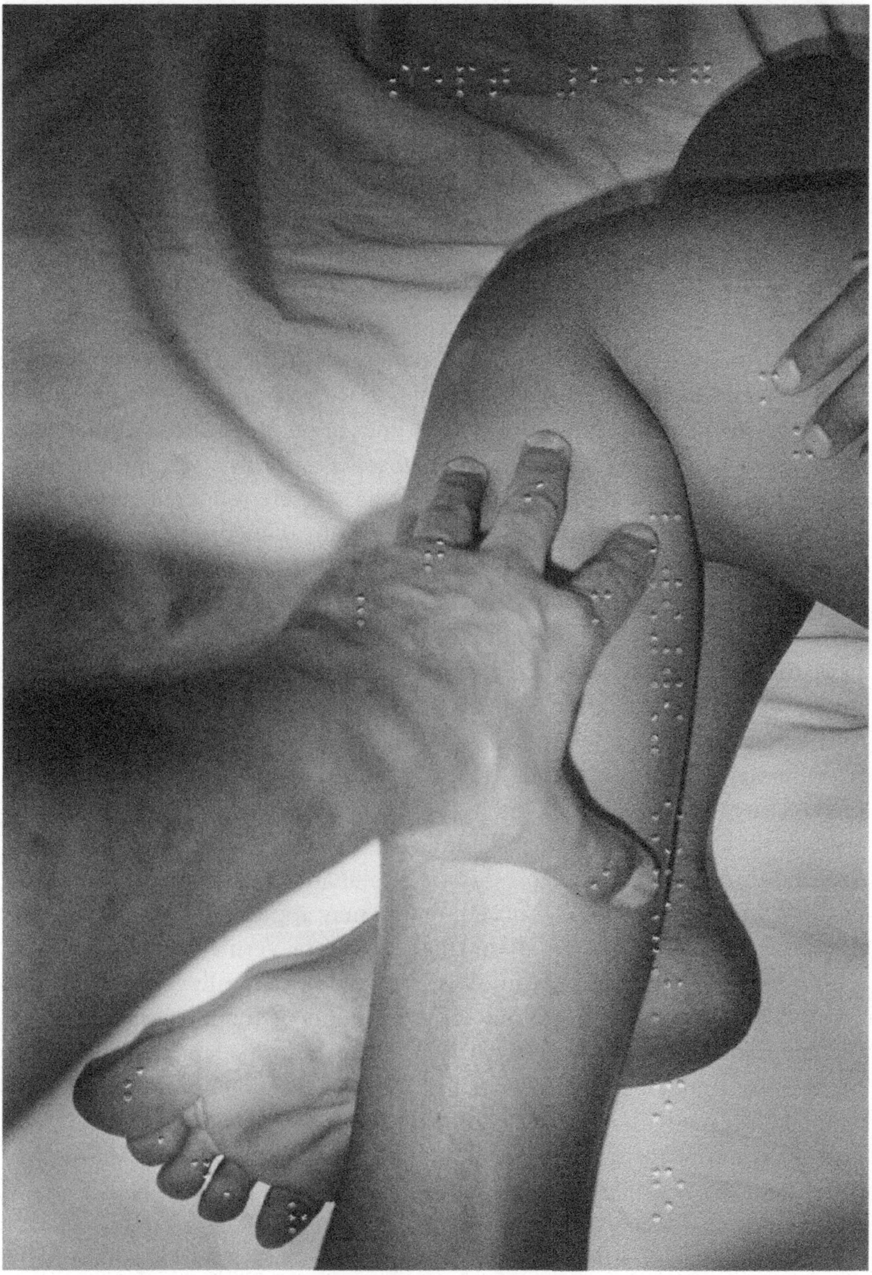

FIGURE 3.2 *Gerardo Nigenda,* Multi-Looks in Corporal Ascension *(2007).*
Courtesy of Plataforma Gerardo Nigenda: gnigenda@yahoo.com.

Alphabet: A Tactile Experience,[12] where each page includes an image from the museum's collection enhanced by raised lines and with a few lines of text in large print and Braille. The front matter suggests that the book is intended to be read by a sighted adult and a blind or visually impaired child. The Braille is uncontracted, Grade I, and so appropriate for a beginner, though some of the language seems a bit above the level of a first grader, as in "N is for noblewoman." So perhaps the intended reader is meant to be somewhat older, even a newly blind adult. The book follows the format of other Braille alphabet books that feature very simple, contour line drawings of objects: "A is for Apple, B is for bell." But here both the images and the tactile enhancements are much more complex. The tactile elements work better in some images than others. On the "Q is for queen" page, with Thomas Sully's portrait of Queen Victoria, raised lines indicate the lines of her head and shoulders, and make it easy to trace the lines for her nose, eyes, brows, and mouth, while more elaborate lines are used to suggest the densely rendered coiffeur. But on the "U is for unicorn" page, with a detail from "Unicorn in Captivity," the form of the animal is traceable, but there is nothing to indicate the enclosure, or the *milles fleurs* background which is a significant visual feature of the tapestry. Similarly, in the detail from Degas's *Race Horses* on the "H is for horse" page, the crisp demarcation of the raised outline seems rather at odds with the hazier visual qualities of the painting. The tactile elements generally communicate that the point of looking at art is to identify what's being pictured. The front matter, which is in Grade II Braille, and so available only to proficient readers, suggests that with older children, the sighted adult can discuss differences in style. Blind children and adults need instruction in tactile drawings. For one thing, there needs to be some explanation that a two-dimensional drawing of an object that is round in reality may appear oval, such as the rim of a bowl, as in "J is for jug," with the detail from Vermeer's *Young Woman with a Water Jug*. Perhaps the book is intended for a legally blind child with enough usable sight to make out some elements of the images, so the tactile features can help confirm what she's seeing, and the large print can help her acquire Braille proficiency. But I think the best audience for this book is sighted children with enough reading ability to read the large print text, and perhaps some curiosity about Braille and blindness. This book will also introduce them to some masterpieces of World Art.

It seems that many elementary school classes include a couple of day's instruction about Braille. Perhaps seeking to serve this market, there is the award-winning *The Black Book of Colors* by Menena Cottin and Rosana Faría.[13] The text consists of ten pages, all of them black, and slick like the pages of a magazine. On the left-hand page there is a sentence or two in Braille at the top, and the same words in white print at the bottom. On the facing page, there is a raised-line drawing illustrating an aspect of the text. For instance, the first page reads, "Thomas says that yellow tastes like mustard, but is as soft as a baby chick's feathers." The facing page has a scattering of raised-line renderings of feathers. The next page reads, "Red is as sour as unripe strawberries and as sweet as watermelon. It hurts when he finds it on his scraped knee." The image depicts unpicked strawberries, but no watermelon or scraped knee. The climax of the story is three pages about the sky, which is first blue, then white when clouds gather, and finally reveals a rainbow when the sun shines through the falling raindrops. The picture accompanying this text assembles a sampling of the objects depicted on previous pages, thus, all the colors. There is no indication whether Thomas, the main character, is blind. On my first reading, I hoped that he is—after all, how many children's books feature a blind protagonist?—and that the book is promoting an understanding that blind people can make analogies between purely visual phenomena such as colors and other kinds of sensory experiences. But he could also simply be a boy with an imagination. The text concludes with the Braille alphabet, and the book jacket says that it is meant to help the sighted reader "begin to imagine what it is like to read by touch." The Braille is Grade I, so appropriate for a new reader, but it is more flattened than is standard, as are the drawings, making it quite hard to decipher, so it would be frustrating for someone just learning to read Braille. Since I mistrust my own Braille fluency, I consulted friends who are more proficient readers, and they too found the flattened Braille difficult and could only make educated guesses about some of the images from clues in the text. While the book raises valuable ideas about sensory analogies that link colors to tastes, smells, sounds, and touch sensations, it also might reinforce the message that Braille is unduly difficult, and that blind people compelled to use it must undergo inevitable hardship requiring a superhuman spirit of courage to accomplish.

A more successful example of a tactile book meant to explain concepts related to visual art is *Des Clés pour Bâtir* (*Keys for Building*) a print/Braille book with tactile images produced by the Cité des Sciences et de l'Industrie in Paris.[14] The Braille here is the equivalent of Grade II, and the language and concepts of the texts seem appropriate for middle-school-aged readers and above. The book opens with the elements: sun, rain, earth—and continues to list building materials—stone, wood, brick, steel. Then it delivers explanations of the physics of various construction elements with illustrations of famous architectural landmarks from the city of Paris. So after the explanation of the physics of the arch, there is a tactile diagram and description of the Arc de Triumphe, with its façade, profile, and footprint. The book progresses through architectural concepts and architectural history: Notre Dame, the Eiffel Tower, the tour Montparnasse, the Pompidou Center, and concludes with a map of Paris where the various monuments are marked. There is even a discussion of the Cite des Sciences et de L'Industrie, where the book was published. There is a certain indoctrinizational bent to all this: the blind reader is meant to come away with a sense of French superiority along with the more general architectural information. Still, the use of Braille and tactile elements is consistent, and one can imagine a blind reader making her way through it without any sighted aid.

In all but this last example, Braille serves primarily to send visible messages to sighted viewers or readers. While the Braille in elevators or on the Helen Keller quarter at least refers, however inadequately, to actual blind people, Graham and Hamilton use Braille as an abstract evocation of the despair and desolation presumed to be synonymous with blindness. Braille is appropriated for sighted purposes, leaving blind people at the margins of society—out of sight and out of mind. Indeed, the struggle to obtain print materials in Braille and other formats remains the major barrier to educational and employment opportunity for blind people. Electronic editions of many periodicals, and the growing number of e-book versions of titles in the public domain increase access to information and literature. But book publishers remain slow to release accessible formats of new titles. And Braille instructions on such public conveniences as ATMs and vending machines, not to mention Braille restaurant menus, continue to be anomalous.

Seemingly in response to the many problematic examples of Braille in public art spaces, British artist David Johnson, who is blind, creates installations that feature large-scale Braille. Here the Braille dots are domes made of poured cement with a diameter of about a foot. They are laid out with standard spacing but still require some ingenuity to be read haptically. The ideal viewer of these installations is perhaps a sighted person who can read Braille visually or else a giant blind person. One of Johnson's pieces was installed on a grassy slope of the University of London's Royal Holloway campus, occasioned by a conference called "Blind Creations" in June 2015. Here it is pictured with the monumental Victorian Founders Building as its backdrop (Fig. 3.3). The title of the piece is *Too Big to Feel*, pointing to the fact that a blind Braille reader will have to resort to unusual means to figure out what it says. In my case, I accomplished this through a combination of clambering around to touch the individual dots, while using my cane to measure the distances between the characters. The result of this exploration was the phrase, "seeing red." There is even a visual hint to the message in that one of the dots in the second word is red. Also, the single red dot among all the white ones made me think of the red stripe that is near the tip of the standard-issue white canes supplied by government agencies. For me, these rehab canes, as they're called, are not as sleek and elegant as others now available, including the one I was using in my exploration of the piece. But this may be an idiosyncratic association. Taken together, the title, the message, and the effort required to decipher it express the annoyance many blind people feel toward how Braille is sometimes used, demonstrated in most of the examples above. It expresses anger, which is not an emotion blind people—or acceptable blind people anyway—are supposed to feel.

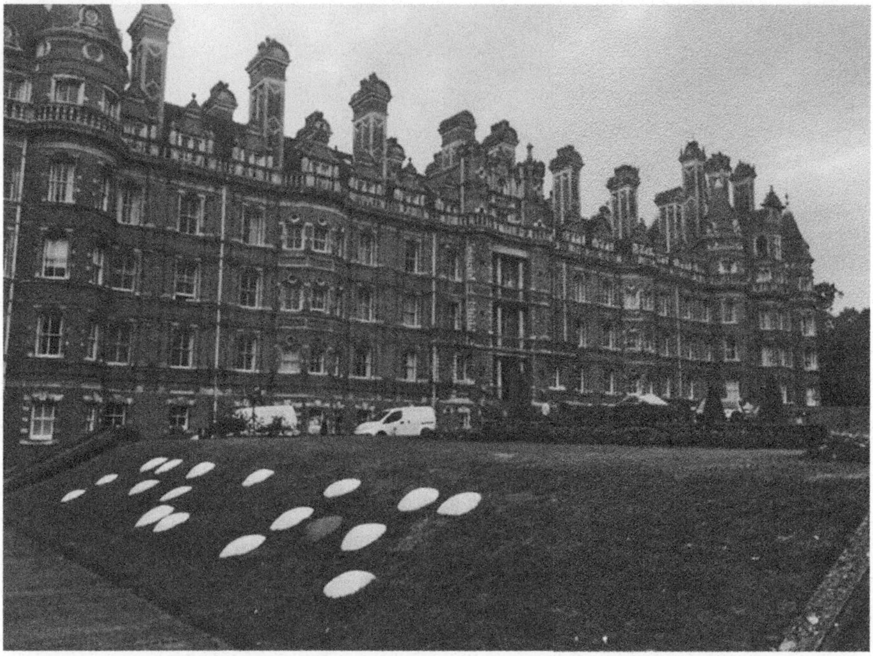

FIGURE 3.3 *David Johnson,* Too Big to Feel *(2015).*
Installation on the campus of Royal Holloway, University of London. Photo by Hannah Johnson.

Blindness, as referenced in the work by Graham and Hamilton, and in many more figurative representations in the history of art, is supposed to denote passivity, mysticism, or possibly a spirit of courage, but certainly not anger. At the same time, Johnson's piece also draws attention to the way that visual metaphors are everywhere. It can be difficult for a blind person to express herself without using language rooted in sighted experience. Thus, the piece references different modes of communication—literal, metaphorical, coded. It invites the touch, but primarily rewards those with the special knowledge of tactile language. What is not visible in the photograph is the unexpectedly pleasing irregular texture of each Braille dot. This is due to the way the dots are produced. Johnson creates a circular hole in a flat surface, lines this with plastic, then pours in a set amount of cement. The surface of each dot retains the creases and dimples of the stretching plastic, which replicates the irregular surfaces of hand-punched rather than machine-made Braille. It gives them an organic feel, enhanced by their setting on this grassy knoll, as if they are the heads of giant mushrooms that sprang up overnight.

In another piece, Johnson creates cement eggs and arranges them in six-slot egg cartons. The eggs and cartons are standard size, and the six-slot configuration simulates the grid for Braille, where each character consists of some combination of one to six dots (Fig. 3.4). This piece is another invitation to touch;

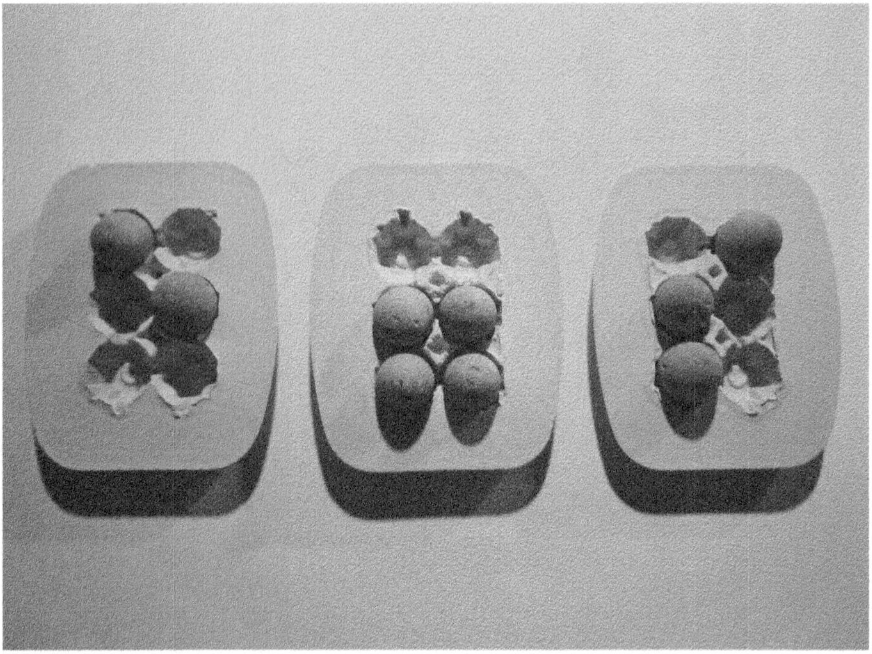

FIGURE 3.4 *David Johnson,* Eggs *(2016).*
Photo by Matthew Brooks.

there are many rewards to touching and handling the eggs. There is a slight disorientation to discover differences in weight and texture, within the familiar, quotidian form, which nestles comfortably in the palm of the hand just like a real egg. There is also a temptation to rearrange the eggs from the original presentation that spells "eggs" to create other messages.[15] Here, the ideal viewer—or to use a term that acknowledges tactile discernment, beholder—is a Braille-reading blind person. And there is an appealing playfulness to the piece, again, an emotion at odds with the stereotype of blind mournfulness and mysticism.

Let us return to the FDR Memorial. On a wall near the statue of Roosevelt in his wheelchair that was added in 2001, there is a new carved inscription of a statement by Eleanor Roosevelt about her husband's disability. Just below it, there is a transcription of the quotation in standard-sized Braille at a comfortable reading height. There is nothing graphically interesting about this Braille. It does not serve as a decorative motif or metaphor for anything, merely as a means for blind people to read the text on the wall. It is still an invitation to touch.

With a little effort, a sighted person could pick up a few of the rudiments of Braille. And if there happened to be a Braille reader present at the monument, conversation might follow. With it, Braille might seem less exotic and blindness less alien and frightening. If the amendment to the original design of the memorial seems a little self-conscious, even grudging, it still serves as a belated recognition that disability exists in the world. It was once, as for Roosevelt, a cause for shame and concealment or the melodrama of metaphor or knee-jerk pieties about the spirit of courage. Now, disability can begin to be understood as just another facet of the human condition, another way of moving through space, reading, communicating, and being in the world. In this context, Braille may seem more mundane and utilitarian, but ultimately a more genuine marker of an inclusive society.

{4}

Touch Tourism

In the previous chapter, I collected instances where Braille shows up in public places, such as historical monuments and art installations, where it is used to signify blindness rather than as a tool for blind people. The association of touch with blindness also has an impact on the ways art museums provide access to blind visitors. And while I would like to dislodge the notion that blind people rely exclusively on touch perception to know the world, I admit that whenever I have the opportunity to get my hands on art, I leap at the chance. When touch tours are done well, they give a person access to aspects of an art work that may not be apparent to the eyes alone.

In fact, I wish the opportunity were available to everyone. I said as much the last time I took a touch tour at the museum of Modern Art in New York (MOMA). "I wish everyone could do this," I said to my docent.

I had my hands on a bronze head by Henri Matisse. It was one of the four pieces in his Jeannette series, produced between 1910 and 1916, and named for Jeanne Vaderin, the woman who served as the model. It was a cold January day at the bitter end of the holiday season, so the gallery was crowded with visitors. Many of them, as I could tell from brief snippets of overheard conversations, were Europeans. But apparently there were a sufficient number who were fluent enough in English that I felt a ripple of interest in my immediate vicinity. I sensed that some of them shared my sentiment and wished that they too could touch the sculpture. At the same time, I felt the docent stiffen, and sure enough, she instantly rattled off the familiar speech about the fragility of works of art and the need to preserve them for posterity. So only a privileged few get to touch them.

I'm glad to be a part of the privileged few and try to make the most of every opportunity. If I had my druthers however, I also wish that I didn't have to wear the disposable plastic gloves—really hand-shaped baggies—that most museums require now. I concede that they are an improvement over the cotton gloves that used to be standard, because they allow for a finer grain perception of texture and temperature. But they're still not as good as going bare-handed.

For one thing, they made my hands sweat. Periodically, I had to peel them off and dry my hands on my jeans. There used to be a good deal of debate about which materials actually are damaged by the natural oils on even the cleanest human fingertips. But now the rule seems to be that it's better to be safe than sorry. Everybody wears the gloves. And gloves or no gloves, there are many works that are deemed too fragile to be touched at all. It has been my experience that artists are a lot less squeamish about people touching their work than are exhibit curators and art conservators. In particular, sculptors who create works meant to be displayed outdoors are scornful of hands-off exhibition policies. If the work can withstand the weather and pollution, what difference should it make if people touch or even climb all over it? But I knew better than to argue these points on this occasion. My docent had her instructions. I took what I could get.

As is the custom at MOMA, I arranged for this tour via the museum's website two weeks in advance of my visit. At the scheduled time, I met my docent at the information desk downstairs. We had a brief discussion about my interests, knowledge, and background and made a plan of action. Since it was the second day of January, we decided to skip the outdoor sculpture garden and focus on some pieces in the permanent collection indoors.

In the perfect world of my wishful imagination, I would be able to be more spontaneous in my museum-going. A few museums around the world have self-guided touch tours. The Metropolitan in New York offers visually impaired visitors the option to pick up an audio or Braille text at the information desk and then touch a selection of sculptures in the Egyptian collection. The British Museum has a similar arrangement for its Egyptian collection and plaster casts of the Parthenon frieze (formerly known as the Elgin Marbles). The Louvre has a tactile gallery with a collection of scale models of a range of works in its collection, which is available for anyone to visit and touch any time the museum is open. These options allow the spontaneity that I crave but are limited in scope. Scale models and plaster casts have their drawbacks. While a scale model can convey a sculpture's overall form, it cannot replicate the proprioceptive experience of standing before a monumental work. The casts of the Parthenon frieze were made before the marbles were transported to England, and so preserve a record of some portions of the originals that were damaged en route. But plaster has a slick, artificial feel with little in common with the cool pleasure of natural stone.

The best self-guided tours direct the visitor's hands to features that may not be visible. For example, the British Museum tour points out subtle changes in texture between the slightly coarser grain of a figure's drapery and the silky smoothness of its skin, while explaining the techniques the sculptors used to achieve these effects. This tour also recommended different touching techniques. The point is not simply to trace the outline and draw a two-dimensional mental image of the three-dimensional sculpture. Different parts of the fingers and hands perceive different aspects. When the audio guide advised me to run my fingers lightly up the extended arm of a Roman discus thrower, the rapidity of the movement erased the element of temperature from my perception. This combined with the smoothness of the marble and the subtle modeling of the form gave me the tingly sensation that I was touching living skin.

Still, the self-guided tours don't offer the versatility of a live docent. There is no opportunity to ask questions or exchange ideas. Ideally, there would be a crew of docents perpetually on site at every museum, ready to go whenever a blind person happened to show up. Of course I recognize the impracticality of this plan. Given the available choices, I prefer the option of a personal docent to guide a tour during regular museum hours as opposed to special tours for large groups scheduled during days when the museum is closed to the public. I'd rather not be segregated in that way. And the advantage of a personal docent rather than a group tour is the ability to customize the tour.

To this end, my MOMA docent and I continued our exchange of personal information in the elevator going upstairs. She was a graduate student in art history finishing her dissertation. We discussed her topic. I told her that I am a writer and English professor, and that my parents were both visual artists. I already knew a lot about art, in particular modern art. I spent a good deal of my childhood at MOMA and the other New York City museums. I confess that I even engaged in some shameless name-dropping, mentioning several mid-century American artists who were in my parents' circle, whose work was on display in that very museum. I wanted my docent to know that she didn't have to start from scratch.

We also touched on my visual impairment. Unlike philosophers who limit their speculations to the total congenital blindness of the Hypothetical, and the cognitive scientists who seek out this ideal as the subject of their inquiry, my docent had a grasp of the complexities of actual visual impairment. She knew that the degree of sight loss along with the age of onset were all relevant factors. Since I have been legally blind since childhood, I am comfortable with what I can and cannot see, and do not strain after visual perception the way an adult who has recently acquired the same degree and type of impairment might. Still, on some touch tours, I've used my hands to confirm something I was perceiving visually. On the touch tour at the British Museum, I was examining a standing Egyptian figure. What I saw when I looked at it was an amorphous hazy column whose color combined the reddish brown of the granite it was sculpted from and a bluish purple. This I assumed to be the color of the shadows or else the complementary hue of the stone. What I knew about the piece came from my general knowledge of ancient Egyptian culture and what I was hearing from the audio description. When I placed my hands on the figure, it seemed to solidify under my palms. Before I even began to feel for the features of its face or the carving representing the drapery of its costume, I was struck by the very solidity of its form. More surprising was the way the color changed. The purple haze vanished, and I saw only the mottled reddish brown of the granite.

But on this particular day at MOMA, I anticipated that a combination of jet lag and the potential distractions of a more crowded environment would make my visual perceptions even less trustworthy than on that earlier occasion. I planned to ignore my eyes and focus on my hands. My docent got the point. She was intelligent, energetic, and a very fast talker. The fast talking came in handy, as there was a lot of ground to cover. She was also very experienced. She had given tours to all sorts of groups and individuals, both blind and sighted, from schoolchildren to potential exhibit sponsors. She included the comments of some of these people in our conversation as we moved from gallery to gallery. I admired the way she amended and enhanced her usual script in response to my observations and comments. We adopted a natural give-and-take as we went along. This was more of a dialogue than a lecture.

There are considerable logistical challenges posed by a touch tour conducted during regular museum hours. In each gallery, my docent had to locate the guard, show her museum badge, and explain what she was doing. Given the crowds, she needed to maneuver us to a place near enough to each work so that I could actually reach them while still hearing her. More importantly, she had to be vigilant to dissuade the other people present from following my example and laying their hands on these works of art. On the self-guided touch tour at the British Museum, a guard followed me at a discrete distance, and shooed away other visitors who showed the slightest sign of reaching toward the sculptures. On other touch tours in the past, I have been asked to refrain from touching until a group of schoolchildren passed through the room. It's one thing to ask adults to refrain from doing what I was doing; it's nearly impossible and possibly cruel to deprive children of this pleasure.

So there we were with these heads by Matisse. The docent told me that these sculptures were a way for the artist to work out ideas about abstraction for painting. In modifying the heads from the fairly naturalistic early ones to the highly abstracted later ones, he was making three-dimensional forms that would help him figure out how to flatten them into two-dimensional projections. I found this fascinating. I was exploring the final head in the series, which is the most abstracted. As I cupped my palms around the massive protrusions of the head's coiffeur, I had the sensation that my hands were resting more or less where the artist's hands had once rested, in the clay versions that preceded the cast bronzes. As I understand it, one of the many pleasures of looking at art is the sensation that in standing before the painting or sculpture one assumes the exact position where the artist must have stood in making the work. One has the illusion of viewing the work, as it were, through the artist's eyes. Here, I had the analogous pleasure of feeling a distant relative of the artist's haptic sensation as he molded the forms. This is why I wish everyone could do this. I felt I was not only in touch with the artist but also feeling something that probably is not apparent to the eyes alone.

In my head, I was trying to work out how the artist would have translated these sensations into the necessary eye-to-hand instructions that would allow him to draft a similarly abstracted portrait on canvas. I scanned my memories for some sort of similar experience. All I could come up with was a memory of the difficult mental exercise required when I first learned to type Braille on a Perkins Brailler. The six dots of the Braille cell that are configured as two vertical columns of three dots are split up from the bottom center to create a horizontal line of buttons on the Braille keyboard. Learning which combination of buttons to press to create the required character was at first a matter of imaginatively moving my fingers from the horizontal alignment of the keyboard to the vertical orientation of the dots in the character I wanted to create.

I said some of this to my docent, attempting to articulate this idea about translation. In the case of my learning to type Braille, it was translating from the horizontal to the vertical. For Matisse, it was the more complex task of translating these three-dimensional forms to two-dimensional images. My docent and I had a brief, rather esoteric, discussion of tactile versus visual perception. I could have quoted Helen Keller's observation:

> Eloquence to the touch resides not in straight lines, but in unstraight lines, or in many curved and straight lines together. They appear and disappear, are now deep, now shallow, now broken off or lengthened or swelling. They rise and sink beneath my fingers, they are full of sudden starts and pauses, and their variety is inexhaustible and wonderful. So you see I am not shut out from the region of the beautiful, though my hand cannot perceive the brilliant colors in the sunset or on the mountain, or reach into the blue depths of the sky.[1]

While classical notions of visual beauty usually turn on symmetry and order, Keller's description of tactile eloquence emphasizes variety, perhaps even disorder. The point is always made that touch is sequential while vision is comprehensive and instantaneous. The hand must move over and around an object, while the eye can take it in at a glance. I refuted this, showing my docent how I could wrap my palms and fingers over and around considerable chunks of the form. My point was that my haptic exploration was not merely to trace the form's outline with my fingertips but rather to envelope the three-dimensional volumes with my palms and fingers. Then I described for her the art class exercise called "Blind Contour Drawing," where the student endeavors to move her eye sequentially around the contours of the object she is drawing and to move her hand holding the charcoal in the same sequence to create the drawing without looking at it. I was making the point that while the eye seeks the outline of the object, the hand does not. The hand embraces the object in its multifaceted complexity.

Then we moved on to ideas about abstraction. The first two heads in Matisse's series are more or less representational. The features of the face are in a naturalistic arrangement and proportion. But in the later ones, the different features are simplified, and their scale relative to each other is radically distorted.

"Does it still feel like a head?" my docent asked me. I think she really wanted to know. Although part of her training to be a touch tour docent gave her the opportunity to don the gloves and do the touching, she admitted that it had been awhile. And since the training, after numerous tours with individuals and groups, she now had many questions about the experience.

Then someone took my picture. In fact, I was aware that several people in our immediate vicinity had their phones out and were aiming them at me.

I was temporarily distracted. Isn't it against the rules to take pictures in a museum? And what exactly were they taking a picture of here? Was it that they also wished they could do what I was doing and so opted for the next best thing—a picture of what they wished they could do? Then I wondered about the future of these images. Had my docent and I become an example of performance art at the museum? Will these images be posted on Instagram, Facebook, and personal travel blogs with some comment about the novelty of seeing this blind woman touching this bronze by Matisse, right there at MOMA? "What will those Americans think of next?" And what will these images say about what the photographers thought I was getting out of this experience?

One thing I know for sure, touching this sculpture did not create an image of it in my mind's eye. I didn't have the foggiest idea what this thing might look like. Even with the more representational early heads, I couldn't say for certain how closely the sculpture might resemble the head of a living woman. In fact, I can't say that I have much of a mind's eye. My imagination is not particularly visual. I know blind people who are better able to create mental images, and others, like Helen Keller, who draw analogies between nature and art to grasp visual concepts:

> It is true, however, that some sculptures, even recognized masterpieces, do not please my hand. When I touch what there is of the Winged Victory, it reminds me at first of a headless, limbless dream that flies toward me in an unrestful sleep. The garments of the Victory thrust stiffly out behind, and do not resemble garments that I have felt flying, fluttering, folding, spreading in the wind. But imagination fulfils these imperfections, and straightway the Victory becomes a powerful and spirited figure with the sweep of sea-winds in her robes and the splendor of conquest in her wings.[2]

Keller's imagination drew on her experience of drapery moving in the breeze to animate the static stone figure. Although Keller could have access to them, she never recorded her reactions to abstract or cubist works like these heads by Matisse. Her celebrity status throughout her life gave her enviable entrée to museum collections wherever she traveled, but it may be that her handlers assumed she would prefer the naturalism of the Classical period. So I was left to my own devices with these works by Matisse and drew on my own idiosyncratic associations.

Unfortunately, in stereotypical and unthinking understandings about sensory perception, touch is described as occupying a less lofty, less intellectual rung of the hierarchy of the senses. Touch is not only associated with sensuality, even sexuality, but also with the emotions. We talk about our feelings, our touching sentiments. So in the photos of me touching these heads was there an expectation that my experience was primarily emotional? In order to make a good photo for these people, should I have tried to squeeze out a couple of tears?

To me, this was very heady stuff. The experience was intensely intellectual—sweaty hands and all. If any of these people behind their camera phones were listening, they might have learned something about three-dimensional versus two-dimensional representation, about visual versus haptic sensation, and a number of other things. Still, I didn't really mind being photographed doing this. It could have been a kind of public service. Someone who knows someone who is blind or visually impaired might see one of these photos and be inspired to arrange a touch tour for them at MOMA or at another museum elsewhere in the world.

In the meantime, my docent and I kept talking. We exchanged our ideas. Her knowledge enriched my experience. And I'd like to believe that my articulation of my experience added to her knowledge of this work. We became a part of each other's future script.

In addition to the many touch tours I have sampled in my travels, I have taken advantage of many other tactile, haptic and kinesthetic opportunities in historical and cultural sites. My late husband was a medieval scholar, and I accompanied him on many visits to European cathedrals and other architectural monuments. In the United Kingdom, the "Cathedrals through Touch and Hearing Program," initiated by the blind author and theologian, John Hull, exists in seventeen cathedrals around the country.[3] Scale models and tactile floor plans, typically set up in Plexiglas cubes with hand holes on either side are available for anyone to touch. Visually impaired visitors can request an audio guide that directs their haptic explorations and supplies historical information.

For me, however, the best way to appreciate a cathedral is to climb its tower. The breathtaking view from the top may be lost on me, but the breathtaking climb up the spiral staircase to get there helps me appreciate the monumental scale of the structure. Also, along the way I have the opportunity to touch much. At Notre Dame in Paris, visitors, both blind and sighted, can touch gargoyles and other carvings. Usually the finest examples of carving and statuary are either roped off or out of reach but tracing a course of ordinary masonry or the flutes of a column reveal the quality of engineering and craft that went into construction.

Another good way to experience a cathedral is to attend a concert or service. The scents of burning candles and incense, and the way the interior spaces shape and disperse the sounds of choral singing, pipe organs, and other instruments, can produce the same awe the architecture conveys visually.

Around the world, there are all sorts of sites that offer blind—and sighted—visitors unexpected opportunities of tactile exploration and appreciation. In Columbus, Ohio, in a park adjacent to the main branch of the public library, known as Deaf School Park, there is a topiary garden representing Georges Seurat's familiar painting, *Sunday Afternoon on the Island of La Grande Jatte*. The sculptor James T. Mason constructed bronze armatures for fifty-four human figures plus three dogs, a monkey, and several boats set in a real pond. The garden was formally dedicated in 1992, and now the evergreen shrubs have grown to fill the forms. There is a plaque indicating the vantage point of the painting, but visitors are permitted to enter the painting to move among and touch the figures. Although it was not designed with this in mind, it is a good place for a blind art lover. There, for the first time, I gained a graphic understanding of pictorial perspective, a concept that I had previously understood intellectually without any personal experience of it. Walking around the garden I could measure my own body against the larger than life figures in the foreground of the painting, and then against the progressively smaller figures as I moved farther into the background. Topiary is an ideal medium for the style and subject of this painting. The prickly texture of the trimmed shrubs creates a nice analogy to the Pointillist technique, and a leisurely stroll around the garden evokes the mood the painting captures.

Obviously, topiary reproduction of painting would not be suitable for every work and would be impractical for museums—though it's appealing to think about. It is, however, becoming more and more common for museums to produce tactile reproductions of paintings. Sometimes, these are simple raised-line diagrams that can convey composition. These have the same limitations of the Metropolitan's Braille alphabet book discussed in the previous chapter. In 2015, the Prado opened an exhibit of six tactile reproductions of famous paintings in its collection.[4] These were an advance on the raised-line diagrams in that they included color, recognizing that many legally blind people retain some color perception. The reproductions began with a high-resolution color photograph. Then a chemical process caused designated portions to swell to varying degrees and allowed for different textures for different areas. So what could be felt was more than simply the outlines of figures but different textures for clothing, hair, skin, and objects. Sighted visitors were also allowed to touch these paintings, with or without blindfolds provided by the museum. The designers of these projects worked closely with ONCE, Spain's national organization of the blind to determine how best to communicate different aspects of the paintings. Each reproduction cost over $6,000, which makes it surprising, not to mention disappointing, that the exhibit was only open for six months.

As with topiary reproductions, these tactile copies only work with figurative or naturalistic styles of painting. For this reason, a few museums offer tours for the blind that feature handling objects to explain other artistic styles and concepts. At the Tate Modern in London, large shards of Plexiglas are used to suggest the fragmentation of Cubism, and a silicone pad, similar to a breast implant, is used to suggest the drapey texture of Salvador Dali's melting watches. In these cases, the point is not to trace the outline or map the composition. Rather, the blind visitor is invited to make a cross-sensory analogy between the object in hand and some visual quality in the painting.

It's worth noting that even before there were legally mandated and official touch tours and tactile reproductions, blind people have benefited from random acts of access. While a blind celebrity like Helen Keller could count on having the opportunity to get her hands on any work of art, ordinary blind people have found ways to gain tactile experiences, usually facilitated by sighted companions to act as lookouts. Sometimes unauthorized access has even been offered surreptitiously by museum staff. A friend of mine told me a story about her undergraduate summer abroad program in Paris. In addition to classroom study, the students had to attend tours at museums and other cultural sites in order to be immersed in the language. This was in the 1980s before there were any organized access programs at museums, so my friend, who is blind, went along simply to improve her aural comprehension of the docents' lectures. At the Rodin museum, she was listening at the edge of the group when a museum guard approached her and asked if she would like to touch one of the sculptures. When she enthusiastically accepted his offer, he took her to *The Kiss*, helped her to climb up on a chair and from there onto the sculpture itself, then stationed himself outside the velvet rope to keep others at a distance. My friend was then free to explore the iconic work tactually, habtically, and kinesthetically. She embraced the nude figures, climbed over and around them, insinuated her own body into the composition. Naturally this drew the attention of her fellow students and perhaps other visitors as well. Perhaps they took pictures of the spectacle she was making of herself.

On a visit to Stonehenge, a guard spotted me with my white cane and asked if I'd like to "come inside the circle." Naturally I leapt at the chance. She asked me to wait until the bus load of visitors who were currently walking the circuit around the monument were done so she wouldn't have to contend with others' requests to have the same privilege. Like the guard at the Rodin museum, she was offering access outside the prescribed practice, which requires blind visitors to request this privilege well in advance. Here's what I learned while I was inside. She directed my attention to the lichens growing on the stones. Then she recommended that I put my ear close and listen. Sure enough, there was an audible rustling and a faint palpable vibration. She told me that this came from the birds who had built their nests down inside deep fissures in the stones. But the thing that struck me most of all was how much warmer it was inside the circle. This was a dreary day in November, brisk though not really cold. There had been a few brief outbursts of sunlight, but apparently the stones had absorbed enough of whatever sunlight there was to radiate faint warmth markedly distinct from the air outside.

When people witness an authorized touch tour in progress, at the very least it functions as a kind of advertisement about available services and raises awareness that blind and visually impaired people can have a meaningful aesthetic, intellectual, and emotional experience in the museum. The next step then, for museum patrons, and for museum service providers, is to recognize that the people who avail themselves of these services have something to give back. Since everyone does not get to touch the art, as much as they might want to, there is a value in hearing what we—the privileged few—have to say about it. The tactile aspect of sculpture is seldom analyzed or even mentioned by art historians and critics. Even scholars with special access to museum collections are constrained by rules not to touch the sculptures. And even if they were offered the opportunity—or surreptitiously snuck a brief touch—would they have the vocabulary to describe the experience? And what about the tactile aesthetics of painting? When scholars discuss tactility in painting, they are usually talking about the ways artists render the textures of different materials—cloth, wood, metal, stone, flesh, fur, or feather. These painted surfaces do not feel like what they represent, of course. Does a Pointillist canvas retain the tactile polka dots of the artists jabbing brush? Imagine the feel of a Jackson Pollock or a Mark Rothko. How does the palpable record of the artist's process add to our understanding?

But I'm letting my imaginative reach exceed my grasp. No one's going to let me get my hands on those paintings. I content myself with the privilege I enjoy. But I think it is a shame to waste the insights of those of us who have this privilege. For this reason, I wish that museum art educators would move beyond the mission of producing a prepackaged narrative for a passive audience. There needs to be an expectation that the blind people on the tour have something to contribute to cultural knowledge beyond gratitude for this gift of inclusion. In other words, we can hope that the future of museum programs for blind people will entail an effort to collect and document our responses to the exceptional access we enjoy. Why not enlist blind docents to describe these experiences to those who do not have the opportunity? Thus touch tours for the blind can become more than just a novelty or second-best solution, but rather a way to enlarge everyone's experience of art.

To this end, in 2016 I joined Australia-based artist Fayen D'Evie in a collaborative curatorial and artistic project called *The Levity, The Gravity*. The

Kadist Art Foundation in San Francisco provided us access to pieces of contemporary art in their collection for us to engage with through touch. Our goal was to compile a vocabulary and taxonomy of tactile aesthetics, and then share our findings in public presentations at the Kadist Gallery. We derived our title from the seventeenth-century philosopher and scientist Robert Hooke, who compiled a list of tactile qualities to be examined in any object: "Gravity, or Levity. Coarseness or Fineness. Fastness, or Loosseness. Stiffness, or Pliableness. Roughness, or Brittleness. Clamminess, or Slipperiness."[5] In referencing Hooke, we were also referencing an earlier period in the history of museums, and the private collections that preceded them, when visitors often touched and handled art and historical objects. As many scholars have noted, this early practice operated with an assumption that invited visitors to a private collection had the refinement to know how to handle these objects correctly and the discernment to derive knowledge from the experience. Once museums opened to the general public, who might have dirty hands and uncouth manners, prohibitions against touching became the norm and collections began to be displayed out of reach and under glass.[6]

Not surprisingly, the great pleasure in this research was having the luxury of more or less unlimited time to spend with these works. Even the best museum touch tour has to keep to a schedule, and there is seldom an opportunity to backtrack and rehandle a previous item. At Kadist, we were able both to examine each piece in minute detail and then move back and forth between pieces to revise and refine our initial observations. The first thing we discovered was that the specific works of art themselves invite or incite different kinds of touch and offer different kinds of rewards. For instance, a small marble cut-out by Daniel Joseph Martinez seemed to encourage a kind of delicate tracing motion with the fingertips, while a wall-mounted piece featuring sections of iron gates by Adrian Wong elicited the impulse to grasp with the whole hand, even to pull with the whole arm and upper body. Other works invited a dexterous manipulation, or a combination of all these techniques enhanced by kinesthetic, proprioceptive whole body movement as with the hanging installation by Jompet Kuswidananto (Fig. 4.1). In the photo, I am joined by Heidi Rabben, a member of the Kadist staff, to examine an element of the construction. What does not show in the picture is the ways our manipulations made the hanging elements wobble and swing. The work seemed to invite movement around and between the various elements, and the slight breeze our bodies produced brought motion into the work.

Our second discovery came when we did our first public presentation. The audience, though attentive to what we were saying, was reluctant to follow our lead and lay their own hands on the work. Even with encouragement, their haptic explorations were tentative and cursory. Clearly, the prohibitions against touching art are so ingrained even for regular patrons of art galleries, that lifting the restrictions did not lead to unfettered haptic exploration. Moreover, we were

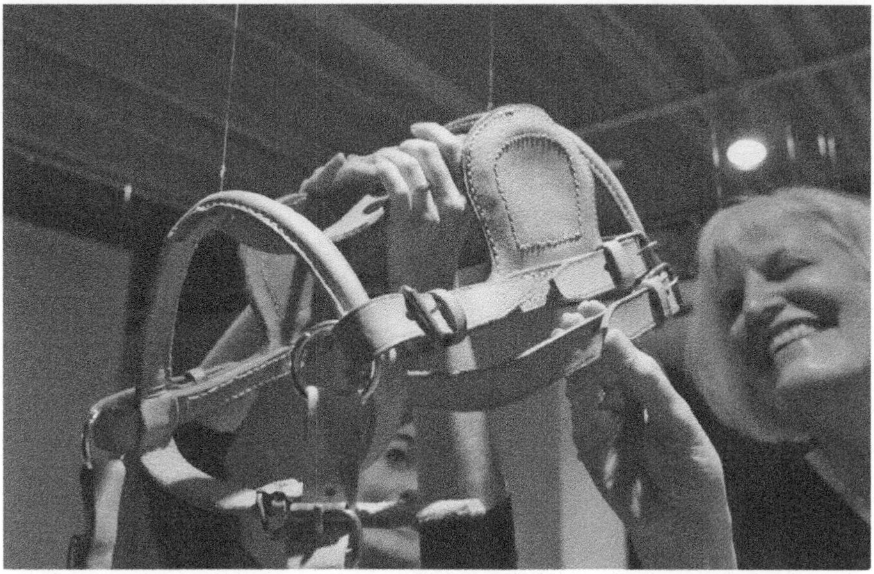

FIGURE 4.1 *Fayen d'Evie and Georgina Kleege (2016).* The Levity, The Gravity: Heidi Rabben and Georgina Kleege Discuss Jompet Kuswidananto's Third Realm, 2011. *Video still.*

Image courtesy of the artists and KADIST.

aware that making a blind person the tactile docent of this exhibit while the sighted attendees looked on with their hands in their pockets risked reinforcing the stereotype that blind people have higher levels of tactile perception than sighted people, and that this could turn the whole event into a kind of freak show. D'Evie has witnessed such reluctance. She has produced works on paper called "Tactile Paintings" that are meant to be touched, but when she has exhibited them, people were not always willing to do so. One man said, "Maybe I'll come back and touch it when there aren't so many people around." For some, apparently touch is something so intimate that it is best done in private. To counter this reluctance, and avoid creating a freak show spectacle, the next phase of our project seeks to develop a choreography or plan for touching. This will not be restricted to sighted people. Though the Hypothetical Blind Man is understood to be all about touch, actual blind people do not necessarily have innate haptic discernment. John Lee Clark, a deaf-blind poet and Braille teacher, has observed that many of his students, even those who have been blind since infancy, are wary to explore things tactually. He promotes "protactile training" meant to liberate blind and deaf-blind people from cultural strictures against touch. [7]

What D'Evie and I hope to accomplish with this project is more than simply suggest how museums and other sites that offer touch tours for the blind might improve their programs. We suggest that tactile information about works of art could add to everyone's understanding and enjoyment. What if a few adjectives describing tactile qualities were added to wall texts and labels in gallery exhibits or in the object files that make up collection catalogues and art databases? We suggest that blind people who are granted this exceptional access could join with the professionals who regularly handle art works—conservators, exhibit installers, not to mention artists themselves—to add another category of aesthetic value.

{5}

Hearsay

As rewarding as some touch tours can be, the vast majority of art works in museums around the world, including the majority of works of sculpture, cannot be touched. So more often than not, art educators tasked with making collections accessible to blind people must resort to verbal description, either in the form of special docent led tours or through recorded texts. But the idea of verbal description of art for a blind audience raises considerable unease. A picture may be worth a thousand words, but the assumption seems to be that those thousand words—or even a million words—will not do justice to the picture. This holds even though ekphrasis, or poetry that describes visual art, has been around at least since Homer. And for centuries, art historians, critics, and artists themselves have described art in reviews, scholarship, lectures, artists' talks, and interviews. But somehow, art educators and access specialists seem to assume that some other method or vocabulary is required if the audience is blind. While it is rarely acknowledged, there seems to be an underlying assumption that blind people lack the ability to conceptualize visual phenomena in ways that will allow them to understand and appreciate visual art.

To begin to grapple with this issue, let me return to Denis Diderot.

In 1760, eleven years after he published his *Letter on the Blind,* Diderot became acquainted with a nineteen-year-old blind girl, Melanie de Salignac, whom he pronounced to be the most surprising blind person who ever existed. She was the cherished child of a family enlightened enough to care about her education and affluent enough to provide her with assistive technologies that were, in the century before Braille was introduced, far in advance of the times. For instance, she had an apparatus that allowed her to write as well as elaborate tactile maps made of wire, fabric, embroidery, and wax. Diderot marveled at her talents as a musician and dancer, and her ability to memorize and recite lengthy poems. To his credit, he even recorded his young friend's criticism of a passage from his *Letter*—the same passage I mocked in chapter 1. She objected to his claim that the blind must be less affected by the pain of others because they cannot see their afflictions, only hear their moans and cries. Or as he put it: "What difference is there to a blind man between a man making water and one bleeding in silence?"[1]. She asserted that, on the contrary, she would feel the most pity for someone suffering in silence because she would know his pain was all the greater.

Diderot does not record any other discussion of his *Letter* or the controversy it generated about his atheist views. (He only touches on theology briefly, when he mentions that Mademoiselle de Salignac's mother was very devout.) For the most part, their conversations seem to have centered on philosophy and geometry. For instance, one day Diderot proposed a thought experiment. He asked Mademoiselle de Salignac to imagine a cube, and then to imagine a point at the very center of the cube with straight lines emanating from it to each of the cube's angles. She found this an easy operation, and before Diderot could pose the next question, she announced that it would yield six equal pyramids with bases the same as the faces of the cube. "But where do you see it?" Diderot wanted to know.

"In my head," she replied, "as you do."[2]

While Mademoiselle de Salignac's response might seem merely playful or pert, in fact she was challenging one of the great thinkers of her day. Her words dispel the age-old image of blindness as a kind of half-life or vacant consciousness, and put her own intellect on a par with the great philosopher's. What impressed Diderot was not merely that Mademoiselle de Salignac could perform this mental geometry, but that she could also do so without imagining the figures in color, since his own imagination depended on color to allow him to keep track of his calculations.

This prompts me to wonder if everyone would imagine this calculation in color. If we could transport Diderot to the twenty-first century, we can imagine his delight in meeting another young blind woman, Sabriye Tenberken, who founded the first school for the blind in Tibet. Unlike Mademoiselle de Salignac, who had been blind since infancy, Tenberken's vision diminished gradually over the course of her childhood. She made a conscious effort to retain a memory of color and even to use color as a way to remember things, by for instance, associating certain colors with certain words, numbers, or days of the week. Early in her memoir, she describes a sight-seeing tour around Tibet. She and her companions visited Lake Namtso, and while the others snapped photos and shouted exclamations at what they saw, she pictured the landscape this way:

> A beach of crystallized salt shimmering like snow under an evening sun, at the edge of a vast body of turquoise water. Farther out, the Namtso changes from turquoise to dark blue, returning to pale blue as it melts into the horizon. The setting sun was painting the surrounding mountains golden yellow, brown, and fire red. A recent downpour had frozen the mountaintops, and

> their peaks were covered with white powder. And down below, on the deep green mountain flanks, a few nomads were watching their yaks grazing.[3]

One of her friends looked up from his camera long enough to notice that she had her face pointing in the wrong direction. What was before her eyes was nothing but barren rock. But, while others always find this anecdote sad, she recalls the incident as proof that she has an imagination.

"But where is this imagination?" Diderot might ask.

"In my head," she would reply, "like yours."

Of course, Tenberken's description is a construction of words, a collection of adjectives culled from the observations of her sighted friends and from written accounts she'd read prior to leaving home. Still, like Diderot, the colors she names link to colors in her memory that she uses to create a mental image of the landscape that she finds meaningful and satisfying.

Diderot surely would have appreciated Helen Keller's treatment of this topic. He would have admired her philosophical precision as she explicates a system of analogies that allowed her to conceptualize purely visual phenomena such as color:

> I understand how scarlet can differ from crimson because I know that the smell of an orange is not the smell of a grape-fruit. I can also conceive that colors have shades, and guess what shades are. In smell and taste there are varieties not broad enough to be fundamental; so I call them shades.[4]

Keller draws on scent and taste to understand the differences between colors. She then elaborates to show her understanding of cultural associations between colors and abstract qualities:

> I have talked so much and read so much about colors that through no will of my own I attach meanings to them, just as all people attach certain meanings to abstract terms like hope, idealism, monotheism, intellect, which cannot be represented truly by visible objects, but which are understood from analogies between immaterial concepts and the ideas they awaken of external things. The force of association drives me to say that white is exalted and pure, green is exuberant, red suggests love or shame or strength. Without the color or its equivalent, life to me would be dark, barren, a vast blackness.[5]

Keller theorizes that her brain retains a five-sensed configuration, which makes it impossible for her to conceptualize objects devoid of visual and auditory details:

> Thus through an inner law of completeness my thoughts are not permitted to remain colorless. It strains my mind to separate color and sound from objects. Since my education began I have always had things described to me

> with their colors and sounds by one with keen senses and a fine feeling for the significant. Therefore I habitually think of things as colored and resonant. Habit accounts for part. The soul sense accounts for another part. The brain with its five-sensed construction asserts its right and accounts for the rest. Inclusive of all, the unity of the world demands that color be kept in it, whether I have cognizance of it or not. Rather than be shut out, I take part in it by discussing it, imagining it, happy in the happiness of those near me who gaze at the lovely hues of the sunset or the rainbow. [6]

Diderot's perplexity over Mademoiselle de Salignac's colorless imagination led him to speculate that in asking her where she saw the cube, he was posing the wrong question. It might have been better, he pondered instead, to ask where she felt it, to speak in terms of a mind's hand rather than a mind's eye.

In this regard, Diderot would have been further enlightened by Dr. Henry Moyes. Born in Scotland in 1750, he eventually settled in Manchester where he lectured on the natural sciences at the Philosophical Society. He traveled widely, including to America, where he gave a lecture at Columbia College on optics, a topic many of his listeners found a surprising choice for a man who had been blind since the age of three. A contemporary account recorded:

> It must be observed that this gentleman's eyes were not totally insensible to intense light . . . The rays refracted through a prism, when sufficiently vivid . . .produced certain . . . distinguishable effects on them . . . The red gave him a disagreeable sensation, which he compared to the touch of a saw; as the colors declined in violence, the harshness lessened, until the green afforded a sensation that was highly pleasing to him, and which he described as conveying an idea similar to what he felt in running his hand over polished surfaces . . . Polished surfaces, meandering streams, and gentle declivities, were the figures by which he expressed his ideas of beauty; rugged rocks, irregular points, and boisterous elements, furnished him with expressions for terror and disgust.[7]

Thus, Dr. Moyes processed his residual perception of color through his mind's hand to create a meaningful system of analogous sensations, a sort of spectrum of textures. For him, mental images might involve color, but the colors registered as tactile rather than visual.

Diderot's understanding of tactile imaging would have been further enriched if he could have met Geerat Vermeij, professor in the Geology Department at the University of California at Davis, who has been totally blind since early childhood. Here he describes his process of examining a group of Asian clams that, though visibly identical, actually belonged to two distinct species:

> The pads of my index fingers traced the outlines of the shells, probed the growth lines for their sharpness and spacing, noted how deeply cupped the valves were, and gathered a dozen other details. With my

> nails I observed the precise shape of the growth lines—were the lines sharp or flattened, reflected or erect, widely separated or close together, and so on. I repeated these observations, all quite unconsciously, with each shell. I picked up the valves again and again, comparing, contrasting, forming hypotheses in my mind, and putting them to the test with additional observations. I had to decide which features were meaningless variations and which might denote characteristics that distinguish one species from another.[8]

Vermeij was able to distinguish one species from the other, an identification that had previously been made only through DNA testing. He would be the first to point out that his skill as a tactile observer was not a supernatural compensatory power, but a technique he had learned and perfected over a lifetime as a working scientist.

I suspect that the idea of a blind conchologist would have made Diderot's head spin. But he would have been impressed by Vermeij's precision about the relative utility of the different parts of his fingers—the pads versus the nails—and the rigor of his method.

While Diderot and Mademoiselle de Salignac did not venture into a discussion of the natural sciences, she did make claims about her own tactile discernment. She told him that if he drew a picture of an object or a face in the palm of her hand she would identify it without hesitation—if the drawing was well done. It is no accident that she should touch on the subject of drawing; Diderot knew a great deal about art and was, at the time he knew Mademoiselle de Salignac, in the process of writing his *Salon Reviews*, what many consider foundational texts in art criticism.

The Salon Exhibitions of the Royal Academy, named for the Salon Carré in the Louvre where they were held, began in 1737. Diderot began writing his reviews in 1759 for the journal *Correspondences Litéraire*, addressing the texts to his friend Friedrich Melchior (known as Baron Grimm), the journal's editor. Diderot attended the exhibits every day of their six-week run, taking copious notes. His texts were written from memory weeks, even months, after the exhibit ended and were published without reproductions of any kind, so require some imagination to appreciate. With over two hundred works in each exhibit, hung from floor to ceiling so many visitors needed opera glasses to view them, it is not surprising that he made errors and omissions. But the majority of his descriptions are astoundingly accurate in every detail. He began from the premise that images do not speak for themselves. Indeed it was a common practice for visitors to the exhibits to enlist or hire docents to tell them what they were looking at. The artists themselves often strolled through the crowd to eavesdrop on these commentaries and correct the assessments of their own work or point out flaws in their rivals'. In his reviews, Diderot's primary technique is to focus on composition:

> I'll describe the paintings for you, and my descriptions will be such that, with a bit of imagination and taste, you'll be able to envision them spatially, disposing the objects within them more or less as we see them on the canvas.[9]

He calls on his readers' imagination—the ability to translate his words into mental images—and their taste—the discernment to judge these mental images against the conventions of academy painting of the day. Readers would have been familiar with these conventions and understood the hierarchy of subject matter: still lifes, landscapes, portraits, and history paintings.

Diderot often points out the difficulties of his task, particularly with larger history paintings depicting scenes from the Bible or classical mythology where scores of figures are distributed around the picture plane. For instance as he describes Jean-Jacques Bachelier's "Hector Rebuking Paris for his Cowardice," he breaks off in the middle to point out that he has only dealt with half the canvas:

> Have you followed all that? Can you picture it in your head? Then you've grasped the left side of the painting. Now for the right side.

Having drawn this map of half the painting in his readers' heads, he shoves it to one side to fill in the rest of the image. Then, as he concludes he congratulates himself:

> Ah! my friend, now I can breathe easier, and you as well. I must have a truly obliging imagination, if it managed to take in all that. And you're hoping perhaps that I'm going to provide a detailed critique of this world? Oh no; you want me to finish, and that would be endless. But rest assured that this description is precise, save a few minor details; a regular *tour de force,* if you will.[10]

He delights in his memory's capacity to absorb so much detail, and then to translate it all into words in order to transfer the image to readers' minds. But this kind of verbal mapping was not his only method. Because looking at art involves more than identifying the objects depicted and their arrangement in space, Diderot frequently abandons this form of description to make up narratives that would explain the images or evoke the same emotional response the image produced in him. In one instance he even invents a dream that turns out to replicate a painting by Fragonard. Frequently he rants against the artists, imagining better versions of the same subjects. Occasionally he records or invents conversations he overheard or engaged in at the exhibits, recreating the crowded, noisy atmosphere and the aesthetic debates of the day. Elsewhere, as in his description of a still life by Chardin, his review becomes a kind of list of instructions the reader could follow to recreate a real-life version of the painting:

> Imagine a squared construction of greyish stone, a kind of window with ledge and cornice. Arrange there with all the nobility and elegance you can

> muster a garland of large grapes extending the length of the cornice and hanging down on either side. Inside the window-jamb place a glass full of wine, a bottle, a broken loaf of bread, other carafes cooling in a faience bucket, a clay jug, radishes, fresh eggs, a saltcellar, two full, steaming coffee cups, and you'll see Chardin's painting.[11]

"But Monsieur Diderot, where will I see the painting? And How?" Mademoiselle de Salignac might ask. "For me, your words evoke mental sensations of texture, temperature, taste and smell. Are these not a part of your response to the painting as well?"

Am I wrong to imagine that Diderot's acquaintance with Mademoiselle de Salignac influenced the writing of his *Salon Reviews*? Although the reviews were written for readers who would have been able to see the paintings for themselves if they had been in Paris at the time of the exhibit, Diderot's methods seem equally meaningful to a blind person. And while others might have thought it insensitive, even cruel, to speak of visual art to a blind person, Diderot was not a man to scruple over such niceties. In fact, he records Mademoiselle de Salignac's explanation of how she understood the properties of mirrors, which she then analogized to drawing, engraving and painting. When she challenged him to correct her explanation, he responded: "To try to teach you any more would be waste of time."[12]

So I picture Diderot, after a long day at the Salon showing up at Mademoiselle de Salignac's home to describe the scene to her, since it was both an artistic and social spectacle. Later, he might return to read drafts of his reviews out loud to her, trying out his different techniques. He might arrange objects on a table top to recreate a still life, He might move around the room to create an aural map of a larger composition. He might even instruct Mademoiselle to assume the pose of one of the figures to see if it helped her feel the emotions the picture projected, though her pious mother might have intervened to prevent her from making too much of a spectacle of herself.

I admit that the image I construct here is a product of my desire—what I'd like to believe rather than anything I can prove. But in support of my speculations, consider how Diderot begins his "Notes on Painting," which was published as an appendix to his review of the *Salon* of 1765:

> Look at this woman who's lost her eyes while still young. The progressive deepening of her sockets hasn't increased the extent of the surrounding pockets. They've sunk into the cavities hollowed out by the organs' absence; they've shrunk. Above, a portion of her brow has been pulled in; below, her cheeks have been slightly lifted. Her upper lip, responding to this movement, has risen somewhat. These alterations have affected all parts of her face, in proportion to their proximity or distance from the principal site of the accident. But do you think that the deformity has been restricted to this oval? Do you think her neck has been completely unaffected? And her

> shoulders and throat? Yes, to your eyes and mine. But summon nature, show her this neck, these shoulders, this throat, and nature will tell you; this is the neck, these the shoulders, and this the throat of a woman who's lost her eyes while still young.[13]

Is this Diderot's verbal portrait of his young blind friend? It is impossible to say. Though Mademoiselle de Salignac was blind since early infancy, there is no record of the cause of her blindness, no mention of an "accident" that might have damaged her eyes or caused their removal. Perhaps the woman Diderot describes was someone else, or merely a figment of his imagination. Still, it is a noteworthy coincidence that he links blindness and visual art in this way.

Whether Diderot had Mademoiselle de Salignac in mind when he wrote about art, he nevertheless challenged himself to understand how her mental processes differed from his own, without exoticizing them. It is no wonder that she had developed concepts about visual phenomena. She lived in the same visual culture as Diderot. She did not grow up in an isolated, all-blind world. She probably knew no other blind people. She lived among sighted people and was accustomed to making sense of their language, customs, conventions, and claims. Like most blind people, she was also familiar with the limits of human vision:

> "I stand," she said, "at the entrance of a long alley; and there is a certain object at its far end. One of my friends sees it moving, another sees it stationary; one says . . . it is an animal, another that it is a man; and on approaching it, it turns out a tree-stump. No one can tell if the tower they see in the distance is round or square."[14]

What about her claim that she could identify a drawing made in the palm of her hand if it was well done. What qualities would make one drawing better than another according to her tactile judgment? Interpreting a drawing on her palm would be yet another familiar occasion of translating a sighted custom into terms she would find meaningful. Here, she would be feeling the drawing with her palm rather than her fingertip and the motion of the drawing finger would be controlled by the other person. In chapter 3, I cited modern research showing that active rather than passive touch is more discerning, and that the speed and pressure of the touching finger also varies perception. Drawing on the palm, as Mademoiselle de Salignac suggested, would require a particular combination of passive and active, static and mobile touching. She was claiming that her mind would follow the motion of the other's hand, forming an image line-by-line in her head. Since the drawing finger would leave no mark on her hand, the person drawing would find himself in somewhat unfamiliar territory, producing a drawing he could not see. Of course, drawing on the palm would have its conventions like all other drawing. If someone wanted to draw the portrait of a person Mademoiselle knew, she would expect him to start with an oval to represent the frame of the face, then add eyes, nose mouth, ears, hair. The drawing would, by necessity, have to be small and simple, more of a miniature caricature than a detailed rendering, highlighting the most prominent feature—a disproportionately large or small nose, a pointy or receding chin, and abundance or dearth of hair. These would be the features she would have known for herself either from having touched the person's face or, more likely given her mother's sense of propriety, from verbal descriptions others had supplied. In fact, she might anticipate that the portraitist would dwell on the distinctive feature and make the identification from that alone.

But Diderot apparently never tried the experiment. In his *Salon Reviews*, he enumerates the qualities that distinguish a good portrait from a bad one. His general advice to artists, as in the passage from his "Notes on Painting," was that they should follow nature more closely, rather than contrive stagey poses and expressions from their imaginations. But Diderot was not himself a visual artist. Could he allow for the possibility of a visual artist who was blind?

If I had the chance, I would use Diderot's own method to describe a work by one such artist for him. The work I have in mind is by Alice Wingwall, titled *Hand Over Dog: Joseph at the Temple of Dendur* (1994) (Fig. 5.1). It is one in a series of images that the photographer and architectural historian produced during the final phase of her sight loss from retinitis pigmentosa. She took her new service dog Joseph to visit her favorite architectural sites around the world. *Hand Over Dog* is a photograph of the Temple of Dendur at the Metropolitan Museum in New York, pictured from the front. In the middle ground of the image, museum visitors stand looking at the temple or walk to and fro. In the foreground, Joseph, a handsome yellow Labrador appears in profile. In the even more immediate foreground, the artist's hand, slightly out of focus, points to the temple, as if directing the viewer's gaze that way. Although the viewer understands that the hand would be above the dog's head in three-dimensional space, in the two-dimensional picture plane the hand is at the level of the dog's nose. But Joseph is looking, somewhat longingly, toward the window. Perhaps his attention has been attracted by some urban wildlife, a squirrel or pigeon. Perhaps he is sitting at attention, awaiting his next command. Or perhaps it is the longing look of a service dog who needs a break. In either case, the image draws on the conventions of fine art photography: with the careful framing and posing of photo portraitists, and the random serendipity of those who photograph street scenes, wildlife, and war. The pointing hand is somehow reminiscent of the convention of the pointing figure in Christian and medieval art. But here the hand plus the dog bring the artist's blindness into the image. Since dogs are not typically allowed in museums, the viewer is lead to understand that this dog must be accompanied by a blind person. The image as a whole represents a complex of ideas about looking and seeing, about showing and meaning. It makes a powerful statement about the role of the artist to organize and direct the viewer's gaze, while

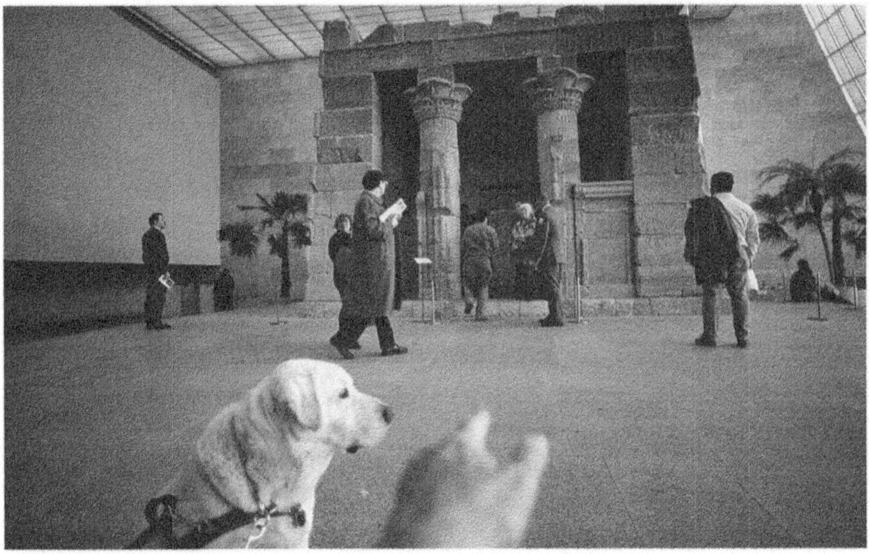

FIGURE 5.1 Hand over Dog: Joseph at the Temple of Dendur *(1994)*.
Photograph by Alice Wingwall, taken at the Temple of Dendur in the Metropolitan. Museum of Art Egyptian Collection, New York, New York.

it humorously debunks the popular myth that the service dog does the seeing for the blind person.

I must bring my own blindness into this image and admit that my whole description is based primarily on hearsay, what I have heard and read about it, rather than direct visual experience. My residual vision only allows me to perceive photographs where the colors are highly saturated and the forms and composition are extremely simple. Here, I needed a lot of help describing the perspective of the image—the precise line-up of hand and dog in the picture plane.

But does my secondhand description nevertheless make an image in your mind's eye? Perhaps, with a little more effort, I can make you want to see it. Again, we hear poor Diderot, his head still reeling with all these new terms—blind artist, service dogs, photography—sputter and ask, "But where is this image, where this desire?"

"In our heads," we say, "like you."

This might not be accurate for all of us. I believe that Alice Wingwall, like other blind artists I know, actually does see this image in her mind's eye. Her visual memory, combined with skills perfected over many decades as a sighted artist and art viewer, allow her to produce mental images that she can then communicate to sighted assistants who help her aim her camera. As I've said before, my own mind's eye is not so acute or reliable. When I try to produce a mental image from my early childhood when my vision was presumed close to normal, the results have the same distortions and lack of detail as my vision today. My description of Wingwall's photograph does not draw a mental image for me. Rather, it produces a sensation in my mind's body. I could lead a tour to the Temple of Dendur, position myself where she stood, borrow someone's service dog and persuade him to pose correctly, distribute the appropriate number of visitors around the space, then shout, "Hold it!" and create a sort of live reenactment of the image, a tableau vivant recreation of the way the words make me feel. Even though I can still perceive color, Sabriye Tenberken's description of Lake Namtso does nothing to my mind's eye. Her words, that center on details of color and temperature—crystallized, turquoise, blue, melting—in contrast with the fiery reds and oranges of the sunset, make me think of a blue popsicle—a sensation in my mind's mouth—a color and a taste, not found in nature.

What Diderot's account of his friendship with Melanie de Salignac reveals is not only his lifelong fascination with blindness, but also his willingness to engage fully with the lived experience of blindness as a way of being in the world rather than a state of deficit or lack. Though he thought of her as exceptional, he knew that her family gave her opportunities for her natural gifts to flourish. As I have noted earlier, it is for this reason, Diderot is often credited with inspiring a move toward education for blind people. But in the centuries since Diderot and Melanie de Salignac carried on their playful debate, the educators and researchers who follow in his footsteps do not always follow his first premises. Diderot valued his blind informant not because she conformed to his previously held theories but because she compelled him to examine all that he took for granted. In comparing his imagination to hers he was not seeking a mirror image. If her mental images differed from his own it did not make them any less vivid or useful. He accepted that Mademoiselle de Salignac would have developed ways to conceptualize the sighted world. His dealings with her suggest that he was teetering on the edge of conceptualizing blind perception, grappling with ideas about outward reality and inward representations, and the complex interplay between words and images.

{6}

Dialogues with the Blind

> Every time a draftsman lets himself be fascinated by the blind, every time he makes the blind a *theme* of his drawing, he projects, dreams, or hallucinates a figure of a draftsman, or sometimes, more precisely, some draftswoman. Or more precisely still, he begins to *represent* a drawing potency [*puissance*] at work, the very act of drawing. He invents drawing.[1]

In the last chapter, I engaged in some willful speculation in imagining that Denis Diderot's writing about visual art may have been influenced by his lifelong fascination with blindness, and more specifically, his acquaintance with blind individuals like Melanie de Salignac. In doing so, I am adding to what could be considered a canon of literary depictions that pair blindness on the one hand and visual art on the other. In chapter 2, I touched on texts that follow the scenario of cases of restored sight, where the newly sighted patients are asked to perform the standard tests of the Molyneux problem. Wilkie Collins's *Poor Miss Finch* also deploys ideas about visual art. As I cited earlier, Collins was well-versed in philosophical speculation about blindness. For example, he raised the same concerns as Diderot about the morality of blind people. Madame Pratolungo, the novel's narrator and the paid companion of the blind Lucilla, frets that she lacks the modesty proscribed for young ladies and draws a metaphor from the art world:

> The female model who "sits" for the first time in a drawing academy, and who shrinks from the ordeal, is persuaded, in the last resort, to enter the students' room by having a bandage bound over her eyes. My poor Lucilla had always the bandage over her eyes.[2]

Lucilla's beloved, Oscar, and his twin brother, Nugent, both engage in artistic pursuits, and their father was a society portrait painter. Oscar has the gentlemanly hobby of engraving ornamental objects he makes from precious metals. In fact, it is Lucilla's tactile examination of his work that first sparks their mutual attraction. She has no trouble deciphering the tactile pictures of ivy leaves and owls on a vase he has made. The leaves are easy, because she has touched them in reality. And while she has never touched a living owl, her table service includes condiment pots in that form. On the other hand, Nugent is a landscape painter—an artist on the grand scale. Madame Pratolungo, who initially prefers Nugent's outgoing personality to his brother's reserve, still mocks the grandiose claims he makes about the power of art to uplift humanity. Significantly, it is Nugent, rather than Oscar, who is most eager for Lucilla to undergo the sight-restoring operation. Oscar is less enthusiastic because he fears how Lucilla will respond to his disfigured appearance from the silver nitrate he takes to control his epilepsy; Nugent hopes she will prefer his unaltered complexion and fall in love with him instead. But there is at least some suggestion that he hopes her restored sight will allow her to appreciate his painting over his brother's handicraft. While the other genres of nineteenth-century painting—portraits and still lifes—are fairly simple to describe to a blind person, and even history paintings with their many figures and complex compositions can be described according to techniques such as those Diderot developed in his *Salon* reviews, landscape painting has the additional complications of such features as perspective and vantage point, and so the landscape painter—the romantic rival in this melodrama—would assume that only a sighted Lucilla would be able to appreciate its seductive power. In the end, however, Lucilla's blindness returns and she marries the right twin, who continues to tinker in his metal engraving workshop, creating tactile ornaments for their domestic bliss. Nugent banishes himself to an arctic painting expedition where he dies alone.

For Collins, blindness is Lucilla's true state. The operation was a misguided attempt to change what didn't need fixing. Thus it is the tactile artisan rather than the visual artist who is the better match for her. The literary examples that follow feature characters who are put in even more direct dialogue with visual art and visual artists. Can we borrow Derrida's assertion in the epigraph and say that these depictions project, dream, or hallucinate a figure of a writer? How do these authors use this pairing to investigate or even invent their own art form, carrying on an old debate about words versus images?

We can find countless occasions when authors use metaphors about the "blindness" of visual artists similar to those I quote in my introduction. For example, the narrator of John Banville's *The Sea* describes his late wife's photography in this way:

> I have always disliked being photographed, but I intensely disliked being photographed by Anna. It is a strange thing to say, I know, but when she was behind a camera she was like a blind person, something in her eyes went dead, an essential light was extinguished. She seemed not to be looking through the lens, at her subject, but rather to be peering inward, into herself, in search of some defining perspective, some essential point of view. She would hold the camera steady at eye-level and thrust her raptor's head out

> sideways and stare for a second, sightlessly, it might be, as if one's features were written in some form of braille that she was capable of reading at a distance; when she pressed the shutter it seemed the least important thing, no more than a gesture to placate the apparatus.[3]

The photographer here is not literally blind, but temporarily sightless in the act of capturing the image. Banville draws on the metaphoric linkages between cameras and eyes, as well as ideas about vision as a kind of long-distance touching that we can trace back to Descartes. Banville employs all these metaphors to enhance the sense of the narrator's ambivalence about his wife's artistic pursuits.

Beyond these clichés about the temporary sightlessness intrinsic to the artistic process, we can find some novels that speculate on the possibility of an actual blind artist. In Rudyard Kipling's first novel, *The Light That Failed*, Dick Heldar is a painter who loses his sight belatedly from a blow to the head sustained in the Sudan. When a friend brings him a gift of some modeling wax, he pokes and prods it for a few minutes, and then asks, "Is it like anything in the world?" But then he immediately abandons the activity, complaining, "Take it away. I may get the touch of the blind in fifty years."[4] He rejects the tacit suggestion that he might switch from painting to sculpture because he is certain that switching from vision to touch will take too long. Instead, he opts for what he considers to be the manly response to his blindness—suicide.[5]

In the century since Kipling's novel, advances in educational and vocational opportunities for blind people may have suggested to one recent novelist that blindness need not lead to such dire consequences. Hilary Norman's thriller *Blind Fear* allows for the possibility of a blind sculptor who is at once very successful and personally fulfilled. Jack Donovan became totally blind at the age of eighteen when he found himself in the path of a bullet intended for someone else. Undaunted by blindness he persevered through art school and achieved international fame for his sculptures of human body parts that he executes with startling sensitivity and exquisite detail. Joanna Guthrie is an English guide-dog trainer and freelance photographer, who comes to Donavan's studio and art school compound to provide him with a new service dog. Apparently, Donavan's artistic moodiness has made him unpopular with the American guide-dog schools. Although Joanna is accustomed to working with blind people, she fatuously admires Donavan's ability to maneuver around his house and grounds, to read people's moods from their voices, and otherwise live independently. He even goes to the movies! He explains that blindness has allowed him to work with fewer distractions, "I've found that all I have to do is *'see'* something one time through someone else's eyes, then add my own impressions—scents, sounds, atmospheres, whatever—and after that I have a mind picture I tend not to forget."[6]

Joanna is attracted to Donavon but feels hostility from a trio of assistants. One, Murdoch Lambert (nicknamed Lamb, though he is anything but innocent) is Donavon's favorite pair of eyes, particularly adept at describing features of their surroundings and strangers they encounter. A sculptor himself, he sometimes constructs scale models of architecture that Donavon can study through touch. More significantly, Lamb also fashions bones out of resin, which Donavon uses as armatures for his work. At least everyone thinks that they are made of resin. People are disappearing in the neighborhood of Donavon's school. And eventually a mass grave is discovered. All the bodies have a part missing, and these parts correspond to pieces of Donavon's famous work. It turns out that the sculptures' armatures are not made of resin but actual human bones covered with gypsum. Joanna suspects the trio of assistants, especially the creepy Lamb. But she frets about the extent of Donavon's hand in the murderous enterprise. The two miscreants are eventually brought to justice, but by the end of the novel, the third assistant Pete, who was innocent of the original scheme, seems ready to take over where the other two left off. He expresses a certainty that it was the bones and not Donavon's talent that made him so successful.

Earlier in the novel, Donavon made a sculpture of Joanna's head, clearly unaided by any bones taken from the living subject. Joanna observes that it

> was a very different creature from the other works she had seen, with little of his extraordinarily lavish attention to minute detail; this piece had clearly been swiftly rendered by a man who had never seen Joanna as others did. And yet it was breathtakingly true to her—to her *essence*—in a way that even the most brilliant photograph could never be.[7]

Significantly, Joanna compares the sculpture to photography—her own artistic medium. While a photograph might be a better likeness, Donavon's sculpture does a better job of capturing her essence, even though (or perhaps because) he produced it from memories of touching her. Still, she recognizes that it lacks the detail that has made Donavon's work famous. So the question remains whether he can match his previous commercial success without the aid of his murderous assistants. The novel allows for the possibility that a blind man could produce art but assumes that he will probably require the slavish devotion of homicidal collaborators. The open ending of the novel not only suggests a possible sequel but also deploys familiar ideas about the moral ambiguity of blind people. Left to his own devices, the blind artist is likely to fall into the hands of evil. His only hope is that he will find himself connected to a virtuous sighted guide, such as the novel's heroine. The art may suffer, but chaos and mass murder will be kept at bay.

It may well be that in every depiction of a blind person—whether or not that person is also an artist—there is some occasion when sighted people are called upon to describe or explain some visual phenomenon. In films, these scenes help highlight the pathos and dependence of the blind character. There is often a kind of plea, the blind person hungrily begging for some verbal description. And since the movie audience can see what is being described, the words are bound to seem woefully inadequate. In Raymond Carver's "Cathedral," a blind man, Robert, asks his sighted host to describe a cathedral pictured on television. The narrator, who has announced that he is not enthusiastic about Robert's visit, and has displayed his prejudices and misconceptions about blindness, attempts a description but finds he lacks the verbal skill and architectural knowledge to do an adequate job. So Robert suggests that he draw a picture instead. Robert follows the motions of his drawing hand and then examines the tactile marks left on the heavy paper. The reader is left with only a sketchy notion of whether this picture is worth the thousand words the narrator cannot supply, much less whether the drawing is meaningful to the blind man. But the collaborative experience is understood to draw the two men together and to give the sighted man the means to overcome his limited understanding of blindness.[8]

While Carver's characters resort to this unusual form of verbal-tactile communication, other depictions tout the virtues of verbal descriptions of visual phenomena. Contrary to the ideal of the Hypothetical, whose blindness is always understood to be total and congenital, in the depictions that follow, blind characters often used to be sighted, and even those who were born blind, live in close contact with sighted people. To varying degrees they have adapted to their sightlessness and draw on visual memories to understand the world around them. But more importantly, they speak the language of the sighted and even sometimes instruct sighted people in the best ways to describe what they see. For instance, in Lorrie Moore's story, "What You Want to Do Fine," the blind lawyer Quilty and his sighted lover Mack go on a road trip. As they visit sites, Quilty calls on Mack to describe what he sees, and then often critiques his descriptions, as here when they visit the St. Louis Arch:

> "Describe the view to me," says Quilty when they get out at the top.
> Mack looks out through the windows. "Adequate," he says.
> "I said describe, not *rate*."
> "Midwestern. Aerial. Green and brown."
> Quilty sighs. "I don't think blind men should date deaf-mutes until the how-to book has been written."[9]

Quilty disparages Mack's first comment because it merely offers an opinion rather than an unbiased translation of visual phenomena. Throughout the trip, Quilty teases his lover about his lack of eloquence. The two men met when Quilty hired Mack to paint his house. Mack's profession might suggest that he has a heightened visual sensibility, but house painting is only one of many temporary jobs, and he is fairly incompetent at it. Quilty's neighbors tell him that Mack has succeeded mainly in painting his bushes blue. At the Art Institute in Chicago, Mack's limited experience of art makes the visit challenging:

> He would rather try to understand the paintings he has seen that afternoon, and has almost understood: the Halloween hues of the Lautrecs; the chalky ones of Puvis de Chavannes; the sweet finger paints of the Vuillards and Bonnards, all crowded with window light and commodes. Mack had listened to the buzzing voice coming from Quilty's headphones, but he hadn't gotten his own headphones. Let a blind man be described to! Mack had his own eyes.[10]

Moore's terse verbal sketches of these works simulate Mack's struggle to articulate his untrained responses. He retains a general impression that somehow evokes childhood associations: Halloween, chalk, and finger paints. Still, he feels superior to his blind lover, who, though more highly educated, is forced to rely on the interpretations of others buzzing through the earphones of the recorded audio guide. His feelings of superiority prompt a charitable impulse:

> But finally, overwhelmed by poor Quilty's inability either to see or touch the paintings, he had led Quilty downstairs to the statuary, and when no one was looking, he'd placed Quilty's hands upon the naked marble figure of a woman. "Ah," Quilty had said, feeling the nose and lips, and then he grew quiet and respectful at her shoulders, her breasts, and hips, and when he got down past the thighs and knees to her feet, Quilty laughed out loud. Feet! These he knew best. These he liked.[11]

Mack's act of compassion has a hint of sexual transgression, as he first checks to see that no one is looking, then guides the blind man's hands to the nude. Again, Mack attempts to assert another kind of experiential superiority. He has been married to a woman, has fathered a child, and had sexual relationships with other women, so he assumes his appreciation of the female form will be of a higher order than what the blind gay man can experience through touch alone. Indeed, Quilty only responds verbally to those parts common to both male and female bodies—the facial features and the feet. The breasts, hips and thighs leave him respectful but speechless. But his silence may also denote his awareness that aesthetic appreciation is not the same thing as sexual titillation. Ultimately, Mack's inability to describe what he sees points to the class difference between the two men. The blind man knows more about art—or at least more about how to behave before art—than the sighted man who can see it.

In *Poor Miss Finch* a similar connection is drawn between the ability to talk about visual beauty and class differences. Lucilla is accustomed to have the natural world described to her, but she laments that her servant is less adept at the practice, suggesting that these values have as much to do with education and background as with vision alone:

> Persons in the lower ranks of life are curiously unobservant of the aspects of Nature. I never (in the days of my blindness) got any information from servants or labourers about the views round Dimchurch. They seemed to have no eyes beyond the range of the kitchen or the ploughed field.[12]

In Moore's story, the dialogues about landscapes and art reveal the two men's basic incompatibility. Similarly, Tracy Chevalier's novel *Girl with a Pearl Earring* presents another kind of friction brought on through debates about art. The novel invents a narrative to explain the origins of Vermeer's famous painting. Griat is a servant in the Vermeer household, who becomes enthralled by the painter's work and eventually poses for the painting that gives the novel its title. Griat is obliged to take the job when her father, a former tile painter, loses his eyes in a kiln accident. His former employment as a visual artisan, if not an artist, means that he already knows and can speak knowledgeably about Vermeer's work. When Griat comes home after her first encounters with Vermeer's painting, her father's leading questions help her recall details that she was unable to articulate on her initial viewings. Her descriptions follow the standard format of the type of taped audio tour that Quilty uses at the art institute, focusing mainly on the figure's pose, the colors of her garments, and the overall composition:

> So I tried to describe the woman tying pearls around her neck, her hands suspended, gazing at herself in the mirror, the light from the window bathing her face and her yellow mantle, the dark foreground that separated her from us.
>
> My father listened intently, but his own face was not illuminated until I said, "The light on the back wall is so warm that looking at it feels the way the sun feels on your face."[13]

Here, she draws an analogy between the visual phenomena and a tactile sensation that she assumes her father will find more meaningful. But as she becomes more immersed in the artist's life, her dialogues with her father become increasingly vexed:

> "The baker's daughter stands in a bright corner by a window," I began patiently. "She is facing us, but is looking out the window, down to her right. She is wearing a yellow and black fitted bodice of silk and velvet, a dark blue skirt, and a white cap that hangs down in two points below her chin."
>
> "As you wear yours?" my father asked. He had never asked this before, though I had described the cap the same way each time.[14]

Her father's question shows his concerns about the growing intimacy between Griat and her employer. To deflect his attention from the style of the cap, she launches into an explanation of the artist's technique to render its whiteness.

> "Yes, like mine. When you look at the cap long enough," I added hurriedly, "you see that he has not really painted it white, but blue, and violet, and yellow."
>
> "But it's a white cap, you said."
>
> "Yes, that's what is so strange. It's painted many colors, but when you look at it, you think it's white."
>
> "Tile painting is much simpler," my father grumbled. "You use blue and that's all. A dark blue for the outlines, a light blue for the shadows. Blue is blue."
>
> And a tile is a tile, I thought, and nothing like his paintings. I wanted him to understand that white was not simply white. It was a lesson my master had taught me.[15]

Griat's father's irritation here has less to do with his blindness and more to do with the apparent range of subtleties available in oil painting compared with the simpler medium of his former trade. At the same time, Griat shows the shift in her allegiance from her father to Vermeer. The painter has expanded her aesthetic sensibility in a way that makes it hard for her to talk to her father whose range of associations has always been so limited. As if conscious of her irritation, he shifts her focus from the use of color to the pose of the figure:

> "What is she doing?" he asked after a moment.
>
> "She has one hand on a pewter pitcher sitting on a table and one on a window she's partly opened. She's about to pick up the pitcher and dump the water from it out the window, but she's stopped in the middle of what she's doing and is either dreaming or looking at something in the street."
>
> "Which is she doing?"
>
> "I don't know. Sometimes it seems one thing, sometimes the other."
>
> My father sat back in his seat, frowning. "First you say the cap is white but not painted white. Then you say the girl is doing one thing or maybe another. You're confusing me." He rubbed his brow as if his head ached.
>
> "I'm sorry, Father. I'm trying to describe it accurately."
>
> "But what is the story in the painting?"
>
> "His paintings don't tell stories."[16]

Despite this final assertion, Griat's description interpolates two different narratives from the figure's static pose. The figure's expression suggests that she is either actively watching something through the window, or else daydreaming with an unfocused gaze. No wonder her father is confused. As if acknowledging her own inadequacy, Griat leaves off her description, stating defensively:

> I did not like him being critical of the painting without having seen it, or comparing it to the tiles he had once painted. I wanted to tell him that if he could only see the painting he would understand that there was nothing

> confusing about it. It may not have told a story, but it was still a painting you could not stop looking at.[17]

While Griat seems to despair of ever being able to explain what the paintings, and the artist, have come to mean to her, it is clear that Chevalier finds blindness a useful device to create and repeat lavish verbal descriptions of the works in question. In effect, she asserts that Vermeer's later paintings invite viewers to compose narratives to explain the figures' poses and expressions. It is as if these paintings function as illustrations for some unwritten text.

As many reviewers have suggested, the international success of *Girl with a Pearl Earring* seems to have inspired Chevalier to repeat the plot formula in her later novel *The Lady and the Unicorn,* including another blind character who functions in a similar way. Here however, the blind character converses directly with the artist and influences the work he produces. Blind Aliénor, daughter of the Belgian weaver commissioned to create the tapestries, is so well adapted to her lack of sight, that Nicolas, the arrogant Paris artist who painted the designs, has trouble at first recognizing that she cannot see. Unlike Griat's father, Aliénor has been blind since birth. She can find her way around her home and the weaving workshop, and can perform all her daily chores unaided. She tends an elaborate garden and advises her father about what kind of flowers to include in the millefleur backgrounds that the workshop is known for. While guild rules forbid women from weaving, she can help with hemming and other sewing tasks, and since she can perform this work without light, she can work at night, which helps the workshop meet its tight deadlines. She has no patience with sighted people who want to pity her or express surprise at her many skills. As she puts it:

> I have other ways of knowing the world.
>
> For instance, I know the tapestries I work on. I can feel each ridge of warp thread, each bead of weft. I can trace the flowers of the *millefleur* pattern and follow my stitches around a dog's hind leg or a rabbit's ear or the sleeve of a peasant's robe. I feel colors. Red is silky smooth, yellow prickles, blue is oily. Underneath my fingers is a map made by the tapestries.[18]

It might at first seem that Chevalier subscribes to the myth of supernatural compensatory powers, where blind people are supposed to have some sort of sixth sense that would allow them to feel purely visual phenomena such as color. In fact what Aliénor is really feeling are the different chemical residues of the different dyes. The oiliness of the blue comes from the woad dye, and Aliénor's dislike of its texture reflects her dislike for the brutish and smelly woad merchant who wants to marry her. Nicolas tries to curry favor by altering his designs so there will be less blue, meaning fewer visits to the workshop from her unwanted suitor.

As in *Girl with a Peral Earring*, Chevalier uses the blind character to point to differences between different artistic media—in this case tapestry versus painting. The painter is startled to learn that the weaver must work from the back of the image, occasionally checking his progress with a mirror held under the threads. Also, the weaver can only see one narrow strip of the image at a time. The whole image is only revealed at the end of the long process when the tapestry is cut from the loom and unfurled. Nicolas exclaims that it is like "painting blind."[19] Like Griat's father, Aliénor wants to have the tapestries described to her. And as with the descriptions of Vermeer's painting, the descriptions attempt to construct a narrative, deciphering symbolic meanings from the various elements in each image. She asks Philippe, the workshop's cartoonist who transfers the designs from the painting to paper, to tell her the story of each design. When his descriptions fall short, she turns directly to the artist:

> "In more detail now. Where is the Lady looking-at the unicorn or at the lion? What is she wearing? Is she happy or sad? Does she feel safe in her garden? What is the lion doing? Is the unicorn sitting or standing? Is he glad to be caught or does he want to get away? Does the Lady love the unicorn?" [20]

Significantly, the details Aliénor seeks are both visual—the postures of the figures, the direction of the lady's gaze—and narrative, defining the emotions of the lady and animals—safe, happy, sad, glad to be caught, in love. Like Leo Steinberg's blind man conversing with Jasper Johns, which I cited in the introduction, Aliénor's questions incite the artist to rethink his ideas. Nicolas seems impressed by the blind girl's demands for details that speak to emotion and motive. Later Nicolas uses her face as the model for the lady in the "sight" tapestry, perhaps a tribute to the ways she has altered his vision.

For Tracy Chevalier, blind characters function not only as a device to prop up and prod the plot of her novels; they also perform in miniature the task of the novel as a whole by soliciting descriptions and constructing narratives to explain enigmatic works of visual art. In Paul Auster's *Moon Palace*, the blind character trains the young protagonist in the art of verbal description as a part of his education to become a writer. The novel's narrator M. S. Fogg goes to work for Thomas Effing, the former painter and purported millionaire, who is now, elderly, blind, and uses a wheelchair. One of Fogg's new duties is to take Effing out for airings in his wheelchair and to describe everything he sees. At first his descriptions are both verbose and imprecise, which incurs the wrath of his irascible employer. But soon he finds a personal value in the exercise:

> Instead of doing it merely to discharge an obligation, I began to consider it as a spiritual exercise, a process of training myself how to look at the world as if I were discovering it for the first time. What do you see? And if you see, how do you put it into words? The world enters us through our eyes,

> but we cannot make sense of it until it descends into our mouths. I began to appreciate how great that distance was, to understand how far a thing must travel in order to get from the one place to the other. In actual terms, it was no more than two or three inches, but considering how many accidents and losses could occur along the way, it might just as well have been a journey from the earth to the moon.[21]

The activity prompts a philosophical meditation—to what extent are seeing and knowing dependent on language? At first, Fogg's descriptions have too much detail and overwhelm Effing with an avalanche of words. But gradually, Fogg develops a different technique:

> The important thing to remember was that Effing was blind. My job was not to exhaust him with lengthy catalogues, but to help him see things for himself. In the end, the words didn't matter. Their task was to enable him to apprehend the objects as quickly as possible, and in order to do that, I had to make them disappear the moment they were pronounced. It took me weeks of hard work to simplify my sentences, to learn how to separate the extraneous from the essential, I discovered that the more air I left around a thing, the happier the results, for that allowed Effing to do the crucial work on his own: to construct an image on the basis of a few hints, to feel his own mind traveling toward the thing I was describing for him.[22]

Initially, Fogg is patronizing in his assumptions about what Effing needs to know. He develops an editing philosophy where less is more, where the silence around his well-chosen words will stimulate the blind man's imagination to fill in the blanks. In so doing, he begins to cast Effing in the role of the blind seer or teacher. The discipline of verbal description becomes a road to his own enlightenment:

> I no longer saw it as an aesthetic activity but as a moral one, and I began to be less irritated by Effing's criticisms, wondering if his impatience and dissatisfaction could not eventually serve some higher purpose. I was a monk seeking illumination, and Effing was my hair shirt, the whip I flayed myself with.[23]

Apparently satisfied with Fogg's progress, Effing sends him to the Brooklyn Museum to look at a painting by Albert Blakelock, giving him these instructions:

> Look at the painting. Look at the painting for no less than an hour, ignoring everything else in the room. Concentrate. Look at it from various distances—from ten feet away, from two feet away, from one inch away. Study it for its overall composition; study it for its details. Don't take any notes. See if you can memorize all the elements of the picture, learning the precise location of the human figures, the natural objects, the colors on each and every spot of the canvas. Close your eyes and test yourself. Open them again. See if you can't begin to enter the landscape before you. See if you can't begin to enter

> the mind of the artist who painted the landscape before you. Imagine that you are Blakelock, painting the picture yourself.[24]

Effing, though blind, clearly retains sufficient visual memory to instruct his sighted assistant in the best way to view art. In fact, I imagine that his instructions would please any artist or art historian, for the way they promote prolonged, systematic contemplation, rather than the glance-and-shuffle that is typical of most museum visitors. Effing's instructions even dictate Fogg's behavior before he gets to the museum. He commands that Fogg should not talk to anyone on his way there, telling him that he should pretend to be "deaf" and should close his eyes while riding the subway and attempt to clear his mind in preparation for his first view of the picture. In effect, his instructions are suggestive of those given by an art teacher.

> Think about your eyes and the extraordinary power you possess to see the world. Imagine what would happen to you if you couldn't see it. Imagine yourself looking at something under the various lights that make the world visible to us: sunlight, moonlight, electric light, candlelight, neon light. Make it a very simple and ordinary something. A stone, for example, or a small block of wood. Think carefully about how the appearance of that object changes when placed under these different lights. Think nothing more than that, assuming you have to think about something.[25]

Here, Effing calls on his assistant to feel grateful for his unimpaired sight. But his instructions are also reminiscent of those given in an art class exercise where the student is encouraged to practice drawing from memory and imagination rather than from life. Typical of Effing's fickle nature, he never questions Fogg about his experience of Blakelock's painting. In fact, all Fogg's training in verbal description seems ultimately a preparation for his true task—to help Effing write his own obituary. This project soon expands to a full-fledged biography where Fogg is called on to paint verbal pictures of landscapes he has never seen for himself. Eventually, piecing together Effing's life story leads Fogg to uncover the mystery of his own paternity. In effect, the novel has at its heart a story about a young writer learning the craft of writing under the tutelage of a blind mystic. In performing the seemingly impossible task of translating visual phenomena into words, the young writer creates his first work of art and simultaneously discovers the key to his own origins.

In the first section of *Moon Palace,* before Fogg has met Effing, his extremely straightened circumstances require him to sell off the library he inherited from his uncle. He feels compelled to read each book before selling it, considering the process a kind of capstone experience to his college education. But the sheer quantity of books, combined with his Spartan diet, make the task quite daunting:

> The closer I got to the end, however, the more trouble the books gave me. I could feel my eyes making contact with the words on the page, but no

> meanings rose up to me anymore, no sounds echoed in my head. The black marks seemed wholly bewildering, an arbitrary collection of lines and curves that divulged nothing but their own muteness. Eventually, I did not even pretend to understand what I was reading. I would pull a book from the box, open it to the first page, and then move my finger along the first line. When I came to the end, I would start in on the second line, and then the third line, and so on down to the bottom of the page. That was how I finished the job: like a blind man reading braille. If I couldn't see the words, at least I wanted to touch them. Things had become so bad for me by then; this actually seemed to make sense.[26]

The starving student fails to make sense of the arbitrary system of symbols on the printed page. His eyes make contact but yield no sensation; the words remain mute. To cap off this bleak image of absolute isolation and failed communication, Auster reaches for the standard simile denoting futility—the blind man. Except that this is a blind man reading Braille. And while Braille is cryptic to the uninitiated sighted reader, the simile foreshadows Fogg's later meeting with his blind mentor. While Effing is not a Braille reader (he hires Fogg to read aloud to him), he is expert in a range of systems of symbolic representation. Auster updates the stock character of the blind seer, at the same time suggesting that the job of the writer is to create images out of words, to make a world visible to a reader who cannot see it.

Returning then to Derrida's formula, we can say that these literary depictions of blind people project, dream, or hallucinate a figure of a reader rather than a writer. Drawing from this random sampling of literary texts, we find that blind characters hold up a mirror where the reader can see herself. When authors speculate on the processes of visual art, a blind character becomes a useful device through which to meditate on the relationship between the reader and the text. The reader can read between the lines like Griat's father, or may crave more detail like Aliénor, or less like Effing. And while the figure of the blind artist may still seem both implausible and dangerous, these dialogues between blind people and their sighted informants serve as an occasion to revel in the transcendent power of language.

{7}

Audio Description Described

In the previous two chapters I explored different treatments of the age-old conflict between words and images, where a blind person acts as a facilitator of inquiry into the nature and value of visual art. In the next two chapters, I turn to the practical, real-world problem of making visual media comprehensible to blind people. Here, I examine standard practices of audio description for film and television. In the following chapter I will discuss how these practices are employed in an art museum.

In April 2015, Netflix, the video rental and online streaming service, announced that its new series *Daredevil* would be available with audio description for the blind and visually impaired. The company also announced that soon it would increase the availability of audio description for all its in-house productions. This step may have been in response to protests from disability activists who remarked on the irony that *Daredevil,* whose title character is a blind superhero, would not be completely accessible to blind viewers. It may have also been a preemptive effort to avoid a lawsuit. In 2012, the National Association of the Deaf won a settlement against Netflix compelling the service to provide close captioning for all its on-demand programming. At the same time, the Federal Communications Commission (FCC) has set mandates compelling television broadcasters to increase the number of programs available with audio description and requiring all movie theaters with digital projectors to offer audio description devices to patrons who request them. What all this means for blind people is that there will be a proliferation of accessible movies and television programs. As accessible offerings increase, it seems an apt moment to review the history of audio description and scrutinize current standards and practices.

Audio description is the umbrella term for techniques meant to make visual media accessible to blind people. These services have been around since approximately the 1980s, when they first began to be offered in live theater performance. The blind audience wore headsets provided by the theater and the describer was positioned backstage or in the sound booth and broadcast brief descriptions about the actors' movements, gestures, facial expressions, and costumes during the natural pauses between the characters speeches. Sometimes more detailed description of the set and a reading of the program were offered before the performance or during intermission. Then, as now, the service is typically only offered for certain performances of the show, and patrons are required to sign up in advance. At approximately the same time that audio description began to be offered in the theater, the service began to be available for television programs and movies. In these cases the description was recorded on a separate audio track accessible to the moviegoer through a headset provided by the theater or via a setting on the television, and then later by selecting the described version on a home videotape or DVD. At the same time, museums began to offer docent-led tours for blind people and/or special taped tours or additional tracks on audio tours used by sighted visitors. Over the years the services have expanded, and the practices have become standardized. While it's understandable that a certain level of consistency and professionalism is necessary, the rules and guidelines that have become codified seem to arise from problematic assumptions about what blind people can understand and should know about visual phenomena.

Until only recently, the standards for audio description have received very little scholarly scrutiny. Literature on the topic is typically written for practitioners and usually only suggest minor tweaks to standard practices or summarize the results of focus group surveys of consumers. Some researchers employ the techniques of narrative theory or discourse analysis to collect data from existing audio-description scripts and to tout the advantage of this kind of analysis without necessarily demonstrating how it will produce better results.[1] One research study used eye-tracking technology on a group of sighted participants watching short excerpts of a film and then used the data to write a descriptive track and compared it with an existing audio description of the same film. Blind participants were then asked to evaluate the merits of the two descriptions. Even the researchers admitted that their findings were inconclusive and that the expense of the technology makes further research of this kind impractical.[2] In disability studies scholarship, when audio description comes up it typically appears in lists of necessary accommodations to promote the goal of social inclusion for people with disabilities, along with closed captioning, sign language interpretation, architectural modifications, and so forth.[3] Scholars advocate for audio description in specific situations, for example, public service announcements for emergency preparedness.[4] But for the most part, in this scholarship as in the literature for producers, there is a kind of tacit acceptance that the foundational assumptions behind the practice are sound and unproblematic.[5]

As will become apparent, I am skeptical about, even hostile to, the current practices. My critique of the standard practices however is blunted by the undeniable fact that I cannot see what I'm missing. So whenever possible

I try to draw the attention of scholars of literature and visual culture to audio description in the hope that the perspective of someone who is neither a service provider nor a consumer could eventually lead to innovation. The increased availability of audio description, such as from Netflix, might mean that sighted people might happen upon it, and discover some utility beyond what was originally intended. In other words, I resort to a familiar tactic of disability rights discourse and draw an analogy between this relatively new disability accommodation and the most familiar one—the wheelchair ramp. The analogy runs that while a wheelchair ramp that was originally intended to provide access to people using wheelchairs and other mobility devices can now be understood to serve anyone, disabled or not, who uses a conveyance on wheels such as a baby stroller, wheeled suitcase, or skateboard. Thus, my goal here is not merely to critique the current practices of audio description but also to speculate on how it might expand beyond a segregated accommodation to create a more inclusive culture.

As a case in point I will focus on the audio-described version of the 2012 Oscar-nominated film, *The Sessions*, written and directed by Ben Lewin, based on autobiographical writing by Mark O'Brian, the poet and journalist who became paralyzed from the neck down as a child and spent the rest of his life dependent on an iron lung. The plot of the film centers on his account of losing his virginity at age thirty-eight when he decides to employ a sexual surrogate. Specifically, I want to describe a screening I attended at Berkeley during a disability awareness event organized by the disabled students group on campus. They were interested in promoting conversation about disability and sexuality. But also, as an awareness raising exercise, they chose to screen the film with the captions and the audio description turned on for everyone in the audience to experience, nondisabled and disabled alike. To increase the audience for this event, I made it an assignment for a class I was teaching, that is, my students were to attend and write a brief account of the event.

My mission here is not to critique the specific example of the audio description of this film. That is to say the description in this instance is no better or worse than in other examples I might have chosen. The audio description of this film was produced by WGBH in Boston, one of the premiere services in the country, and so can be said to represent the industry standard. This occasion gave me a rare opportunity to compare my observations with those of my students, who in this instance were all sighted, and thus allows me to bring some problematic aspects of standard practices to the fore. More significantly, the observations of my students suggest other applications and other audiences for audio description and prompt me to speculate on future innovations that could improve the medium.

Before I get to *The Sessions*, I should say something about my experience of visual media. I am old enough that my viewing practices predate the advent of audio description. Like many blind people in the industrialized world, I go to the cinema, screen films at home, and listen to television programs. And like most moviegoers, I almost always know something about a movie in advance, either from reading reviews, hearing a preview or advertisement, or talking about it with friends. This anticipatory description typically gives me at least a general outline of the plot. For the most part, I can usually follow the action from dialogue and sound effects, and only rarely require some additional information from a viewing companion. For me, less is more. Usually the only thing I ask when I'm in the cinema is to have signs, letters, or any other text that is shown on the screen read aloud to me. If a character says, "Stop waving that in my face," I might ask, "What is he waving in her face?" though this may be obvious from context. The most frequent question I ask is, "Why is that funny?" This comes up when the humor turns on some sight gag or visible element. Sometimes I am content with what I call retrospective description. In the inevitable conversation that follows going to a movie with a friend, I may ask about some detail that did not make sense. But often this is part of a give-and-take conversation, where I am as likely to remark on some feature of the sound track, or subtlety in an actor's vocal performance, as to need visual details explained. So generally speaking, I don't require much in the way of audio description and rarely choose it when it's an option on a DVD I might be screening at home.

But while my preference would be for less rather than more detailed description, other listeners might have other preferences. The blind and visually impaired audience served by audio description is diverse, including people born with absolutely no visual experience, to people who have lost some degree of vision late in life. Audio description must take all this diversity into account. And in the case of a movie, the description needs to be scripted and timed to fit in the silences between lines of dialogue and other aspects of the soundtrack.

One of the main imperatives of the standard practices for audio description is that the content must be neutral and objective. For example, in an instructional YouTube video, Rick Boggs, founder and manager of Audio Eyes, another leading producer, includes ten principles of audio description, and the first is "describe what you see."[6] Other guidelines advise that the describer should answer the journalist's classic who-what-when-where questions, and refrain from imposing any evaluation or interpretation: "Describe objectively without personal interpretation, censorship, or comment. Descriptive adjectives are important in enhancing a scene, but must not reflect personal view."[7] In extreme instances, the imperative to refrain from interpretation means that a character will be described as turning up the corners of her mouth rather than smiling. Guidelines also dictate that the describer should avoid any technical cinematic vocabulary, even terms that are in common parlance:

> Generally it is appropriate to avoid filmmaking jargon and reference to filmmaking techniques—e.g., "close-up" or "fade to black." Most film or

> television is naturalistic; that is, the intent of the creator is to have the audience engage in the willing suspension of disbelief. Just as with live theater, the area surrounded by the proscenium (the film or television screen) is considered the "fourth wall" of the area in which actors are playing. This technique helps consumers feel as though the action is "real." As noted earlier, when a describer calls attention to the artifice of filmmaking, he or she "breaks the fourth wall."[8]

Leaving aside the generalization about the naturalism of most films and television programs, the guidelines promote an image of blind people as less interested in or even aware of the artifice of film. The rules seem based on an assumption that a film is mostly a matter of narrative, where plot elements supersede anything to do with a filmmaker's particular visual aesthetic.

The insistence on objective neutrality seems to come from an assessment that sighted viewers enjoy an autonomous, unmediated experience of visual media, which is more or less the same from viewer to viewer. Therefore, if the describer simply chooses the correct words, an image will be transmitted directly to the blind person's mind's eye where she can form an independent, aesthetic judgment about it. As I've already said, I am not sure that I have a mind's eye, or if I do, its vision is impaired precisely to the same degree as my physical eyes. I am not particularly adept at forming mental images to illustrate words I hear or read. Part of my objection to the term "mind's eye" is semantic. Like other scholars of representations of blindness in literature and culture,[9] I have noted the many instances of figurative language which equate blindness with ignorance, prejudice, and obliviousness. I also note the prevalence of metaphors equating sight and vision to intelligence, wisdom and prescience as the flipside of the same problem.[10] When cognitive functions are linked to the eyes in this way it denigrates other ways of knowing. More often than not, when people talk about a blind person's mind's eye it seems a misguided attempt to make us feel better for our lost vision: "You may be blind but you still have an imagination just like a normal person." Other blind people will differ both in their sensitivity to this and other metaphors of sight and blindness, and in terms of the way they might represent their own mental processes.

Without digressing into a lengthy discussion of the cognitive processes linking words to images, I still have to quibble with the notion that absolute objectivity is possible or even desirable. Language inevitably comes with connotations and associations that differ from speaker to speaker. A contributing factor is that audio description is not attributable to a single author. Sometimes the person speaking the description actually wrote it; sometimes the text was a collaboration, or authored by another individual or team. So while a scholarly treatment of a text, painting, or film may be scrupulous in sticking to a neutral description, the reader can ascribe the particular word choices to the subjectivity of the author, with audio description the illusion of objectivity is reinforced because the description is delivered without authorship, as if it represents some unassailable truth.

The rule about objectivity even affects the vocal performance of the describers. There is a certain tone of voice that all the professional describers tend to assume. The tone is at once neutral and perky. The voices are calm, controlled, but also cheerful. The vocal performance evokes the sense of a viewing companion who is there to offer commentary without judgment, to participate in the viewing experience without being affected by it. Sometimes this is radically at odds with the content of the film. The neutral cheerfulness is the same whether the action on screen shows a violent murder, a thrilling car chase, or a steamy love scene.

Guidelines are not specific about matching the describer's voice to the content of the film in terms of gender, age, or regional accent. In the case of *The Sessions,* the describer is female. The choice has practical benefits since the film opens with several instances of voiceover from Mark O'Brien's perspective. We hear his voice, but the female describer announces that his lips are not moving. If the describer were male, identifying one disembodied voice from another might have been more difficult.

Since I've never screened *The Sessions* without the description on, it's impossible to know what I would have missed or misunderstood without it. But the first thing I was aware of is how the whole movie is about description. In all the sex scenes, the sex surrogate, Cheryl, played by Helen Hunt, describes what she's doing, while she's doing it. Mark O'Brien played by John Hawkes, later describes what happened in the sessions to his priest, Father Brendan, played by William H. Macy. In other scenes, Cheryl tape records reports of the sessions, using more clinical language. Even Mark's assistant, Vera, played by Moon Bloodgood, describes what's supposed to be going on between Mark and Cheryl, as she waits in another room. So in my experience of the film, the audio description became just another layer of anticipatory or retrospective description of the action.

Given the fact that the dialogue is already describing the main physical action, a good deal of the descriptive track focuses on subtler aspects of body language and facial expressions. Since he is playing a character who could not move his body below his neck, John Hawkes does a lot of acting with his face. There are many references to eye, eyebrow, and mouth movements. In fact, all the characters' facial expressions are highlighted. The most elaborate gesture described is the priest's shrugs. The priest shrugs in every scene. Although he tells O'Brian that he thinks God will give him a free pass for his sessions with the sex surrogate, he still finds the arrangement challenging to church orthodoxy and to his own beliefs, so the shrug seems an apt gesture to convey all this. But it is mentioned so often that it begins to sound like he must have some sort of uncontrolled physical tick. I'm not sure this would have been as noticeable to a viewer not hearing these subtle body movements identified each time as shrugs.

There is very little reference to costumes. Though the film is set in the 1980s, apparently the costumes are similar enough to contemporary styles so as not to merit mention. There are, however, two scenes when Mark and one of his assistants go shopping for shirts. In one instance he selects one that is described as a dark paisley button up. The student sitting next to me felt compelled to enhance this description by saying, "and it's really ugly." Later, during the session with Cheryl, she comments on the shirt, prompting Mark to ask, "Is it racy and sophisticated?" and she replies, "You took the words out of my mouth." The intent of the shirt-buying scenes is clear; Mark's growing interest in Cheryl makes him more conscious of his appearance and more inclined to take care about his sartorial choices. But the failure of the describer to make an aesthetic judgment about the paisley shirt made it hard to assess the characters' banter about it.

Since standard convention is that the describer should not use cinematic terminology, the temporal movement from scene to scene is indicated with the word, "now." When the scene cuts from one of the sessions to a later scene between O'Brian and the priest, or to a simultaneous scene between Vera and the motel clerk, the description announces the time or space switch with "now in the church," or "now in the motel lobby." Then when there's a cut back to the main action of the session, the describer says, "back in the motel room." Since the characters' reactions to each other during the actual scenes are muted or not articulated, these movements to later instances where they are able to relive and narrate the events provide a kind of retrospective revelation of motivation and interiority. But the repetition of the word "now" is potentially confusing, unless it is understood as referring to the temporality of the viewer. In effect it's saying, "now we are looking at X," rather than attempting to define the different time frames of the characters' experience.

The imperative about neutrality means that often audio description withholds information in a way that can draw undue attention to it. For instance, Mark's respirator tube, which he uses during the day when he is out of the iron lung and moving from place to place on a wheeled gurney, is first referred to as a "white plastic tube," and then just as a tube. It is not until after the scene when Mark explains his iron lung to Cheryl that the tube becomes the respirator tube. I understand the logic. To call it a respirator tube would be an interpretation, supplying information that a sighted viewer might not know. From the responses of my students, I know that there are viewers who might not be able to surmise the function of this bit of plastic. But for me, this withheld information made me question my initial surmise in a way that was potentially distracting.

There's an even more significant bit of withheld information about Vera's race. When she's first introduced she's described as "a young woman with glasses, her hair in a braided ponytail." There is no mention of the hair color or anything else about her appearance. By contrast, Cheryl is initially described as a middle-aged blonde, and Amanda, another of Mark's assistants, is described "as a raven-haired young woman." Then in a scene when Mark asks Vera about her first sexual experience, he goes on to ask, "Was he a Chinese boy?" She explains that she always dated white boys in high school to annoy her parents. This prompted a laugh and I had to ask the student sitting next to me to explain that Vera appears to be Chinese-American. Audio-description guidelines about racial or ethnic characteristics have evolved over the years. It used to be that race was never mentioned, but current standards recommend including this information:

> Identify ethnicity/race as it is known and vital to the comprehension of content. If it is, then all main characters' skin colors must be described—light-skinned, dark-skinned, olive-skinned. (Citing the race only of non-white individuals establishes "white" as a default and is unacceptable.)[11]

In the case of *The Sessions*, the audio description is caught between the two practices. I'm told that there are several characters who could be described as African American, but this information is apparently deemed irrelevant to the plot, even though, for sighted viewers, it may well play a role. And while Vera's race is not mentioned at her first appearance, later the motel clerk, with whom Vera has a mild flirtation, is described as "an Asian male clerk." I'm left to wonder over the politics of these choices. Is it that once Vera's race is made a topic of conversation between the characters, then it is acceptable to mention the race of the new character with whom she is thrown together?

But the most significant bit of withheld information involves Helen Hunt's nude body. In the sex scenes, Cheryl disrobes and there are numerous full frontal shots of Hunt's naked body. Though the descriptive track narrates the removal of her garments, and the various positions she takes in bed, there is no description of her naked body. In fact, from the descriptive track it would be possible to surmise that these scenes are shot in such a way that the viewer cannot see her breasts and genitals. In reviews of the film and interviews with Hunt, much is made of the nude scenes. Hunt was praised for her courage in baring her forty-nine-year-old body. And I have to assume that her nudity and her age have an impact on viewers who are mostly accustomed to seeing only young nude bodies on screen. This points to what seems to me a somewhat misguided attempt on the part of the descriptive service to leave something to the blind viewers' imagination that is explicit to the sighted viewer. This felt unduly paternalistic to me, as if I needed protection from this central element of the film's content. It also led me to wonder whether this aspect of the film prompted the choice of the female describer. Is it based on the heteronormative assumption that a female viewer would be less likely to be aroused by a nude female body, making the female voice seem more detached and objective?

It's not that I wanted a lurid or detailed assessment of Hunt's physique, but I wanted to understand the effects on viewers. I questioned my students about Hunt's body and received giggling and stony silence. Undeterred, I threw them a few adjectives, asking for a simple agree or disagree answer. Since she was initially described as a middle-aged blonde, and she is the mother of a teenaged son, I asked, "Is she well-preserved?" A female student told me, "Better than that." But that was all I could get out of them. I consulted with a friend of mine, who I guess could be described as a middle-aged woman, though not a blonde. She said that Hunt has "a Hollywood body" and went on to elaborate that her body is symmetrically proportioned, with nothing sagging, no stretch marks, no unusual scars or birth marks—in other words, an idealized version of a woman's body. I asked if there was any evidence of surgical enhancement, but she could not say.

While my students were reluctant to comment on the effect of Hunt's nudity, they were struck by how much else was left out of the audio description. They listed numerous visual details they thought should have been mentioned. Others complained about the absence of cinematic terminology. But despite these flaws, I was surprised by the many students who responded favorably, saying that the description fit so well with the plot of the movie that they couldn't imagine it without it. Several made the point that I made above about how it drew their attention to the temporal and spatial shifts between scenes and highlighted the retrospective content of the narrative. Several students made the wheelchair ramp analogy, imagining that audio description might be a useful enhancement to anyone, providing greater insights into characters' motives and the actors' craft. One student described his own movie-viewing practices and imagined audio description as a useful tool. The student pointed out that he, like most of his peers, seldom watches movies in the cinema anymore, but at home on one screen while simultaneously doing something else on another, and so he imagined that the audio description could allow him to multitask more efficiently. His ears would be primed to listen for certain key words to alert him to lift his eyes from his video game or Facebook page, to watch a scene of interest in the film. In this case, I assume he would be attending to any mention of body parts, nakedness, and so forth.

But the possibility that sighted people might consider audio description as a useful tool or enhancement of their viewing experience gives me hope. Another cause for optimism comes from filmmakers themselves. At the 2013 Edinburgh Film Festival, I spoke on a panel where the organizers took the novel approach to pair sensory access, such as audio description and captioning, with linguistic access—dubbing and subtitling. The audience was made up of independent filmmakers primarily from non-English-speaking countries. It was imperative for them to improve linguistic access as a way to enlarge the audience for their films. This made them unusually receptive to ideas about audio description as another facet of this goal. My co-panelist and I urged them to think about access from the outset of their projects rather than something added on in postproduction by the professional agencies that might have little awareness of their goals or intentions. Someone suggested assigning someone to be "access producer" in charge of these matters. Another facet of the wheelchair ramp analogy points out that access works better and is more aesthetic if it is part of the original design rather than bolted on later.

An even more encouraging development comes from a more mainstream source. In December 2015, Pixar Animation Studios launched an initiative to produce audio description for their films in-house rather than delegating it to one of the external service providers. As part of this initiative, Pixar is working with Disney to develop a smart phone app which would allow blind users to access the audio description directly from the app. This would eliminate the problem that many blind movie goers experience when the device that the theater is supposed to provide doesn't function correctly. And since the phone app is available to anyone with a smartphone, there's a possibility that any user, blind or not, could turn on the audio description to enhance their viewing of the film. This in turn opens up the possibility that the filmmakers might deliberately use audio description as a narrative feature of the film.

How might such a narrative device work? A friend told me about an experience her elderly father had with audio description of a DVD he watched at home. He inadvertently turned on the audio description, not realizing it was intended for blind viewers. When she asked him how he liked the film, he responded that initially it seemed a fairly conventional narrative, but then there was commentary delivered by a disembodied voice, not associated with any character. He described this as a very modern device, something new he had never encountered before. At first, he was perplexed, but eventually he began to interpret this track as a sort of free-floating omniscient narrative voice, noting facial expressions and gestures in such a way to draw his attention to them, and thus compel an additional layer of interpretation.

Of course, this is an example of an accidental misuse of audio description, but it suggests that audio description might appeal to people who are not blind. Audio description is sometimes touted as a useful option for sighted people wishing to listen to a film or TV program "eyes-free," while driving for instance.[12] It is also beginning to find application in educational arenas, such as for English-language learners and students with learning disabilities besides visual impairment. As users diversify, it can be hoped that demand for improvement and innovation will change the medium.

In 2013 the Video Description Research and Development Center of the Smith Kettlewell Institute in San Francisco launched YouDescribe.org, an experimental platform where nonprofessionals can add audio description to YouTube videos. Joshua Miele, the director of the project, is blind himself and so all too aware of the shortcomings of the current standards. Initially, the project envisaged primarily pedagogical applications. A video assigned for a middle or high school science class could be described by a blind student's teacher, parent, or friend and then made available to other blind students across the country. But beyond this educational context, the idea is that anyone can supply information about visual material that will be useful to people who can't see it, and if the volunteer describers are unfettered by the professional standards, and in more direct consultation with blind people, they will innovate new techniques. For instance, they could experiment with different vocal performance styles, or pitch the description more directly to a specific age group. Among other features, the site allows for the possibility that there will be multiple descriptions of the same material, allowing a user to choose the one most in line with her taste or else build understanding through hearing multiple subjective interpretations. A user can select a favorite describers profile and access all the videos that person has described. Eventually it may be possible to request a favorite describer for a particular video. The technology also allows describers to add in-line description during pauses in speech as in the professional manner or to pause the video for lengthier description. Ultimately it may be possible for describers to add different levels of description, and users could choose whether to access it. These experiments in audio description have direct implications to such new developments as the Disney smartphone app, allowing users to customize their viewing and listening experience. Additional content could be accessed before or after the screening of the film, so that users could enhance the experience with anticipatory or retrospective description.

Whether experiments such as YouDescribe will have an impact on the professional services remains to be seen. Joel Snyder, who literally wrote the book on audio description, expresses defensiveness and a certain condescension: "This crowdsourcing idea — Y'all come [try it], you don't need to know how' — that's just crap . . . Josh might say, 'Well, crap's OK!' and God bless him, but being blind doesn't make you an expert in audio description." [13]

In Snyder's comment I hear a tone familiar from decades of encounters with professionals in special education and rehabilitation, who are benign as long as their methods and assumptions are unquestioningly appreciated, but become hostile when a recipient of their services critiques, complains, or suggests another way. For my part, I recognize that crowd-sourcing has its pitfalls: for instance, people might add ironic description, deliberately misrepresenting or exaggerating what's going on, for the amusement of sighted viewers, thus destroying the utility for blind audiences. Nevertheless, new voices and new eyes have something to contribute. I have devised writing exercises using YouDescribe to develop students' critical thinking and interpretative skills.[14] My goal is not to inspire them to seek careers in audio description. It is not currently a particularly lucrative or stable profession, though if demand increases this might change. Still, many of my students enjoy the exercise and have taken up YouDescribe as a kind of hobby. Beyond these experiments,

I imagine a future where filmmakers, screenwriters, and actors collaborate on an audio description track that is more in keeping with the film's aesthetics, and film scholars and critics contribute descriptive commentary that enriches anyone's viewing experience. In other words, I hope that audio description can be elevated from its current status as a segregated accommodation outside the general public's awareness and launched into the new media—a literary/interpretative form with infinite possibilities.

{8}

What They Talk About When They Talk About Art

As I have said, since the vast majority of any museum's holdings cannot be touched, access programs for the blind rely on verbal description of painting, drawing, prints, photography, and the majority of sculpture. In the last chapter, I suggested that audio description for film, television, and theater could be considered a new literary, interpretative genre with the potential to enhance the experience of sighted people who choose to access it. In the fine arts setting, audio description is an extension of the docent lectures and gallery talks that have long been a mainstay of museum education programs. Typically, the service providers have a background in art history or art education and adapt their offerings to specific individuals and in response to consumer feedback.

Still, even with this direct communication with blind consumers, some of the rules of audio description seem based on a limited understanding of blind perception and imagination. Here, as for film and television, one of the first rules of audio description is the imperative that the describer should only supply objective facts. For example, the New York-based organization, Art Beyond Sight (formerly Art Education for the Blind) has published guidelines for audio description of the fine arts. The basic instructions are to read the label, giving the painting's title, the artists' names and dates, and the dimensions of the work. The text goes on to advise objectivity so that the blind audience can form an independent opinion:

> After the general idea of the work is conveyed, the description should be more vivid and particularized. Describe pertinent details, and focus on different parts of the work. Remember that the listener is depending on you to give an accurate description. Try to use objective references rather than ones that might sway a blind person's point of view. Give enough information so that listeners can form an image in their minds, and come to their own opinions and conclusions about a work of art.[1]

While the advice is to be objective, there's still an acknowledgement that a degree of subjectivity is necessary to determine which details are pertinent, what kind of language will be vivid and particularized, and how much information is enough. Even deciding where to begin a description—with the most significant element in the composition or the peripheral details that supply context—requires subjective interpretation. Nevertheless, the idea seems to be if the words are chosen carefully enough, they will produce a detailed image in the blind listener's mind's eye that will allow her to form an independent aesthetic judgment about it. For example, here the description of Jean-Honoré Fragonard's *The Swing* (1766) strives to create a detailed and vivid sense of the painting while refraining from passing judgment about its quality:

> The scene is set in a lush, overgrown garden. Billowing clouds of leaves on the twisted branches of ancient trees almost overwhelm the composition. Greens and blues lit by golden sunlight fill the canvas. The girl is dressed in a pink silk confection. She sits on a very plush swing, which has a gilded wooden seat upholstered in red velvet. One of her tiny feet kicks off a small, pink mule, sending it flying into midair. This gesture reveals her plump legs covered in white stockings, which are fastened by a pink garter. Only the young man, lying in the undergrowth with a rapturous expression on his face, can see any more. Perhaps she has kicked her shoe into the bushes as an excuse to join the young man. The only other witnesses to the scene are statues. A cherub crouches on the pedestal behind the young man. He holds a finger to his lips, urging two smaller stone *putti* to keep their silence about the young man's presence. The smaller *putti* nestle among the bushes underneath the swinging mistress.[2]

The description complies with the rule about objectivity by stopping short of defining the effect the painting has, or is expected to have on a viewer. The lushness of the garden, the plushness of the swing, the plumpness of the girl's legs, the rapture of the young man's expression certainly all derive from a subjective interpretation. And there's an implicit interpretation in the speculative statement about the girl's motives for kicking off her shoe. The lavishness of the description is in keeping with the luscious extravagance of the painting, and the way all the details coalesce to suggest a narrative. The listener gathers that the viewer is meant to find the image pleasing and sweetly titillating, without the describer's explicit statement of this effect. But how does this text differ from what might be found in an art history textbook? There, we might find the word rococo, and some of the details might be identified as symbols, for instance, the lost shoe as a symbol of lost virginity. The sighted student of art history is understood to need this supplemental information to appreciate the painting, but the blind listener to the objective description is left to imagine the painting as cut off from historical context or artistic convention.

So the question is, do blind people really need a different kind of discourse to understand visual art? For a direct comparison of description meant for the blind with texts meant for the sighted consider the audio guide at the Museum of Modern Art in New York. Like most of the world's major museums, MOMA rents devices with recorded audio tours of its collection. MOMA's device features a number of different tours: one for the mainstream public, called "Modern Voices," one for children, and one for the blind and visually impaired, called "Visual Descriptions." Anyone who rents the device, or downloads the smartphone app, can listen to any or all of the tracks. In fact, when the Visual Descriptions tour first became available, consumer feedback showed that even visitors without visual impairments found it useful. It may be that the particular demands of modern art, especially works that are not representational, make some detailed descriptive orientation helpful to novice viewers. At the end of each track on the Visual Descriptions tour there are instructions for how to dial up the mainstream Modern Voices text about the same work. Thus the Visual Descriptions can be understood to lay a descriptive groundwork, while the Modern Voices track gives the next level of information. Incidentally, if an adult listener is willing to disregard the sound effects and music meant to make the children's tracks more entertaining, there are specific viewing instructions that could be helpful to a museum visitor of any age. Unfortunately, there is not perfect overlap between the three tours. Fewer than thirty works are described for the blind or for children, while there are scores of tracks for sighted adults. But theoretically, anyone who has listened to the whole Visual Descriptions or children's tour has a kind of primer to make the Modern Voices tracks more meaningful.

The most significant difference between the three tours has to do with authorship. In the mainstream track, the words are spoken by and attributable to an individual, usually a museum curator. In some instances, there are recordings of statements by an artist, or an art collector, and there are additional tracks describing conservation and restoration practices. For the most part, there's the feeling that these are impromptu observations, rather than a reading of a written text. Still, the listener knows that these are an individual's opinions, based on personal experience or academic training, but nevertheless subjective. The tracks for blind people and children are delivered without attribution, as if the words are indisputable facts.

Let us compare the three different descriptions of Henri Matisse's *The Red Studio* (1911). I choose this painting because it was one of my mother's favorites. When I was a girl, my orthodontist's office was near MOMA, and it was often our custom to meet there after my appointments. This was in the days when museum entrance was free. Our usual meeting place was *The Red Studio,* which my mother never tired of looking at. She had a fascination with studio and gallery painting, where artists display their virtuosity at rendering miniature versions of paintings by other artists, or, as in this case, their own work. She never specifically articulated her response to the painting, but she nevertheless communicated that one could never tire of looking at a particular work, that one could wish to view it multiple times, and engage with it more than once.

So I'm hoping that the descriptions will somehow give me an insight into her response to this painting. Here is the opening of the description for the blind:

> This is the painting of an artist's studio without the artist. Paintings and frames are propped against the walls. Sculptures rest on stools, and compositions hang at various heights around the room. Most striking is the color. Matisse floods the canvas with red, a rich, deep red, like tomato soup. This overall red surface creates a sense of flatness with little sense of depth.[3]

This opening gives a general overview of the painting. Although the goal is objective neutrality, the simile to tomato soup seems somewhat idiosyncratic. Why tomato soup? Why not just tomato red? Nevertheless, I appreciate the assessment of the effect of the redness—that it creates a sense of flatness without depth. So I gather that Matisse is not adhering to any conventions of naturalism. The viewer is aware that she's viewing a representation of a three-dimensional space but is not meant to be taken in by the tricks of perspective drawing. The track then goes on to map all the objects in the painting beginning in the lower left and moving in a clockwise sequence. The description about the table in the lower left and the objects on it is very detailed:

> A white plate on which Matisse has painted a blue nude woman. A white box of blue pencils, sketchily painted in with visible sweeps of the brush. An empty wine glass, roughly outlined in pale blue against the red of the table top. A green glass vase with a round body and a tall narrow neck. Out of the vase flows a long vine, with round green leaves. The plant creeps around a sculpture by Matisse of a nude figure which sits near the far end of the table.

For me, this systematic, detailed sequence feels unnatural, and is a bit hard to follow. As each new object is named, its significance is amplified only to be diminished as the next object is identified. My sense of the whole composition keeps slipping out of my grasp. By the time the description maps the left and back walls of the studio and gets to the upper right of the painting, it's as if even the describer runs out of steam and the description becomes more general: "Dotted about the wall, are more of Matisse's paintings, all in his simplified, colorful style."

Is this really the way a sighted person experiences this painting? I can understand how an inexperienced viewer might appreciate having some of the smaller objects named, and to know that the paintings and sculptures depicted are all by Matisse. But I'm left to wonder, where does the viewer's eye go first? Is there something that draws the eye, and, in that drawing, is there significance?

> The track from the children's tour encourages me to believe that I'm onto something for the way it begins with an instruction to scan the whole painting for information:
>
> Take a moment to look all around this painting. Where do you think we are? How do you know? See all the paintings in this painting? Don't forget

> to look on the walls and on the floor. There are a few sculptures too. Try to find them. And what about on the table? Did you see a ceramic plate and a white box of blue crayons?

Note that the questions are somewhat leading. It begins with the instruction to look around the painting, but then supplies the answers to what the child is supposed to see. Also, while the description for blind people tours the painting in a systematic clockwise sequence, these instructions invite first a general scan and then a kind of hunt-and-find approach, where the viewer's gaze would zigzag from point to point, finally zeroing in on one of the smallest elements—the box of crayons. The description instructs the child listener to "look closely" a couple of times and concludes with "a secret to share with your grown-up," that Matisse's actual studio was white and that he tried several different colors before settling on the red. Viewers are told that they can detect these earlier versions by looking closely. Here, there is a slight deviation from the description for blind people where some of the blue and yellow lines are identified as "gaps in the red" or "underpainting." I'm left to wonder if the red was applied over a layer of yellow and a layer of blue. Or did Matisse use these colors as outline, applied on top of the red?

I hope for clarification from the mainstream track, but this issue does not come up. This description is spoken by the influential emeritus curator, John Elderfield. He begins with general historical commentary:

> This painting was made in the summer of 1911 and shows the studio which Matisse was then using in a suburb of Paris. We see examples of Matisse's own works of art, a presentation of his career to date almost. If we look to the left of the clock in the center of the picture—interestingly a clock without any hands—we can see at the bottom of the clock a little landscape, one of Matisse's very earliest paintings. The big figure painting to the far right was done in 1907, and the white sculpture underneath it is a very recent work.

We are oriented relative to the grandfather clock, and then instructed to look first one way then the other. Like the description for children, Elderfield suggests that looking at a painting involves a more random sequence of eye movements to light on and identify objects—a series of saccades rather than a systematic inventory. He also makes the point that Matisse made the images of his paintings and his materials (the box of crayons) stand out from the red surroundings, to heighten the viewer's sense of their significance. Or as the description for children puts it: "Making the paintings stand out is one way that Matisse lets us know that making art was important to him." The description for blind people does not offer this interpretation. It refers to Matisse's "simplified, colorful style," without commenting on the way the paintings apparently appear to stand out, or float above, the surrounding red. Elderfield only comes back to Matisse's use of color toward the end:

> For Matisse, color was an agent of expression, but he also obviously used it as a way of organizing the space of his pictures. Here color has this quality of functioning a bit like the medium of time, where all these things are floating but open up into different worlds.

Having begun his description with a reference to the clock without hands, he concludes with this simile linking the all-pervasive red to the medium of time. I am compelled to go back to the description for the blind where the simile is to tomato soup. Is there an assumption that blind people will respond more readily to a reference to a nonvisual sense, taste, specifically the homey wholesomeness of tomato soup, while sighted people can make the figurative leap to the medium of time?

Still, taken together, the three descriptions enhance the impression I already have about this painting. For me, what stands out is the redness. Since I can still perceive color, especially large expanses of highly saturated color as there is here, when I am actually in front of this painting, I have a distinct sensation of the redness sweeping over me, though it has nothing to do with the taste of tomato soup or any sensation associated with the medium of time. After that, I can force myself to detect the non-red elements of the painting, and to observe that they might appear to float, or stand out from the red, but my residual vision lacks the acuity to tell for sure what objects are being depicted. I know that there are miniature versions of Matisse's paintings, because I understand the premise of the work. I am awed by the artist's skill to render these miniatures. For instance, I know that the large nude on the left side is not only a much-reduced version but also pictured at an angle, as if propped slant-wise against the wall. What did Matisse have to do to pull this off? The docent who provided the touch tour I chronicle in chapter 4, mentioned in passing that one theory about the redness of *The Red Studio* is that Matisse was attempting to recreate the visual phenomenon of the retinal after-image that regularly occurred when he came into his white studio from the lush green garden outside. This corresponds with my own experience of such retinal effects. My own damaged retinas regularly cause me to experience after-images and unexpected light shows that sweep over my visual field, something happening inside my eyes rather than an accurate perception of the world outside them. So it's as if the painting captures that split second of ocular illusion, except that the colors of the miniature art works are untainted by the redness, and so meant to seem outside ordinary perceptual experience, and so outside time. Is this what Elderfield meant?

With *The Red Studio*, we are dealing with figurative representation. However flattened the perspective, the painting still depicts recognizable objects in a discernable context. What about paintings that are not representational, such as Jackson Pollock's *One: Number 31, 1950*. While the descriptions for Matisse differ in terms of the way the viewer's gaze is directed, where the blind viewer is taken on an orderly tour around the image, and sighted viewers seek out recognizable objects to derive meaning from them, with Pollock, the three tours follow more or less the same method. The description for the blind begins with a reference to the huge size of the painting (8 ft. 10 in. by 17 ft. 6 in.), and then continues with some general observations:

> The picture hanging on this wall is painted on a very large, wide canvas. If you stand in the middle, it seems to expand indefinitely on either side of you. It's an abstract work without any hint of representation. Its colors are somber: black, blue, gray, brown, and white, on an off-white background. It's painted in Jackson Pollock's famous drip technique. And there's no better way to describe the way it looks than to explain how it was painted.

We are given a specific vantage point—the very center of the painting so that its surface extends beyond the viewer's peripheral vision in every direction. I am left to wonder how it feels to have one's entire field of vision taken up with this painting, beyond a kind of awe at its monumentality. But I am grateful that there is no attempt to map it systematically. Then we are given a summary of the method that produced this painted surface. The track goes on to describe Pollock's drip method of painting where, rather than standing before the canvas on an easel, he spread an unprimed canvas on the floor, and then moved around it, dripping, dropping, splattering and flinging paint onto it. This appeals to me. I know what it feels like to drip, drop, and fling paint. This description of the process provides me a distinct sensation in my mind's body, and a sound in my mind's ear. As if to affirm this association, the track for sighted children, includes sound effects meant to simulate the sound of splattering paint. This would make me judge my own response as naïve, but the track for sighted adults, spoken by MOMA's curator of painting, Ann Tempkin, describes this process too, specifying that "drip" does not quite do justice to the range of physical actions the artist performed. Like Elderfield, Tempkin puts this painting in historical context, mentioning that Pollock started his career painting in a more conventional manner.

While the blind viewer is told to imagine a stationary vantage point at the center of the canvas, the track for children directs the viewer first to step away from the canvas, then later, to move in close. It also gives the child viewer guidance in viewing an abstract painting:

> Now, look at the most important part of the painting. What, you can't see one? In most paintings the artists shows us what's most important. But here, the colors and paint are spread all around, so your eyes roam all over.

While the child looking at the Matisse was told to look around for meaningful objects, here she is encouraged to allow her eyes to roam with no definite goal. So the child learns to move both her body and her eyes.

The three tracks begin with the same method of describing how the painting was made rather than to identify what it looks like. And all three conclude with reference to the tactility of the painting. The description for blind people invites the viewer to engage her mind's hand:

> One can imagine the experience of running one's hands over its nobly surface and following the trails of paint with one's fingertips.

Similarly, the description for children, invites an imaginative tactile exploration:

> Okay, now walk up closer and choose one thread of paint. Don't get too near! But use your finger in the air to trace where your thread is going. Follow it as far as you can. Can you keep track of it under all those layers? Or do you get lost in the tangle?

Coincidentally, the child is receiving instruction in proper museum etiquette here: get close, but not too close. Trace the lines of paint, but don't touch the painting. Ann Tempkin concludes the mainstream track with a slightly different emphasis:

> This was a very physical kind of painting. It wasn't a painting that one could do sitting down, or that one did without a tremendous expenditure of energy. And that energy is actually transferred onto the canvas in a way that's very direct and immediate.

So while children and blind people are encouraged to imagine their own corporeal interaction with the painting, sighted adults are invited to imagine the artist's body, to put themselves in his physical experience, and thus to perceive the painting as a record of that expenditure of energy.

For me, MOMA's descriptions for the blind are the most revelatory when the work is the most abstract. For instance, the description of Barnett Newman's *Vir Heroicus Sublimis* (1950–1951) a monumental, monochrome red painting measuring 7ft. 11 in. by 17 ft. 9 in., dwells on the precise shade of red, comparing it first to the red of a sports car and then to the liquid red of blood, rejecting the first as too bright and the second as too dark. (I note in passing that there is no mention of tomato soup.) The description then offers a statement about the viewer's perception: "such a large, flat expanse of red can seem to change, even as you look at it." So I get the point that the painting is meant to create an ocular effect in the viewer's eyes, that prolonged contemplation produces a perceptual experience for the patient viewer, that the artist elicits an active collaboration with the viewer. By contrast, the description of Henri Rousseau's *The Dream* (1910) maps the whole composition from the lower-left quadrant in a clockwise sequence, as with the Matisse. If I had slightly more residual vision, I might appreciate having the different animals and human figures identified, because I gather that some are semi-hidden among the dark foliage. But as with the Matisse, the detail of the description gets in my way.

I assume that the pale skin tones of the nude woman draw the viewer's gaze, and that the other figures only reveal themselves as the viewer moves her gaze around. I'm left to wonder about the effect. Is this slow exploration meant to replicate a dream state?

Occasionally, the Visual Descriptions track violates the rule about neutrality and delivers specific interpretations. For example, after a detailed description of the wheel and kitchen stool of Marcel Duchamp's *Bicycle Wheel, New York* (1951), the description explains, "Yet these two simple objects were a bomb thrown at the conventional art world. Duchamp exploded the idea that the work of art has to be the unique creation of the artist's hand." Thus we move rapidly from unbiased description to an interpretation of the artist's intentions. This coincides with the mainstream track that begins with a recording of Duchamp speaking about the work in 1946, followed by Ann Tempkin, elaborating the same idea about the philosophy of his "ready-mades." The children's track invites the listener to speculate on what makes this a work of art and concludes with another secret to share with "your grownup," that Duchamp had originally wanted viewers to be able to spin the wheel, breaking the rule that art is only supposed to be appreciated visually.

In general, the more abstract or conceptual the work, the more closely the three tracks adhere to the method laid out for the Pollock:

> "There's no better way to describe the way it looks than to explain how it was painted." The emphasis is on the artist's methods and philosophy. I wish the same rule applied when describing more figurative works. My imagination tends to get bogged down with the careful enumeration of details; I'd rather hear more about the artist's method and intentions or more about how the work was received by contemporary viewers. When this historical or interpretative information is withheld from me it feels unduly paternalistic, only one or two steps removed from the leading questions of the tracks for children.

I could fault the way the track for the blind tends to infantilize the listener, but since the device gives me the opportunity to listen to the mainstream version as well, I feel less slighted. But since all this audio can be found on the museum's website and smartphone app, why should a blind person go to the museum? While a sighted person can expect that viewing the work of art in person will be better than viewing even the best high-resolution reproduction, what's the point for blind people? This is where docent tours for the blind come in. Obviously a docent led tour opens up the possibility that the blind viewer can request specific types of information. The majority of the world's museums now offer some kind of programming along these lines. MOMA allows the option that a blind visitor can arrange a tour with a private docent, as with their touch tours. Other museums offer group tours and regularly scheduled activities for the blind. Some deliberate effort is made to taylor the usual docent lecture to the specific needs of the blind visitor. In some instances, museum volunteers are enlisted to help blind people navigate through the galleries. On one such tour I attended at the Metropolitan, the volunteers outnumbered the blind people. We made a stately processional with our canes and dogs and our sighted assistants who carried folding stools so we could be seated while listening to the docent. This arrangement seemed intended for recently blind people, unaccustomed to navigating independently, and the people I talked to on that occasion were regular attendees, motivated as much by the social aspect as the cultural enrichment.

While the lectures may be governed by the same problematic rules for audio description, there is still the opportunity for blind group members to ask questions and perhaps elicit the type of information that they prefer. Experienced museum educators have benefited from this and learned to adapt their lectures accordingly. Georgia Krantz, formerly the art educator at the Guggenheim, developed the Mind's Eye program for blind and low-vision visitors. In the beginning, she endeavored to give highly detailed descriptions of each art work, but when one blind visitor complained that the detail was getting in the way of his comprehension, she learned to give description on a need-to-know basis.

> My solution has been to provide a carefully considered but bare-bones description of a work, followed directly by the question: "What else can I describe to help create a more complete picture?" The visitors themselves unpack the details of the description through their questions about further details and their observations about what has been described. The verbal imaging description itself becomes a platform for collective participation where everyone's imagination and abilities are given space to unfold.[4]

There's a monthly program at the Museum of Fine Art Houston, called Art Beyond Sight, where blind and visually impaired visitors spend an hour with a single work of art and engage in a group activity of participatory description. The sighted facilitator begins with some basics, and then the participants ask questions, soliciting more detail, and discuss amongst themselves to build knowledge about the painting of the day.[5]

From time to time in my classrooms I engage my students in a kind of participatory audio description. I have them look at something, an image related to what we're reading, even an image on a book cover, and then ask them to describe what they see. Someone will say something, and almost immediately someone else will chime in, either adding detail or contradicting a previous statement. Then someone else will elaborate to explain the discrepancy. I ask questions to elicit more clarification and debate. What begins as an act of generosity—students describing something to the blind professor—evolves into a complex discussion of the image. The questions I ask compel them to look more closely and choose their words with greater care. I endeavor to lead to questions about their emotional, aesthetic, and intellectual responses to what they see. Where does your eye go first? What is it that draws your attention? What is the image trying to say to you? How do you know?

In my classroom, I am typically the only blind person present, but I am also the professor, therefore using this activity of group description for some purpose meant to benefit everyone. In museum docent tours, this scenario is reversed. The sighted docent is the one with the specialized knowledge, and the blind participants are the ones seeking information. Krantz acknowledges that her experience with the blind participants has enhanced her general teaching strategies:

> It is remarkable how much I have learned from Mind's Eye visitors about the perception and experience of art, which I not only formalize into teaching strategies, but also regularly share with sighted visitors.[6]

Still, these specialized programs segregate blind visitors, when presumably the same methods could be instructive for anyone. Who wouldn't benefit from an hour-long contemplation of a single painting? Why not open up these programs to include sighted people? As with the example of MOMA's audio device, much can be gained from multiple descriptions of the same work of art. For this to work however, museum educators need to avoid recreating a freak show scenario, where the blind person asks naïve, winsome questions for the entertainment of a sighted audience. There needs to be an awareness of the power dynamic in who asks the questions and who has the answers.

Increasingly, museums employ blind and visually impaired people, along with people with other disabilities, in their access and education departments. The majority of institutions that offer programming for the blind conduct surveys of consumers and assemble focus groups to evaluate their services. The next step it seems to me would be to solicit the advice of blind and visually impaired artists. Having adapted their art practice to vision loss, and having learned to communicate their intentions to sighted assistants and to process others' descriptions of their work, they would be particularly adept at recommending methods of verbal description.

For instance, the blind photographer, Alice Wingwall, described two private docent tours at the Centre Pompidou in Paris. She was critical of the description of a Harlequin by Picasso where the attempt to render the details got in the way of comprehension. By contrast, the description of a monochrome blue painting by Yves Klein gave her the opportunity to question the docent about the precise qualities of "International Klein Blue" and to get up close and describe the brush strokes. Wingwall had seen these paintings, or similar works when she was sighted, so she was seeking description that would refresh her memory rather than to introduce her to something unknown. For her, the failure of the description of the Picasso was not merely in the overwhelming preponderance of detail but also in the docent's unwillingness to deviate from his script and answer her questions about the artist's techniques. The docent describing the Klein was not only willing to answer her questions but also allowed herself to be led by those questions to engage in a more detailed examination of the painting.[7] Wingwall frequently gets her descriptions of art from her husband, the architect Donlyn Lyndon. Their shared background in architectural terminology and history gives them a shorthand vocabulary that make his descriptions meaningful to her, though not necessarily to others. Once I heard Lyndon describe a small sculpture by Louise Nevelson using chiefly architectural and landscape terms. He was not making a simile to describe what the abstract construction looked like or reminded him of; he was delivering an impromptu assessment of angles and grades, and interpretation of how the piece was put together. At the same time, his tone took on an excitement that conveyed another level of interpretation. Lyndon's description was not only highly subjective but also highly specialized, tailored to Wingwall's preferences and background.

British sculptor David Johnson prefers live description to recorded audio tours and finds a virtue in even inept description:

> I've had a wealth of experience of audio descriptions in art galleries and art related locations. Nearly all of these experiences have had something positive to offer. Poor descriptions can tell you more about the describer than the art and this is sometimes amusing and interesting in itself!
>
> However, in general, I like live descriptions of art where a three-way "conversation" emerges between the art, the describer and myself. I guess I like to try and get behind what the artist might have been getting at, and I like to hear about the effect that the art is having on the describer there and then. I don't really like too much contextual information and I don't like too many long, technical terms which, again, can tell you more about the describer than the art![8]

Johnson's emphasis is on a three-way conversation between the describer, himself, and the art work. In other words, he understands the art work as something active and mutable. There's something to be gained even from a flawed description, and the possibility that the describer's perceptions may evolve through the very act of description. He perceives his role as an active part of the process and the describer as more than an objective conduit to some fixed truth. Johnson makes a distinction between the description provided by people he already knows and description delivered by a museum docent:

> I really like going to galleries etc. with family and/or friends for the same sort of reasons just stated. The "conversation" I mentioned above is far more likely to emerge with friends or family than otherwise. Having said that, I do enjoy going to galleries with relative strangers for the possibility of getting new and unexpected perspectives. [9]

Carmen Papalia, the Canadian social practice artist, has created a number of projects around the theme of blind access to museums. For his project, *See For Yourself*, he solicited friends to describe iconic works of art, then commissioned contemporary artists to create a new work of art from the verbal description. Finally, audio description of the new piece is produced. The project becomes a visual art equivalent to the children's game of telephone, where the final version hardly resembles the original. Obviously the project has more to do with raising awareness than proposing practical instructions that others could follow. And Papalia points out that his prior knowledge of both the describer and the artists doing the visual translations contribute to his appreciation:

> In some way, I know the work as an insider too—since I have personal relationships with everyone who translated and since I can recognize their personality in their process / approach . . . Then there are the artists who made their translations specifically for me (with inside jokes and all) and who made visual choices that would offer a particular experience to me as a viewer through visual description . . . like my good friend Rozzell Medina, who slipped a Canadian flag into his parody of The Raft of the Medusa! That piece is most certainly intended to get a response from me!![10]

If I can derive any specific recommendations from the comments of these three artists and from my own experiences as a museum-goer, it would be to abandon the pretext of objectivity. It is impossible and beside the point. The blind listener knows that there's some interpretation involved in even the most basic description, and often the systematic cataloguing of depicted objects is more information than anyone wants. Once the pretense of objectivity is abandoned, it could be replaced with descriptions of the artist's techniques, as well as the effect the work has on the viewer, recognizing that this will differ from individual to individual. For the blind artist, it is this information that has the greatest benefit. Like me, Johnson's preference is for description that centers on the specific impact that the work has on the viewer:

> One of my preoccupations is trying to understand better what it is that "turns our head" or holds our attention when viewing art (and anything else come to that!). I'm pretty sure that what grips us when standing in front of great art is more than just trying to fathom the ambiguity of facial expression or the identity of historical figures in a painting, or the meaning of symbols used in a work; it also has a lot to do with the fascinating, complex, mysterious and more elemental interplay of the effect on us of colour, juxtaposition, light, space, time, and emotion.[11]

{9}

Blind Self-Portraits

STUDIES IN BLUE AND BRONZE

Concluding this book with a discussion of a few contemporary blind artists provides me the opportunity to put into practice some of the techniques proposed in the previous chapter, particularly forms of participatory description. As will become apparent in what follows, my description of the art work here is a compilation of others' descriptions drawn from criticism and reviews, from conversations with friends whose eyes I trust, and, in most cases, from my conversations and correspondence with the artists themselves. My compilation attempts to preserve what I generally find most interesting about these conversations—how viewer's eyes may be caught by something initially and then move to other elements in the image to enhance, elaborate, or even re-assess first impressions. The process affirms my belief that looking at art is a dynamic, accretive, and mutable process, which runs counter to the standards of audio description of art for blind people. It has been necessary for me to enlist this testimony of others' eyes because the art work here is primarily intended for a sighted viewer, though I will also consider and possibly show a bias for work that is equally accessible to a sightless beholder such as me. As I say in the introduction, I only look at a very small sample of contemporary blind and visually impaired artists working in the world today, and for the sake of concision and cohesion I have chosen, somewhat arbitrarily, to discuss only their work that falls into the genre of the self-portrait. I do this for several reasons. In comparing the ways this group of artists, working in a range of media—painting, photography, film, social practice, and sculpture—handle this time-honored genre, I hope to get away from the discourse of exceptionalism. My point is not to marvel at the fact that these artists produce art without sight. Rather, I'd like to understand how their solutions to the problem of self-representation challenge and possibly dismantle the image of blindness previously embodied in the mythological figure of the Hypothetical Blind Man.

In *Memoirs of the Blind: The Self-Portrait and Other Ruins*, Jacques Derrida draws a parallel, indeed traces a kind of familial lineage between drawings of blind people and self-portraits. He observes that in both cases, the eyes are pointed in one direction, while the hands are aimed in another. The blind people's hands stretch out, searching, groping for unseen objects, while the vacant eyes are downcast or cast skyward, the body often contorted in two directions, drawing the viewer's gaze. Similarly, in the self-portrait, especially those that depict the artist at an easel or holding a sketch pad, the eyes gaze out at the viewer, while the body faces away, the hands often partially obscured by the canvas or page.

Derrida analyzes depictions of blindness from the eighteenth and nineteenth centuries, but his observations are equally applicable to a twentieth-century example such as Pablo Picasso's *The Blind Man's Meal* (1903) (Fig. 9.1). Like many artists, Picasso did not always title his paintings, so one might wonder whether the interpretation of blindness comes from someone else. But here's how the artist describes the image: "I am painting a blind man at the table. He holds some bread in his left hand and gropes with his right hand for a jug of wine."[1] When I solicit a description from friends and pose my favorite question—where do your eyes go first?—sure enough everyone points to the hands, specifically the right hand reaching for the jug. The hand is extended, the wrist bent upward at approximately a forty-five degree angle, the elongated fingers on the verge of making delicate contact. Picasso describes this gesture as "groping"—the characteristic gesture of blindness. I recognize this gesture but think of it as more deliberate than "groping" denotes. If you're reaching for an object you can't see and don't want to knock it over (after all, the wine constitutes half the man's meal), this angle of approach makes sense. Certainly it's safer than the way a sighted person would do it, thrusting the extended fingers forward as if about to shake someone's hand. The other element that attracts the viewer's gaze to this part of the composition is the color of the jug—a dull golden ocher in contrast to the blue of the rest of the painting. There's even a small patch of white denoting light glinting off the glazed surface to add to the effect.

The painting is from Picasso's blue period, so everything else in the painting—the figures clothing and cap, the wall behind him and the table before him—all share variations of the same blue. Even his skin, though lighter than his clothing or surroundings, has a bluish cast to it. Someone described the colors to me as various shades of denim. This comparison works for me because I know how denim fades, and it is even more apt when we remember that while denim is now ubiquitous, even in high fashion, in the era of the painting it would have been exclusively associated with laborers. My painter friends debate the precise combination of pigments Picasso must have used—cobalt, Prussian, cerulean. In any case, I know from general cultural associations, that the effect of all the blue is apparently morose and mournful. I gather

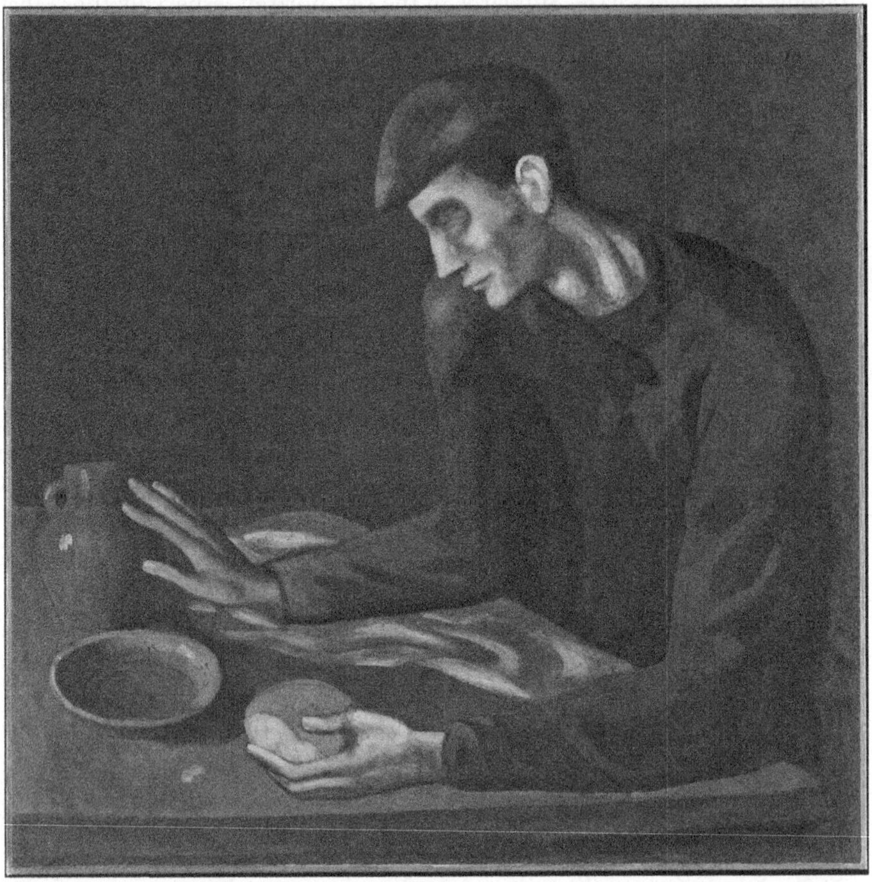

FIGURE 9.1 *Picasso, Pablo (1881–1973)@ARS, NY.* The Blind Man's Meal *(1903). Oil on canvas. H. 37–172 in., W. 37–1/4 in. (95.3 x 94.6 cm). The Metropolitan Museum of Art, Purchase, Mr. And Mrs. Ian Haupt Gift, 1950 (50.188).*

The Metropolitan Museum of Art.

that this is the blue of dusk, the waning of the light. The emotional effect is reinforced by the gauntness of the figure. His body, arms, and hands are all elongated and thin. The cords of his neck and his cheekbones are sharply delineated. His trunk seems somewhat hunched forward, contorted slightly to the left, as the hand reaches to the right. The unexpected angle of the hand combined with the contrasting color of the jug draw the viewer's gaze there first, and then this unusual starting point seems to make the viewer direct her gaze to the figure's eyes in an almost instinctual way, as if to find some explanation there. The eyes have been described to me as deep-set, deeply shaded by their sockets, the lids lowered over the eyeballs so that little more than slits are visible. The eyes do not appear to be looking at anything; certainly they are not looking at the groping hand. And they are not looking outward as a conventional portrait's might be expected to do. The viewer's impulse to find meaning in the eyes is thwarted and the man's blindness becomes legible. Still, it is in the groping hand and its atypical position that the blindness shows first and most prominently.

Derrida claims that in attracting the viewer's attention to the hands in this way, the artist is reflecting the gaze back onto himself:

> If to draw a blind man is first of all to show hands, it is in order to draw attention to *what one draws with the help of that with which* one draws, the body proper [*corps propre*] as an instrument, the drawer of the drawing, the hand of the handiwork, of the manipulations, of the maneuvers and manners, the play or work of the hand.[2]

In the portrait of the blind man then, the artist draws attention to the hands both to show the blindness and to suggest his own artistry. So is the picture of the blind man a kind of self-portrait? It might be said that every painting is a kind of self-portrait, showing not necessarily what the artist looks like, but how he sees or feels. Did Picasso feel some sort of affinity for this blind man? In showing the blind man's hands—one grasping, the other groping—is the relatively young Picasso saying something about his own artistic process where he clings to the conventions of his classical training while groping toward the unknown experiments of his future career? Certainly we can assume that he was not displeased when, fifty years later, the documentary by Henri-Georges Clouzot *The Mystery of Picasso* refers to him as a "blind genius."[3]

Derrida also points out that in the self-portrait there is also a depiction of blindness. It's something about the eyes. In depictions of blindness the eyes are looking the wrong way, rolled back in the head to show too much white, or simply hard to read, as in Picasso's blind man. The self-portrait's eyes look out of the picture plane and meet the viewer's gaze in a particularly disarming way. There is often the look of someone caught in the act of something—the artist caught in the act of being an artist. As Derrida describes it, the characteristic look of the self-portrait's eyes comes from the standard artistic practice of drawing from one's reflection in the mirror. The artist must catch his own gaze in the reflection, then look back to the drawing to make the marks that will represent the eyes. In the split second of shifting from the reflection to the drawing, the artist experiences a millisecond of blindness, when he is not seeing what he's looking at. He's drawing from life but also drawing from memory, even though the elapsed time between sighting the reflection and transferring it to paper is less than the blink of an eye.

The self-portrait has a long tradition in the history of art. Even when artists could not afford to pay a model, the genre meant they could always have someone to paint, and the mirror method allowed them to display a particular kind of virtuosity—a complex feat of eye-hand-brain coordination. Today, an artist could draw a self-portrait from a photograph. A painter friend, who teaches drawing, tells me she can always detect when a self-portrait is drawn from a photo, because the eyes lack the dynamism of the mirror method. I wonder if self-portraitists ever use the blind contour drawing method, keeping their gaze stuck on the mirror and moving the hand around to trace the contours on the paper without looking at it. Would the result have the same stasis in the eyes as drawing from a photo, I wonder. And what if the artist is actually blind rather than metaphorically blind, or made temporarily blind in the shift of the gaze from reflection to drawing? How do artists create portraits of themselves if they can no longer see what they're doing, much less their reflection in the mirror? In his memoir about going blind, *Touching the Rock*, John Hull describes how when he wants to remember what someone looks like, he tries to remember an old photograph of the person. But gradually his memory of the image begins to fade. He invokes an image of a gallery of photographic portraits, where one by one the photos are removed, leaving blank spaces on the wall. The loss extends to his memory of his own appearance:

> I find that I am trying to recall old photographs of myself, just to remember what I look like. I discover with a shock that I cannot remember. Must I become a blank on the wall of my own gallery?[4]

But John Hull is a theologian, not a visual artist. I am compelled to believe that visual artists develop habits of mind that allow them to manipulate and retain mental images better than the average person. Once, applicants to art academies were required to demonstrate an equal ability to draw from memory as to draw from life. If, as Derrida claims, the self-portrait always involves memory, is the blind artist who retains both a mental image of herself and a memory of her craft really at a disadvantage?

Consider the example of British painter Sargy Mann (1937–2015). He had a variety of vision problems throughout his career and said that his experience of cataracts and retinal detachments gave him a long apprenticeship to prepare for the total blindness that came when he was age sixty-eight. In other words, he was accustomed to making adaptations to his painting practice to accommodate his visual impairments, and so even total blindness simply occasioned more adaptations rather than ending his practice.[5] Shortly after losing all his residual sight, he reported that, as an experiment, he took out his paints and brushes, which he already kept meticulously arranged so he could lay his hands on what he wanted without having to see it. When he loaded his brush and applied blue to his canvas, he saw blue in his brain. Then he chose to add magenta and again saw this color in his mind's eye. He asked his daughter to look at what he was doing, and when she approved he decided to continue. This experience is often touted as miraculous, but it seems to me that Mann, like other painters, had habituated his brain to anticipate the appearance of paint before he applied it. He also said that his early education in mathematics and engineering helped him learn to keep complex spatial arrangements in his mind, and he also likened his mental painting process to playing chess without seeing or touching the board. He developed techniques to measure out the angles of light falling on his subjects, and the sight lines from the subject to the canvas, using long sticks he called "rays of light." Then he marked the canvas using blue tack and rubber bands so he could find where he wanted to apply the different colors. His wife, who is also a painter, helped mix paints to duplicate the colors he had mixed the day before, and he questioned her and other family members to ascertain if the colors and shapes were conveying what he wanted. His dealer and many celebrity collectors perceived little change in his work post-total blindness.

Throughout the history of art there have been many artists who developed some degree of sight loss late in life: Claude Monet, Edgar Degas, Mary Cassatt, and Georgia O'Keeffe, to name only a few familiar examples. There are those who believe that Rembrandt developed cataracts late in life, because his later self-portraits have a certain fuzziness versus the crystal clarity of his early ones. It can be risky to diagnose visual impairments posthumously, and a self-portrait is not a good diagnostic tool, since artists may be striving to achieve effects beyond the simple documentation of their own visual perception. After all, no one believes that the Impressionists all shared blurry vision, any more than the artists who decorated ancient Egyptian tombs shared a lack of depth perception. Many artists who lose sight give up art, or switch from one medium to another—painting to sculpture, for instance. But other artists, like Mann, innovate techniques to continue working. In so doing they may be striving to produce work that is indistinguishable from what they did when their sight was average. In other words, they make an effort to conceal the blindness. In fact, for every artist who acknowledges the development of some visual impairment, there must be many others who strive to keep it a secret. Even those who admit to a loss of vision may avoid association with other blind people and group exhibitions with blindness as a theme. Sometimes their dealers or collectors advise these artists to avoid association with other blind or disabled artists, since belonging to this category may be assumed to diminish the quality, and therefore the value, of the art. Sometimes these adaptations are lauded as heroic overcoming, and the avoidance of association with other blind people as a valiant resistance to succumb to blindness, even if viewers criticize the work in pitying tones behind the artist's back. But here I will consider artists who make blindness a theme of their work. How do they make the blindness show? And in showing the blindness, do they conform to or deviate from classical depictions of blindness like Picasso's?[6]

For Picasso, like many other artists who have depicted blindness, the image evokes sorrow, even desperation. The blind man is alone, in austere surroundings. In fact, the blindness can be understood to stand in for the general array of human misery: poverty, social disenfranchisement, solitude. A certain amount of this bleakness comes from the mournful denim blue of Picasso's pallet at the time. But he also deploys the familiar play between the hands and eyes—the groping hand, the unseeing eye—to denote the blindness. It is yet another image of the Hypothetical Blind Man—who is all hands, especially when shown by the visual artist, who is all eyes. But is this the only way to represent blindness? Do the self-portraits of blind artists evoke the same sense of isolation and loss? Do they emphasize hands over eyes?

Though not a conventional self-portrait, in Alice Wingwall's *Hand over Dog: Joseph at the Temple of Dendur* (see Fig. 5.1), which I described in chapter 5, the artists hand brings her blindness into the image. The viewer is compelled to wonder what the dog and the hand are doing in the photo, and then to look from them to the temple and the other figures in the scene, to piece together an array of ideas about how the artist directs the viewer's gaze. Wingwall says that when she was a sighted photographer she was reactive—seeing something and then capturing its image. Now that she is blind she has become a proactive photographer, anticipating the images she wants, then arranging herself and her camera to capture them.[7] *Setting Sun over the Gulf of Mexico* (2013) (Fig. 9.2), as the title indicates, is a color photo of the sun setting over a body of water. The artist's left hand dominates the left side of the photo. The hand holds a pair of sunglasses. The glasses have a strap or ribbon attached to the branches, presumably to be hung around the neck. There's the suggestion that the photographer whipped off her sunglasses to aim the camera, but then was unaware that they were still in the image. At first glance, it might appear to be a tourist's snapshot gone wrong. But the deliberate composition suggests otherwise. Like other self-portraits, this is an image of the artist caught in the act of making art. The viewer is compelled to look at the glasses, with the artist's hand's firm grasp on them, and then through their shaded lenses, or past them to the sunset. The deliberate inclusion of the protective lenses reminds the viewer both of the artist's embodiment and the artifice of photography. The artist's eyes were behind these dark glasses—a traditional attribute of blindness like the white cane or service dog. The photographer shows the dark glasses that would distort the colors of the sunset. The gesture

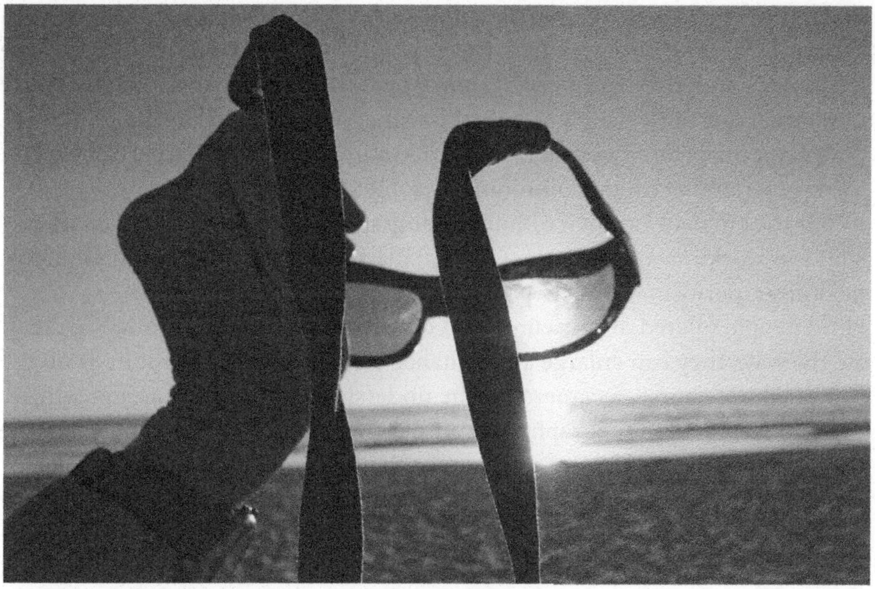

FIGURE 9.2 *"Setting Sun over the Gulf of Mexico" (2013).*
Photograph by Alice Wingwall, Anna Maria Island, Sarasota, Florida.

suggests a desire to remove the blindness to regain sight in order to appreciate this iconic image of natural beauty. At the same time there is a self-referential wit here, a mocking simulation of the kind of failed snapshot the stereotypical blind person would likely make.

For Wingwall, like other photographers such as John Dugdale and Kurt Weston, who all had a professional art practice prior to becoming blind, it might seem that a conventional self-portrait would be a comparatively simple task, setting up the camera to face the photographer, measuring out the distance and adding light according to established formulae. Even without any of this special knowledge, an amateur blind photographer can produce a selfie like anyone else, aided by assistive technology that is now a standard feature of many smartphones. I can aim my phone at my head and the screen reader will announce, "face detected," and then "large face," and then, "face near bottom edge," and finally, "face centered." It assumes that what I want is a nicely centered head shot and lets me know when I have everything lined up correctly. Conveniently, it also announces that it has detected faces when I aim it outward at friends, even at cats and dogs when I can get them to sit still for the purpose. The same technology allows me to deposit checks to my bank account, telling me to "get closer," and then "hold steady," before it snaps the shot for me. When I aim the camera at anything else—a beautiful landscape, an historical monument, a crowded street scene, or any of the other things people take pictures of—the screen reader says nothing. In those instances,

I'm on my own. Moreover, the screen reader only recognizes a face when both eyes and the mouth are visible. If my face is in profile, it says, "zero faces." The technology seems to have been designed to allow blind users to take the genre of photograph most people usually take. It assumes that what I want to produce is an image of myself that conforms to normative standards, rather than a self-portrait that might communicate something else.

For the amateur or novice blind photographer the camera might be understood to works as a prosthetic, which replaces functions their impaired eyes no longer perform. In fact, participants in photography classes for newly blind people offered at museums and other arts organizations often appreciate the ways they can enlarge and enhance images in the dark room or on the computer. Of course, a camera can be understood to function as a prosthetic even for a sighted photographer because camera lenses can do things that the human eye cannot. It is no accident that the inventors of photography analogized parts of cameras to parts of eyes—the film to the retina, the lens to the lens. But for a professional photographer accustomed to anticipate the different effects that can be achieved through composition, lighting, focus, printing, and so forth, the medium does more than simply replace lost vision. At first glance John Dugdale's *Spectacle* (1999) (Fig. 9.3) appears to be a conventional head shot of the artist. His face takes up almost the entire image. It is lit from the right so the left half is in deep shadow. Short dark hair frames the pale skin of his face, and dark stubble surrounds the lips and covers the chin, jawline, and neck. He wears eyeglasses. His right eye is visible through the lens but the left eye is completely in shadow. Balanced above these glasses is another pair of glasses. Light glints softly off the curvature of these lenses suggesting that they have a high level of magnification. Visible through these lenses are portions of the skin of his forehead. According to some descriptions, there is a reflected image on the surface of these lenses, but interpretations vary on what this might be. It's the image of what his eyes would be looking at but cannot see. Dugdale pictures himself with the assistive devices he used to produce and assess his work, drawing the viewer's attention to the multiple levels of lenses he employed to make this image. Similar to the way Wingwall photographs her sunglasses, Dugdale draws attention to the photographic medium itself, the ways lenses reveal and obscure reality.

He also references the history of photography. The actual photo has a squarish format and is smaller than life size. One imagines holding it in one's hand, like other old-fashioned photographs, such as daguerreotypes, which gives the image a kind of intimacy. The entire image has a bluish caste to it. It is a cyanotype, an alternative photographic process, invented in the 1840s that Dugdale adopted to detoxify his practice. The blue here is a bit brighter than Picasso's blue, though some find that it also gives the image a similarly mournful tone, or else an historic feel, like a photograph in sepia. But the expression on Dugdale's face strikes most viewers as neutral, not smiling, but not

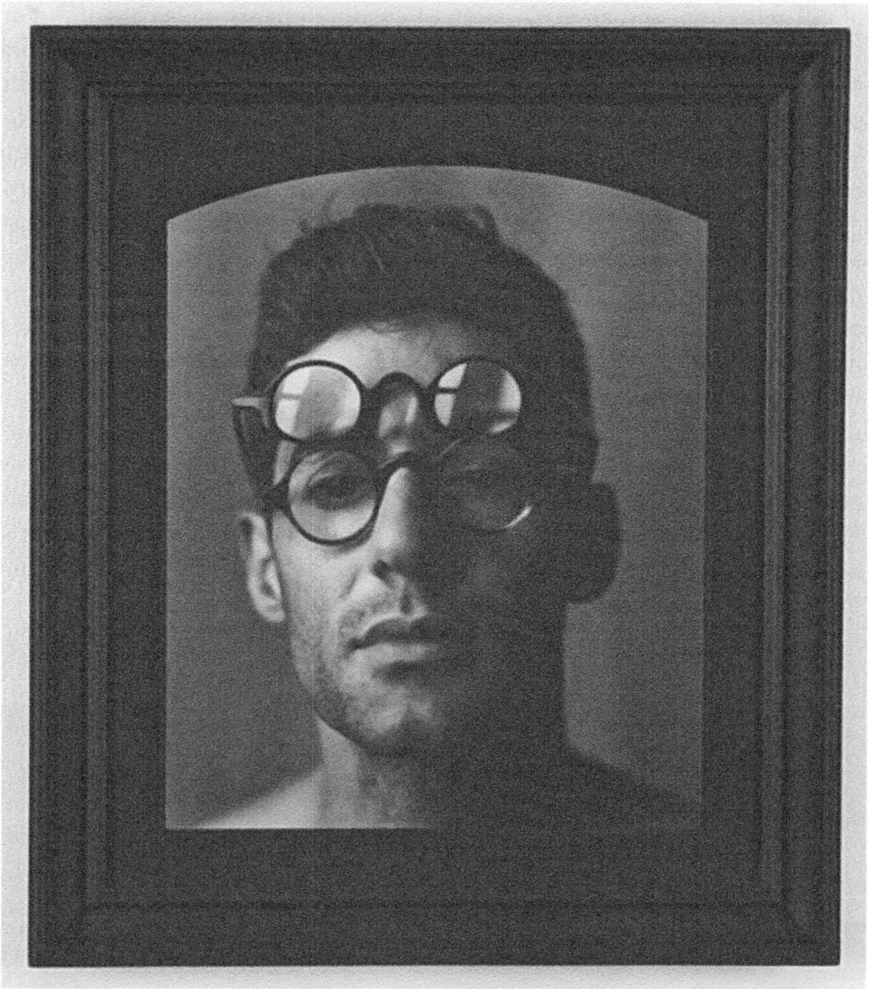

FIGURE 9.3 *"Spectacle, Morton Street, NYC" (1999).*
© John Dugdale.

frowning either. His one visible eye is lined up to meet the viewer's eyes, but the lens covering it, and the shadow around it, make it difficult to read its gaze. The expression has been described to me as "frankly appraising," and "a little hostile," but also "contemplative." The image asserts the artists agency even while showing the mediation of assistive devices. And it invites a direct engagement with the viewer, the artist staring back.

Kurt Weston did a series of self-portraits called "Blind Vision," that also shows the blindness by drawing the viewer's attention to the photographic process. He used a scanner in place of a camera and says of his process: "I felt the extremely shallow depth of field and stark black backgrounds were a perfect way to represent my visual impairment. The scanner became a tool of self-reflection, and an exploration of creating images, rather than finding them."[8] So like Wingwall, he became a proactive rather than reactive photographer. For instance, *Losing the Light* (2004) (Fig. 9.4) is a black-and-white photograph showing the artist's face in profile. It also shows his hand, to the left of his head, splayed as if pressed up against the surface of the image as if breaking his fall against it or fending something off. The background is completely black, so the artist's pale skin stands out in stark contrast. The glass surface of the scanner seems to have been smeared with a clear but sudsy liquid that appears as horizontal streaks across the image, somewhat obscuring elements of the face. It creates white outlines around some of the fingers and a blob around the nose. Some viewers view this as dry and feathery like cobwebs, while others describe its fluidity. While this feature might be understood as a stylized recreation of the streaky distortions and floaters of a visual impairment, it also makes the separation between the artist and the viewer palpably prominent. The effect is striking, slightly violent, as if his face has been forcibly pressed up against or slid across the surface. The head is disembodied, as if floating up out of the darkness. The image denotes the artist's sense of loss, and the violence of that loss, as well as his disorientation.

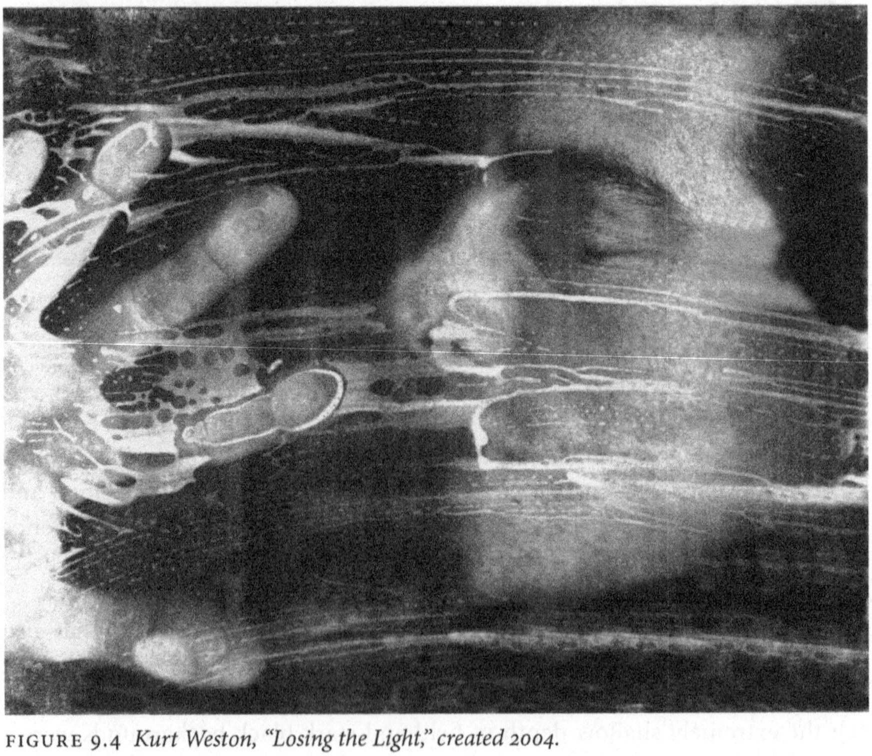

FIGURE 9.4 *Kurt Weston, "Losing the Light," created 2004.*

As in the previous example, and Picasso's portrait of a blind man, the blindness is suggested through something atypical in the image. The viewer is compelled to look and then look again. The instinct to look at the eyes is thwarted—because they're closed in Weston's self-portrait, and simultaneously obscured and duplicated in Dugdale's. But still, to extend Derrida's description where the hands are the artist's primary instrument, here, as with Wingwall, the photographers draw attention to the instruments of their medium. Weston makes the transparent "fourth wall" of the photographic surface visually apparent, while Dugdale and Wingwall show lenses as devices that can both reveal and distort.

These photographers had established careers before losing vision and their self-portraits foreground adaptations and tools that allowed them to continue their art practice. Sargy Mann's self-portrait (Fig. 9.5, which is also the cover image) is somewhat atypical of his characteristic style because at first glance it might appear to be an abstraction, a play of complementary colors with swirls of dark blue and violet in the center of the composition, and yellows, greens, and oranges in the surrounding areas.[9] But most viewers readily recognize the shape of head and shoulders in the central area as a silhouette, as if he's picturing himself in front of a bright landscape or window with the light source behind him. There is a suggestion of eyeglasses protruding slightly at the sides of his head, and the contour of brow and nose. Some viewers describe shadowy repetitions of the silhouette as if in a photograph with multiple exposures. Others perceive a dark drapery over the face, as if a black scarf had been

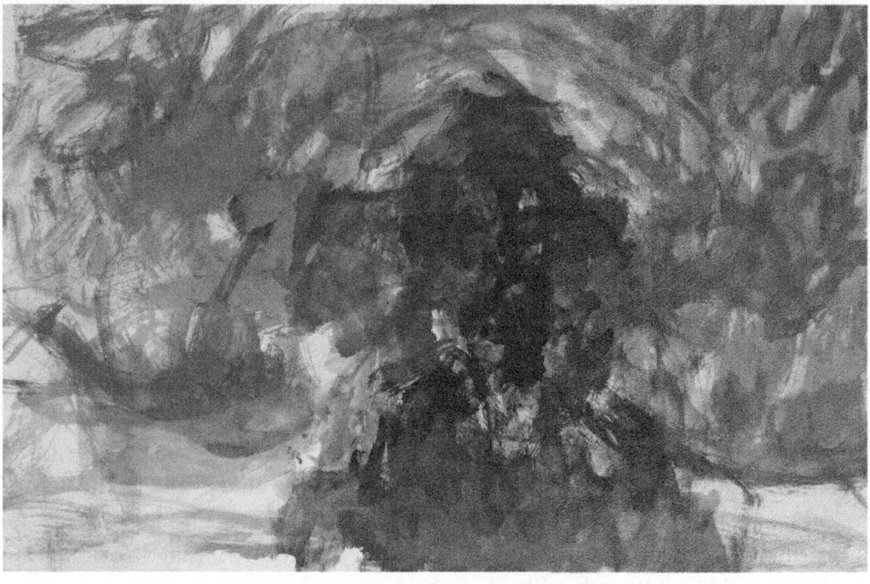

FIGURE 9.5 *Sargy Mann,* Self-Portrait, Borgo Pace *(undated).*
Gouache on paper, 15" x 22" (38 cm x 55.9 cm).
Image courtesy of Cadogan Contemporary, London.

draped over his head. There's the sense of horizontal brush strokes at about eye level as if smudging out or scraping off that section of the image, as if erasing it to apply a new version. The black and blues here may denote mournfulness, as in the Picasso, or the stark shock of lost vision as in Weston's black backgrounds. At the same time, the handling of the paint may be an attempt to render in a less emotional more matter-of-fact way a specific aspect of his impairment, where a loss of central acuity effaces detail and gives shadows a denser materiality.

While Wingwall, Dugdale, and Weston show their blindness by foregrounding different facets of the photographic medium, Mann handles paint in a way to simulate the loss of visual acuity. Derek Jarman's *Blue* (1993) is an autobiographical meditation on the artist's lost vision that also can be understood to simulate the experience of blindness. But rather than using his medium to replicate the distortions of his impairment, he represents it in terms of an emotional response. Jarman set out to make an autobiographical film without using images of himself—or images of anyone else for that matter. Part of this reticence was in opposition to the proliferation of images of gay men with AIDS that were so prevalent at the time. Jarman, like others, felt that these images showing gaunt and disfigured young men seemingly meant to evoke sympathy, actually risked serving a conservative, heteronormative warning against homosexuality. *Blue* is a seventy-six minute film that consists of a continuous display of a highly saturated blue accompanied by a soundtrack featuring the artist and other actors reading from Jarman's journals and poetry along with bits of music, gongs, chimes, ambient sounds from the street and the hospital. The soundtrack includes passages of Jarman's soft-spoken observations about his daily life at home, in doctors' waiting rooms, and the hospital infusion suite where he received treatment. Interspersed are passages, seeming excerpts from, a fantastical narrative, featuring a blue-eyed boy protagonist named Blue.[10]

So while Jarman's film narrates something of his experience of lost vision, it also metaphorically simulates the experience, by depriving the viewer of images, and perhaps simulating the artist's own frustration with this imageless state. But the film is also a kind of radio play; indeed it was once simulcast on British television and radio, so that the audience could have a more immersive sonic experience. As with a radio play, different settings are indicated with ambient sounds: the whoosh of car tires on wet pavement, the clatter of dishes in the café, the pings and rattles of medical equipment. The more abstract sections feature bells and gongs and echoey alterations in the actors' vocal performances. Some of the text is chanted or sung. Though there is no linear narrative, the attentive audience can overcome any initial disorientation and follow along. Like other blind artists, Jarman simulates blindness by denying the viewer the images she expects, even craves, in the cinema. At the same time, the film recreates the artist's re-orientation from image to sound.

The blue here is not the mournful blue of Picasso's blind man. It is in fact International Klein Blue. Jarman was influenced by Yves Klein's color theory and aesthetic philosophy. I have never had the opportunity to watch this film in a cinema, and I wonder what it would be like. I imagine that it would be akin to standing before one of Klein's monochromes, except that there would be no visible brush strokes, and the viewer would not be free to move to the next gallery when she had her fill. It would be a sort of enforced meditation, then. Everything I have read about the film focuses on the text. I have never found a description of what it's like to sit there and stare at the blue screen for over an hour. If it were shown now, I imagine the dark theater pierced by small illuminations as viewers pulled out their smart phones desperate for something to look at. As it happens, blue is the color I can perceive most readily, especially this vibrant ultramarine (more so than Picasso's darker blues), and so I admit I have a special feeling for it. The thought of sitting in a dark theater with a large screen drenched in this blue all but makes my mouth water. For this reason, my reading of the film is rather more positive than the average viewer's. Early in the film the artist proclaims, "in the pandemonium of image, I present you with the universal blue," and it resonates with my own relief that for at least the duration of this film I will not need to struggle to comprehend what I cannot see. Aural comprehension is elevated from its usual secondary status, and for once I feel myself at an advantage over other viewers. I appreciate the fact that this film that is about blindness, repeating rebellious statements such as: "From the bottom of your heart, pray to be released from image," and "the image is the prison of the soul," is also accessible to a blind viewer. This is not to claim that Jarman had a blind audience in mind any more than any other filmmaker. My sense of a transcendent attitude is a bit of a misreading. Though the film includes his encounters with other visually impaired patients in the doctor's waiting room, it is far from a declaration of blind allegiance. The overall tone is elegiac; a recurring motif is the repetition of a list of men's names, apparently of friends or lovers who had recently died of AIDS. And the filmmaker does not flinch from references to his own mortality. Still, there is an exploration of the blind condition that extends beyond the loss of sight into a realm of different perceptual and artistic possibilities.

While Jarman's simulation of blindness deprives viewers of images to reorient them to other modes of knowing, Carmen Papalia, the social practice artist mentioned in previous chapters, focuses on the experience of blindness in social contexts. Several of his projects simulate the experience of a recently blind individual who feels himself the conspicuous object of others' gazes—making a spectacle of himself. These performances suggest a range of different emotional responses. When he replaces his standard white cane with the marching band (see Fig. 1.1) or with an excessively long version (Fig. 9.6), he emphasizes this conspicuousness but with a sense of humor. Typically, the white

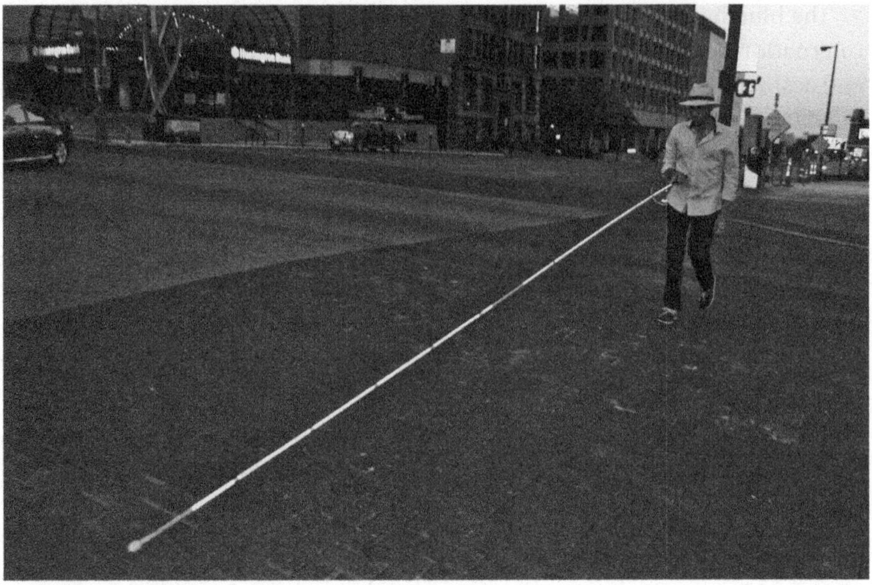

FIGURE 9.6 *Carmen Papalia, "Long Cane" (2012).*
Photo by Kristen Rochelle Lanz.
Courtesy of Carmen Papalia.

cane is supposed to be in proportion to the blind person's height. In this image, Papalia strides forward, wearing one of the hats that are always a part of his performance costume, the fifteen-foot-long cane extending halfway across a city street. The excessively long cane not only denotes the feeling of taking up too much space on the urban landscape but also seems to comment on the phallic implications of the cane, referencing the idea that the length of the cane is compensation for the loss of masculinity that blindness is supposed to bring.[11] In the video *White Cane Amplified*, Papalia replaces his white cane with a megaphone and takes a walk through a suburban neighborhood. In the opening, he tries to use the megaphone to amplify the sound of his tapping cane, but soon finds he can't manage the logistics (Fig. 9.7), so he drops the cane and strikes out without it. As he travels, he speaks the messages the white cane is intended to communicate nonverbally: "I'm visually impaired. If I bump into you I'm sorry." When he comes to an intersection, he broadcasts, "I need help crossing the street. Is there anyone there who can help me cross?" Eventually, a couple of children help him across. At the next intersection he repeats his general inquiry and a driver yells, somewhat angrily, "No, it's not clear to cross. Go to the cross walk." For a long stretch of sidewalk, he repeats, "I can't see you; hopefully you can see me," and then just, "I can't see you" (Fig. 9.8). His tone becomes stressed and plaintive. The experience of watching this video, or in my case, listening to it, is harrowing. The performance foregrounds his resourcefulness but also his frustration and vulnerability as he attempts to navigate an environment that was not designed with blind pedestrians in mind.

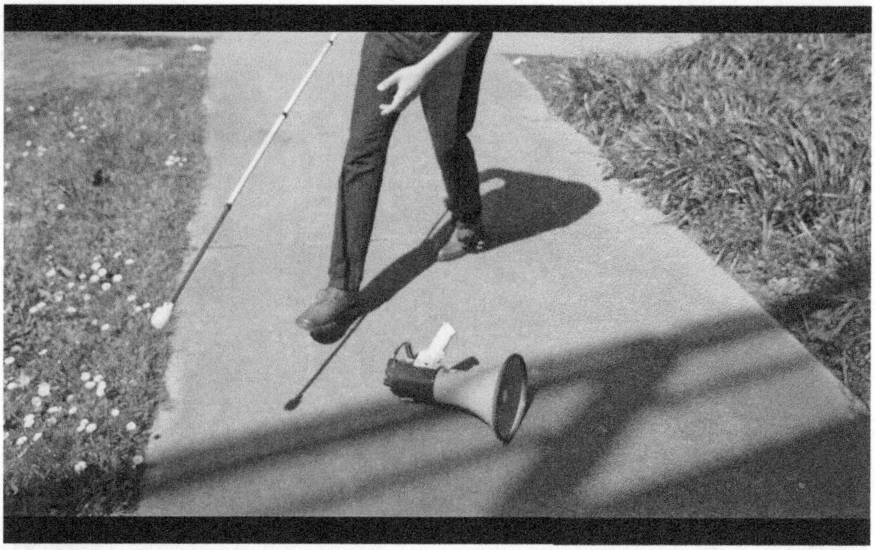

FIGURE 9.7 *Carmen Papalia, "White Cane Amplified" (2015).*
Video still by Phillip Louie.
Courtesy of Carmen Papalia.

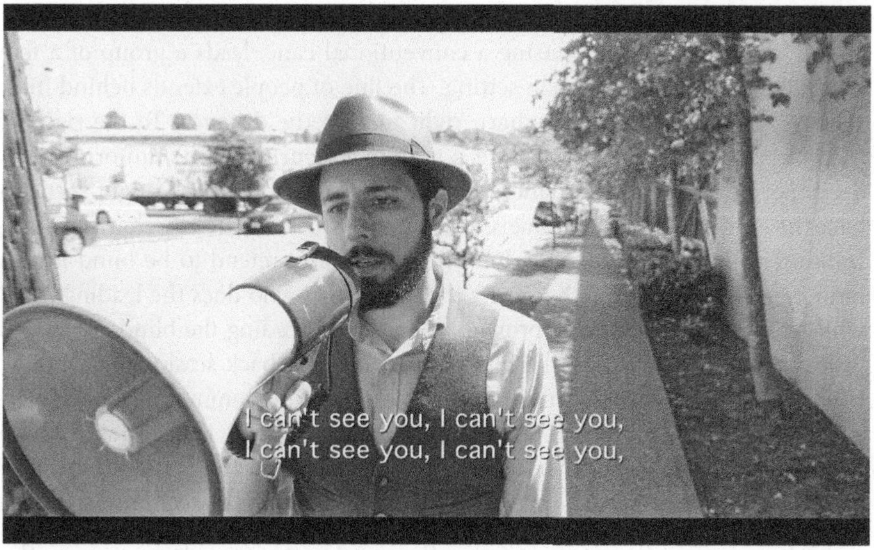

FIGURE 9.8 *Carmen Papalia, "White Cane Amplified" (2015).*
Video still by Phillip Louie.
Courtesy of Carmen Papalia.

By contrast, Papalia's *Blind Field Shuttle* performances (Fig. 9.9), evokes a different range of emotions. During these site-specific performances, he takes a group of people on a walk where each person closes her eyes and puts a hand on the shoulder of the person in front of her. In the performance documented

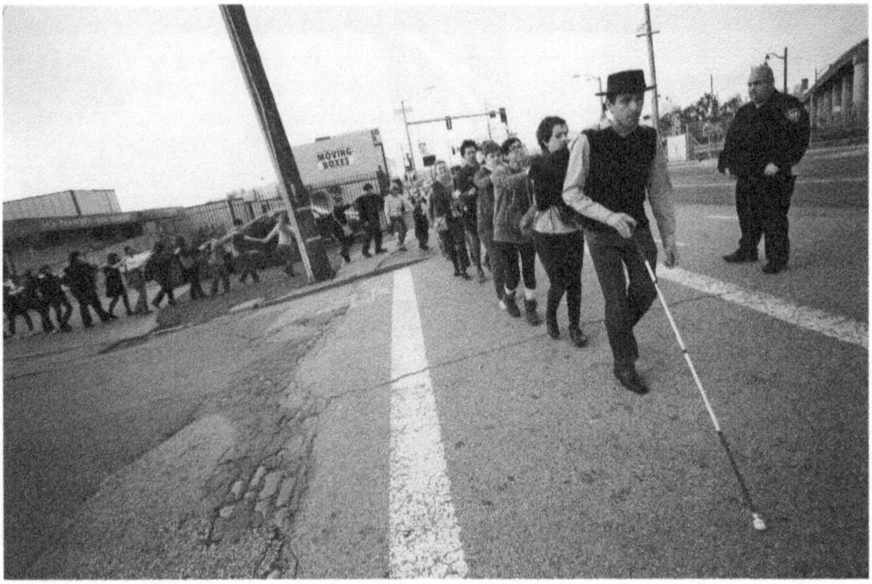

FIGURE 9.9 *Carmen Papalia, "Blind Field Shuttle" (2012).*
Photograph by Jordon Reznick.
Courtesy of Carmen Papalia.

in the image, Papalia, now using a conventional cane, leads a group of a few dozen participants in an urban setting. The line of people extends behind him, showing the group making a sharp right turn in the distance. To the right of the image, near the front of the line, a man in a security guard's uniform, looks on in perplexity or consternation. At first, these performances might seem to have the quality of a simulation exercise, such as ones initiated by charity organizations, where sighted people don blindfolds and pretend to be blind for an hour or a day. Except that here, it is the blind man who does the leading. And while this may allude to the proverb of the blind leading the blind, or in this instance, the blind leading the blindfolded, the talk-back sessions that follow these performances often center on issues of trust and community rather than a formulaic solicitation of an empathetic response. While the participants are all in contact with each other and indirectly with the artist at the front of the line, there's an emphasis on proprioception—a whole-body tactile perception. The experience foregrounds way-finding techniques, the anticipation of changes underfoot through contact with the walker in front, and even the recognition of aural landmarks. And like the project with the marching band, the blind man is in community with others rather than in the mournful isolation of typical representations.

While I have to admit that the accessibility of Jarman's *Blue* may be merely a serendipitous coincidence, Papalia's interest in museum access compelled him to think about how his "Blind Field Shuttle" performances should be documented and displayed in gallery spaces. As is typical of social practice and performance art, at first the work was documented by photographs and videos, but Papalia was bothered that work produced by a blind artist, that refers to blindness, would not be accessible to a blind audience, not even the artist who produced it. So in 2012, he collaborated with sound artist Kai Tilman to create an aural reproduction of these walks. In a gallery corridor, speakers were mounted at head height (Fig. 9.10). Exhibition visitors walked through the corridor and heard the recorded sounds of two of these walks playing on a loop.[12] So the reproduction was at once sonic and also kinesthetic.

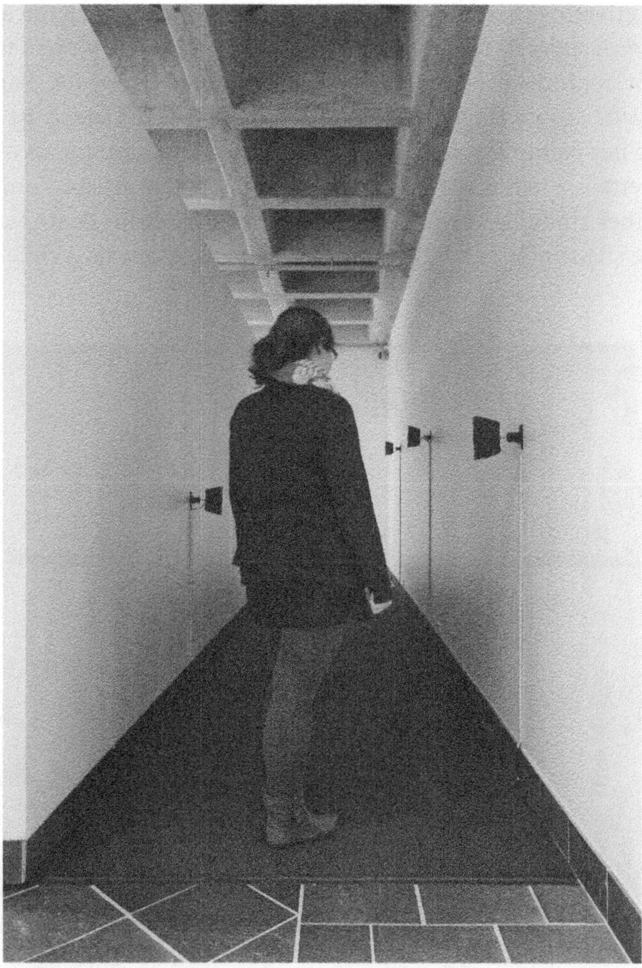

FIGURE 9.10 *Carmen Papalia with Kai Tillman. Documentation from "Blind Field Shuttle" on Saturday, June 16, 2012 and Sunday, June 17, 2012. Multichannel sound installation.* Image courtesy of Lisa Boughter.

Though at a much earlier stage in his career, Papalia is like Sargy Mann in that his visual impairment has been a part of his art practice since the beginning. But unlike Mann, his work takes blindness as a theme. British artist Aaron McPeake came to his art practice after a career as a lighting designer for the theater and opera. On the side, he also did painting, photography, and video work as well. As he became blind, he took up sculpture in cast bronze. Much of this work has direct autobiographical references, especially to the experience of loss. He was inspired when a friend gave him a gift of a gong from Tibet. He cast gongs out of objects related to deceased loved ones and his own lost childhood. This work not only invites touch but can be said to also require it. It is only when the viewer strikes the gongs with the wooden sticks the artist provides that the prolonged doleful note of the bell bronze is released, activating their elegiac quality. At the same time, tactile exploration of these pieces suggests the loss of the originals; the bronze preserves the forms but cannot reproduce tactile and other nonvisual elements. For example, *Eileen's Palette* (2007) (Fig. 9.11) memorializes McPeake's late artist mother by preserving her painting palette, replete with the blobs and smears of paint. An artist's palette is a telling artifact, particularly to fellow artists. I am reminded of my mother studying the palette of her teacher after his death, scrutinizing the precise shade of green he had mixed for his last canvas. While McPeake's

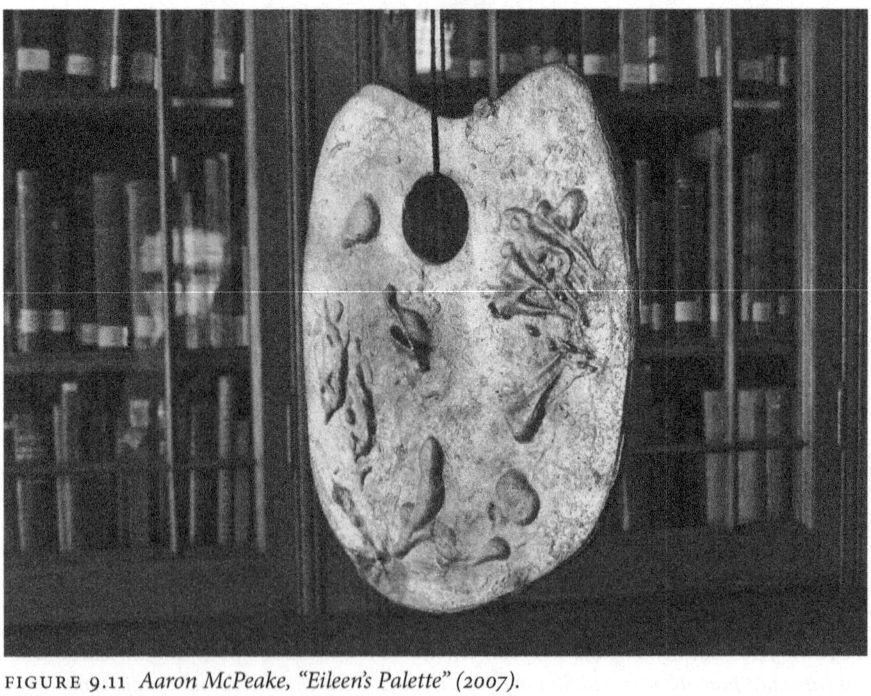

FIGURE 9.11 *Aaron McPeake, "Eileen's Palette" (2007).*
Image courtesy of the artist.

gong suggests an artist legacy passed down from mother to son, it also effaces not only the colors of the paints but also their viscous texture and telltale odor. *My Teddy Brownie* (2007) (Fig. 9.12) preserves the somewhat droopy form of the much handled child's toy but tactually denotes the loss of its comforting fuzzy squishiness. *Breast Cancer Radiation Mask* (2008) (Fig. 9.13) at first glance appears to be a pliable sheet with holes pierced through it, but a closer examination—visual or haptic—reveals the woman's torso it was formed to protect from the harmful side-effects of cancer treatment. The perfectly circular holes, suggestive of a manufactured object, are in tension with the fragility of the human form underneath, and suggests both the struggle of the cancer patient and the helplessness of her partner witnessing it.

McPeake also references the loss of his own sight. *Once I Saw It All* (2008) (Fig. 9.14) reproduces the familiar Snellen eye chart, with its array of alphabet letters diminishing in size from top to bottom, is a literal memorial to the artist's loss of perfect visual acuity.

Blind Narcissus Invents his Own Mirror (2007) (Fig. 9.15) is a gong reproducing the artist's head and shoulders. He took a photograph of his own shadow, then used the two-dimensional silhouette to create a three-dimensional form to make the cast. Here the form of the face is somewhat abstracted. This is not a death-mask reproduction of the artist's face, but the general form of a head with ears and a configuration of facial features is recognizable. The bronze is coated with a highly polished mirror surface, where the sighted viewer can see

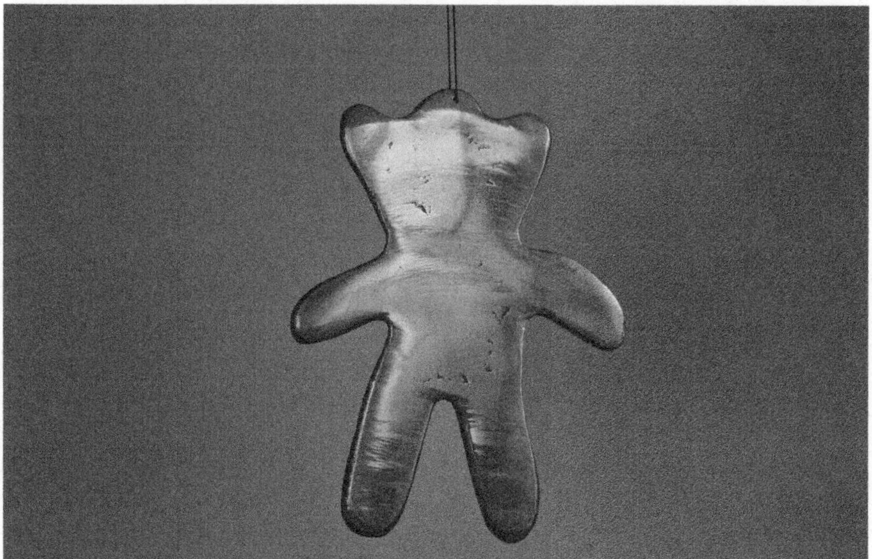

FIGURE 9.12 *Aaron McPeake, "My Teddy Brownie" (2007).*
Image courtesy of the artist.

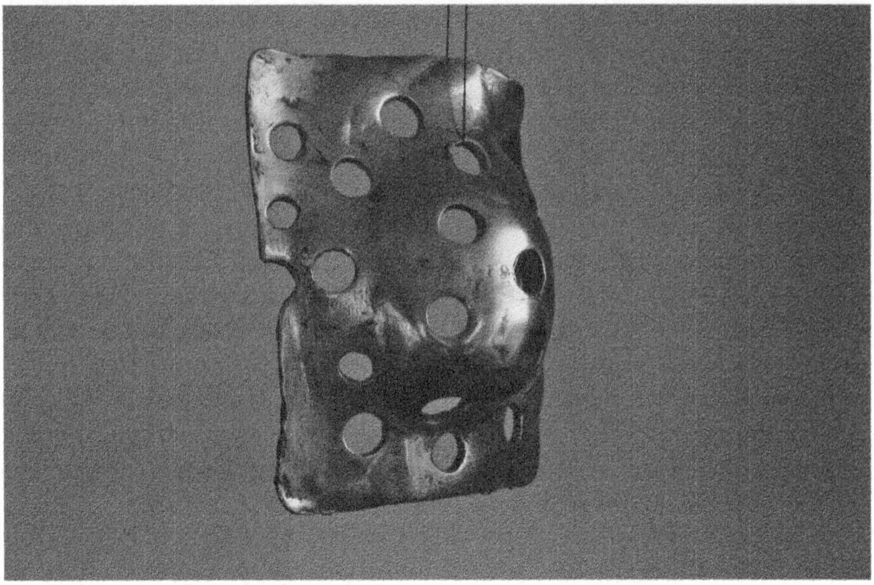

FIGURE 9.13 *Aaron McPeake, "Breast Cancer Radiation Mask" (2008).*
Image courtesy of the artist.

a distorted funhouse reflection of herself. The self-portrait is elegiac of his lost vision but also transcends that loss by suggesting a re-orientation to nonvisual senses. When struck, the gong emits a particularly prolonged note, which oscillates slightly as the piece swings in the air. It invites a meditative pause for reflection and announces a shift in sensory appreciation. If, as Derrida tells us, the sighted self-portrait requires a mirror, the blind artist invents other modes of self-representation, and other modalities of perception.

In addition to these gongs, McPeake also makes cast bronze bowls, called *Singing Bowls* in reference to their remarkable sonic qualities (Fig. 9.16). These range in size and shape from rounded forms that fit nicely in the cupped palm, to much larger, straight-sided versions as tall as the viewer, which are meant to be displayed outdoors. The finishes range from highly polished to more granular, and the colors range from shiny gold to dark, coppery brown. They are appealing visually, tactually, and aurally. In presentations and gallery talks, the artist encourages a kind of playful engagement with these pieces, describing, among other things, the sonic changes that occur if there is water in the bowl. He also notes that prolonged handling leaves a distinctive scent on the beholder's hands. He was pleased to hear that children who encountered a larger piece in an outdoor setting enjoyed pressing their faces against the cool metal on a hot day. He speculated that they might have even licked the surfaces when no one was looking. So they are pieces that appeal to all the senses—separately and in juxtaposition. Handling some of these bowls at a 2015 exhibit, I found the

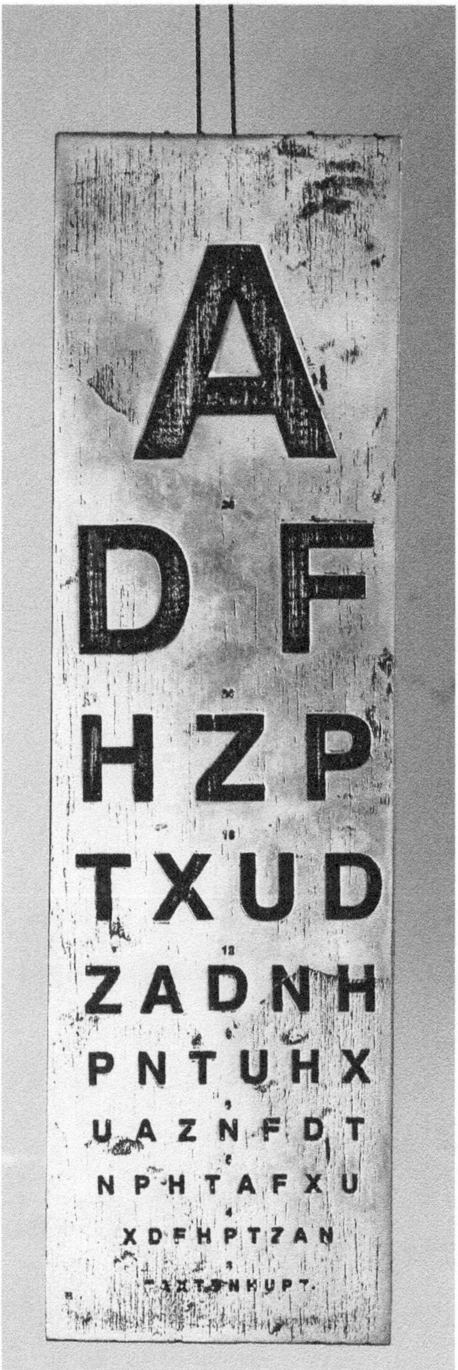

FIGURE 9.14 *Aaron McPeake, "Once I Saw it All" (2008).*

Image courtesy of the artist.

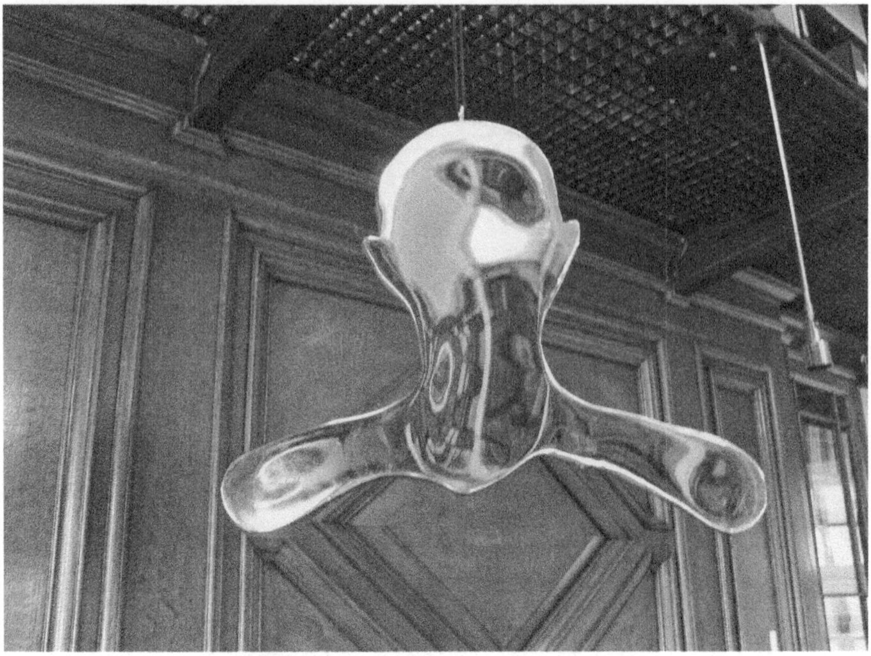

FIGURE 9.15 *Aaron McPeake, "The Blind Narcissus Invents His Own Mirror" (2008).*
Image courtesy of the artist.

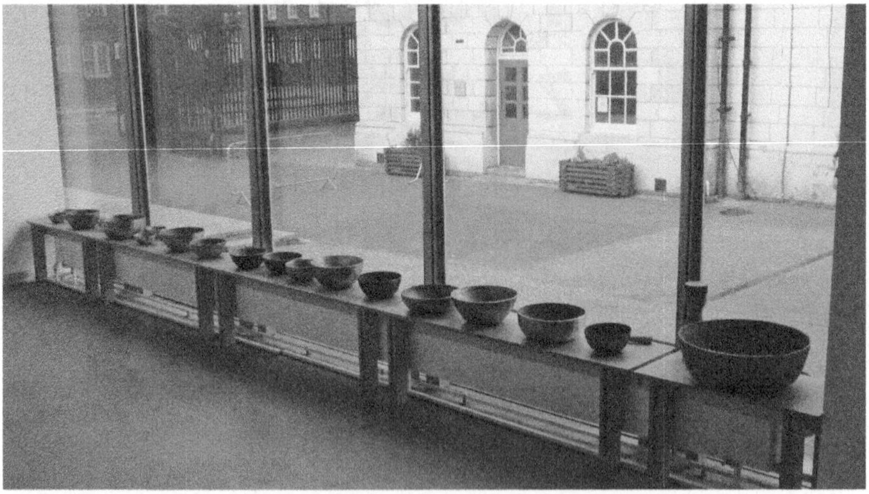

FIGURE 9.16 *Aaron McPeake, "Singing Bowl Chamber Orchestra" (2012). Installation view in line, @Chelsea Space, London.*
Image courtesy of the artist.

forms and surfaces tactually interesting. The artist's hand is apparent in the range of shapes, finishes, and textures. I struck one of them and listened to the long sustained note; and at the point that I could no longer hear it, I touched the edge with my finger and found it still vibrating at a very high frequency. The surface felt fizzy under my touch, and reminded me of something I know but do not often think about: sound and touch are intimately linked. Sound waves are vibrations felt by the ear. But here they were also felt by my fingertips. Though the *Singing Bowls* do not reference the artist's blindness or other personal history as the gongs do, they propel the beholder to reshape notions of beauty.

Of course, McPeake's work also challenges art display practices. Displayed behind glass or out of reach, the bowls and, to a lesser degree the gongs, would merely be well-crafted ornaments, without interest beyond the look of them. It is only through touch and sound that their full aesthetic impact is released. Visitors to a display of McPeake's work who adhere to the strict hands-off policy will miss out. However, there's an equal risk that a crowd of beholders, released from these strictures, all striking the gongs simultaneously, will create a kind of cacophony that might miss the point as well. Also, prolonged handling of these pieces will alter their finishes. The mirrored surface of the *Blind Narcissus* has begun to grow dull, and the artist is undecided about whether he should restore its original luster or allow this change to make a statement. There are sacred sites and public monuments around the world that bear a record of repeated touching, stroking, even kissing. Think of the Blarney Stone or the bronze statues of Hans Christian Anderson and *Alice in Wonderland* in New York's Central Park. The changes in the patina of these works become a part of the story they tell.

Fayen D'Evie, mentioned in chapter 4, who expressed a bemused frustration that people refused to touch her *Touchable Paintings*, has created, in collaboration with Sophie Takách, a series of works in wax and bronze, called *Tactile Dialogues*, that are meant to change over time through repeated handling. She creates casts by placing silicon between her own palm and someone' else's while clasping hands. The casts preserve the negative space created between the two palms—a unique moment in time between two individuals. They are at once self-portraits and portraits, retaining the lines, creases, and pores of the two palms, and the convexities and concavities of minute variations in pressure and release during an ephemeral tactile encounter. She makes a cast in wax, which she distributes to others with the expectation that their handling of these over time will change them. She also casts them in bronze, which will retain its shape longer, even while its surface will bear traces of handling over time. While they appear to be small, abstract sculptural forms, they are appealing little objects to handle (Fig. 9.17). Figure 9.17 shows three of these pieces nestled together on a bed of fine leather. Light highlights the protrusions and reveals the lines and creases of the two palms.

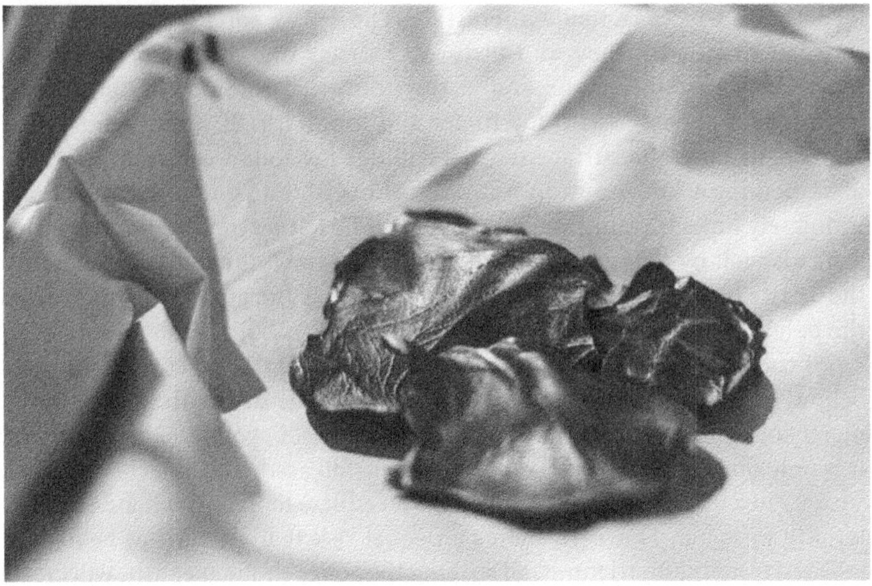

FIGURE 9.17 *Fayen d'Evie and Sophie Takách,* Prologue to Handling *(2016). Bronze cast of three tactile dialogues, vegetable tanned hide, and steel. (Detail).*
Image courtesy the artists.

They are reminiscent of other organic forms, such as leaves or shells—fossils of a past interaction between two people. What doesn't show in the image is their appealing heft and the variety of textures from smooth and sharp, to rough and granular. They warm to body temperature and release their bronzey scent. It is hard to resist the temptation to attempt to fit them into the corresponding spaces of one's own palm. Comparing the different examples invites speculation about the specifics of each encounter—a kind of retrospective two-sided palmistry.

Like McPeake's gongs, these *Tactile Dialogues* challenge standard display practices, since their meaning is only activated through handling. The typical museum plinth would overwhelm their small size and turn them into ornaments. As an alternative, in one exhibit, they were suspended in a kind of hammock made of fine leather and then hung from weighted pulleys. A light touch lowered the leather hammocks to each beholders preferred handling height, where they could be unwrapped and examined (Fig. 9.18). The soft texture of the leather was a reminder of the skins that made the impressions, and the unfolding of this covering compelled a kind of reverence for the preciousness of the encounters each piece records.

Like other artistic innovations, these works by D'Evie and McPeake challenge the conventions of museum display and teach beholders new ways to think about art. It is intriguing to speculate how this training may influence the

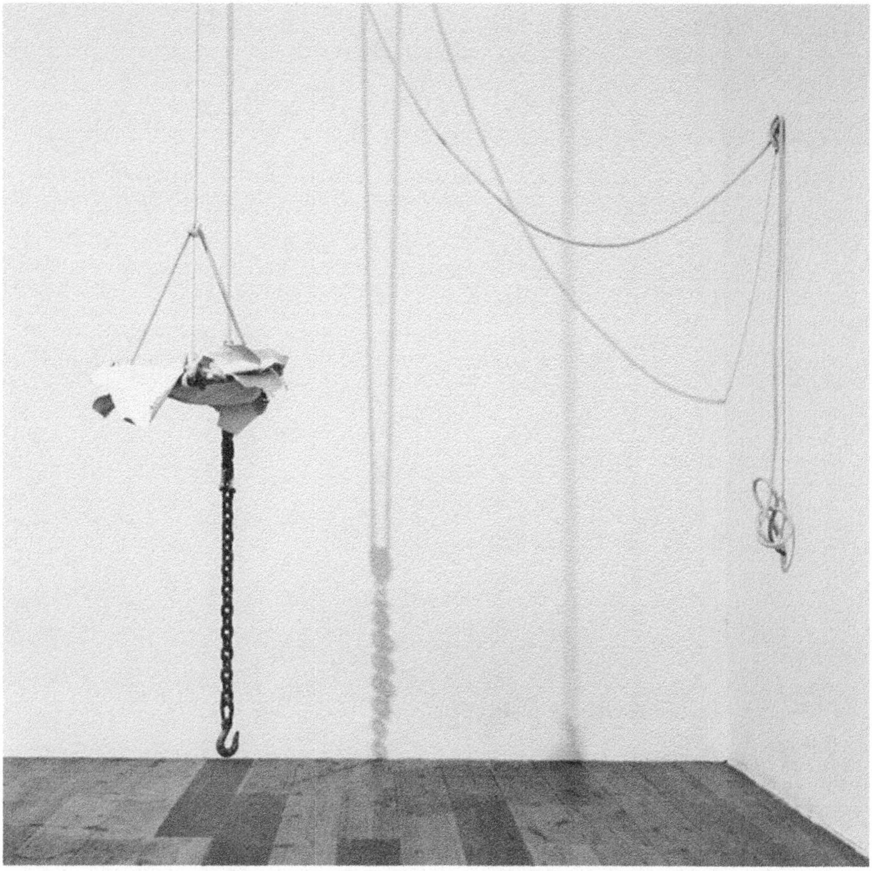

FIGURE 9.18 *Fayen d'Evie and Sophie Takách,* After Hooke *(work in progress) (2016).* Bronze cast of three tactile dialogues, vegetable tanned hide, steel, and rope. (Detail). Image courtesy the artists.

perception of sculpture by other artists—something to look forward to. Taken together, the self-portraits of all these artists show a diversity of responses to the experience of blindness, from grief to playfulness, from frustration to a savvy irony about the conventions of their chosen artistic media. Even while these artists expose vulnerability and sadness for lost sight, gone is the otherworldly isolation of the Hypothetical Blind Man. They acknowledge the traditional linkage of blindness to tactile perception, even while they break from that tradition to explore other sensory modalities. They insist on their status as insiders rather than outsiders to visual culture, and foreground the complex three-way communication that takes place between the artist, the art work, and the beholder.

{ NOTES }

Introduction

1. Leo Steinberg, "Jasper Johns: The First Seven Years of his Art," in *Other Criteria: Confrontations with Twentieth Century Art*. London, Oxford, New York: Oxford University Press, 1972, 48.

2. *The Mystery of Picasso*, dir. and prod. by Henri-Georges Clouzot, 1956.

3. James Elkins, *The Object Stares Back: On the Nature of Seeing*. San Diego, New York, London: Harcourt, 1996, 233.

4. Barbara Pierce, editorial note on Amalia S. Levi, "Beyond Vision: Integrating Touch into Museums, the Tactile Museum of the Lighthouse for the Blind, in Athens Greece," *The Braille Monitor*, 48, no. 6 (2005), https://nfb.org/images/nfb/publications/bm/bm05/bm0506/bm050606.htm. Accessed September 2, 2016.

5. American Foundation for the Blind, "Blindness Statistics: Educational Attainment," http://www.afb.org/info/programs-and-services/professional-development/experts-guide/faq/1235. Accessed September 5, 2016.

6. American Foundation for the Blind, "Blindness Statistics: Employment," http://www.afb.org/info/living-with-vision-loss/for-job-seekers/employment-statistics/125. Accessed September 5, 2016.

Chapter 1

1. Elizabeth Gitter, *The Imprisoned Guest: Samuel Howe and Laura Bridgman, the Original Deaf-Blind Girl*. New York: Farrar, Straus and Giroux, 2001, 51.

2. For a comprehensive treatment of this topic see Mark Paterson, *Seeing with the Hands: Blindness, Vision and Touch after Descartes*. Edinburgh: Edinburgh University Press, 2016.

3. Rene Descartes, "Optics," in *Discourse on Method, Optics, Geometry, and Meteorology*, trans. by P. J. Olscamp. Indianapolis, IN: Hackett (1637) 2001, 67.

4. Ibid., 68.

5. John Locke, *Essay Concerning Human Understanding*, ed. Peter H. Nidditch. Oxford: Clarendon Press (1609) 1975, 146.

6. William Cheselden, "An Account of Some Observations Made by a Young Gentleman, Who Was Born Blind, or Who Lost His Sight So Early, that He Had No Remembrance of Ever Having Seen, and Was Couch'd Between 13 and 14 Years of Age," *Philosophical Transactions*, 402 (1728): 448.

7. Dennis Diderot, *Thoughts on the Interpretation of Nature and Other Philosophical Works*, ed. David Adams. Manchester: Clinaman Press (1749) 1999, 151.

8. Ibid., 153.

9. Ibid., 156.

10. Ray Charles, interview on *The Today Show*, NBC, October 4, 2001.

11. Diderot, *Thoughts on the Interpretation of Nature*, 172.

12. Ibid., 159.

13. Thérèse-Adèle Husson, *Reflections: The Life and Writing of a Young Blind Woman in Post-Revolutionary France*, ed. Catherine J. Kudlick and Zina Weygand. New York and London: New York University Press (1825) 2001, 25.

14. Ibid., 141.

15. Helen Keller, *The World I Live I*, ed. Roger Shattuck. New York: New York Review of Books (1908) 2003, 19.

16. Ibid., 29–30.

17. Ibid., 45.

18. Ibid., 45–46.

19. Bryan Magee and Martin Milligan, *On Blindness*. Oxford and New York: Oxford University Press, 1995, 46.

20. Ibid., 104.

21. Ibid., 56.

22. Ibid., 97–98.

Chapter 2

1. John Howard Griffin, *Scattered Shadows: A Memoir of Blindness and Vision*. New York: Orbis Books, 2004, 219.

2. William Cheselden, "An Account of Some Observations Made by a Young Gentleman, Who Was Born Blind, or Who Lost His Sight So Early, that He Had No Remembrance of Ever Having Seen, and Was Couch'd Between 13 and 14 Years of Age," *Philosophical Transactions*, 402 (1728): 449.

3. Ibid.

4. There are many accounts of this case. I have relied primarily on Zina Weygand, *Vivre Sans Voir: Les aveugles dans la societé française, du Moyen Age au siècle de Louis Braille*. Paris: Éditions Créaphis, 2003.

5. Oliver Sacks, "To See and Not See," in *An Anthropologist on Mars*. New York: Alfred A Knopf, 1995.

6. Brian Friel, *Molly Sweeney*. New York: Dramatists Play Service, 1996, 53.

7. Wilkie Collins, *Poor Miss Finch*. Oxford and New York: Oxford University Press (1872) 2008, 220.

8. Ibid., 418.

9. Mike May, "Mike's Journal," 2001, http://web.archive.org/web/20040401192741/www.senderogroup.com/mikejournal.htm

10. Project Prakash 2003. http://www.projectprakash.org/

11. T. Gandhi, A. Kalia, S. Ganesh, and P. Sinha, "Immediate Susceptibility to Visual Illusions After Sight Onset," *Current Biology*, 25, no. 9, (2015): 358–359.

12. B. Balas and P. Sinha, "Observing Object Motion Induces Increased Generalization and Sensitivity," *Perception*, 37, no. 8 (2008): 1160–1174.

13. John M. Kennedy, *Drawing and the Blind*. New Haven and London: Yale University Press, 1993, 423.

14. Ibid., 156.

15. Ibid., 325.

16. Nicholas Howe, *Writing the Map of Anglo-Saxon England*. New Haven and London: Yale University Press, 2008, 140.

Chapter 3

1. American Foundation for the Blind, "Blindness Statistics: Educational Attainment," http://www.afb.org/info/programs-and-services/professional-development/experts-guide/faq/1235. Accessed September 5, 2016.

2. American Foundation for the Blind, "Blindness Statistics: Employment," http://www.afb.org/info/living-with-vision-loss/for-job-seekers/employment-statistics/125. Accessed September 5, 2016.

3. Frederic K. Schroeder, "Braille Usage: Perspectives of Legally Blind Adults and Policy Implications for School Administrators," https://nfb.org/braille-usage. Accessed December 4, 2016.

4. Ruby Ryles, "The Impact of Braille Reading Skills on Employment, Income, Education, and Reading Habits," *Journal of Visual Impairment and Blindness*, 90, no. 30 (1996): 219–226.

5. Karl Vick, "Memorial's Braille Letters Pose a Sizable Problem for the Blind," *Washington Post*, May 20, 1997. Posted on the National Council on Disability Articles Archive, file:///F:/Blind%20ART/visible%20braille/National%20Council%20on%20Disability%20Document%20Archive%20-%20Archives.htm.

6. Ibid.

7. Emerson Faulke, "Braille," in *The Psychology of Touch*, ed. Morton A. Heller and William Schiff. Hillsborough: Lawrence Erlbaum, 1991, 219–234.

8. Mary Katherine Coffey, "Histories that Haunt: A Conversation with Ann Hamilton," *Art Journal* (Fall 2014): 12.

9. Lynne Cooke, "The Ann Hamilton Experience—Installation Artist—Interview," *Interview*, July 8, 1999.

10. Ibid., 8.

11. Yoshiko Murakami, *Les Mains Pour Voir*. Paris: Actes Sud/ Foundation CCF pour la Photographie, 1999.

12. Ileana Sánchez and Rebecca McGinnis, *Art and the Alphabet: A Tactile Experience*. Puerto Rico: Creativo Creative, 2003.

13. Menena Cottin and Rosana Faría, *The Black Book of Colors*, trans. Elisa Amado. Toronto and Berkeley: Groundwood Books, 2008.

14. C. Bessigneuil et al., *Des Clés pour Bâtir*. Paris: Éditions de la Cité de Sciences et de L'Industrie, 1991.

15. While *eggs* requires four characters in the Roman alphabet, it only needs three in Braille. The double *g* is indicated by moving the character for *g* from its usual location at the top of the Braille grid to the lower level.

Chapter 4

1. Helen Keller, *The World I Live In*, ed. Roger Shattuck. New York: New York Review of Books (1908), 2003, 12.

2. Ibid., 15.

3. See: http://www.johnmhull.biz/cathedrals%20through%20touch%20and%20hearing.html.

4. Raphael Minder, "At Museo del Prado, Blind Visitors Can Touch Masterpieces," *New York Times*, March 6, 2015. http://www.nytimes.com/2015/03/07/arts/design/at-museo-del-prado-blind-visitors-can-touch-masterpieces.html?_r=1.

5. Robert Hooke, *The Posthumous Works of Robert Hooke*. Farmington Hills, MI: Gale Ecco, 2010, 36.

6. For a history of touch in museums see Fiona Candlin, *Art, Museums and Touch*. Manchester: Manchester University Press, 2010; and Constance Classen, "Touch in the Museum," in *The Book of Touch*. New York: Bloomsbury Academic, 2005, 275–287.

7. John Lee Clark, "Metatactile Knowledge," http://johnleeclark.tumblr.com/.

Chapter 5

1. Dennis Diderot, *Thoughts on the Interpretation of Nature and Other Philosophical Works*, ed. David Adams. Manchester: Clinaman Press (1749) 1999, 156.

2. Ibid., 197.

3. Sabriye Tenberken, *My Path Leads to Tibet*. New York: Arcade, 2003, 44–45.

4. Helen Keller, *The World I Live In*, ed. Roger Shattuck. New York: New York Review of Books (1908), 2003, 67–68.

5. Ibid., 69.

6. Ibid., 70

7. James Wilson, *Biography of the Blind*, ed. Kenneth A. Stuckey. Washington, DC: Library of Congress, 1995, 357.

8. Geerat J. Vermeij, "Teaching Exploration: Correcting a Glaring Flaw in the Education of Blind Children," *The Braille Monitor*, 47 (2004): 9, http://www.nfb.org/Images/nfb/Publications/bm/bm04/bm0410/bm0410tc.htm. Accessed August 23, 2016.

9. Dennis Diderot, *Diderot on Art*, vol. 1: *The Salon of 1765 and Notes on Painting*, ed. and trans. John Goodman. New Haven and London: Yale University Press (1765) 1995, 6.

10. Ibid., 58.

11. Ibid., 62.

12. Diderot, *Thoughts on the Interpretation of Nature*, 199.

13. Ibid., 191.

14. Ibid., 194

Chapter 6

1. Jacques Derrida, *Memoirs of the Blind: The Self-Portrait and Other Ruins*, trans. Pascale-Anne Brault and Michael Naas. Chicago and London: University of Chicago Press, 1993, 2.

2. Wilkie Collins, *Poor Miss Finch*. Oxford and New York: Oxford University Press (1872) 2008, 59–60.

3. John Banville, *The Sea*, 2006, 128.

4. Rudyard Kipling, *The Light That Failed*. New York: Carroll and Graf (1891) 1986, 234.

5. For a more detailed reading of *The Light That Failed*, see Georgina Kleege, *Sight Unseen*. New Haven and London: Yale University Press, 1999, 72–74.

6. Hilary Norman, *Blind Fear*. London: Piatkus Books, 2000, 58.

7. Ibid., 186.

8. Raymond Carver, "Cathedral," in *Stories*. New York: Alfred A. Knopf, 1983, 209–228.

9. Lorrie Moore, "What You Want to Do Fine," in *Birds of America*. New York: Picador, 1999, 158–159.

10. Ibid., 152.

11. Ibid.

12. Collins, *Poor Miss Finch*, 371.

13. Tracy Chevalier, *Girl with a Pearl Earring*. New York: Plume, 1999, 47.

14. Ibid., 90.

15. Ibid., 90.

16. Ibid., 90–91.

17. Ibid., 91.

18. Tracy Chevalier, *The Lady and the Unicorn*. New York: Dutton, 2004, 95.

19. Ibid., 115.

20. Ibid., 96.

21. Paul Auster, *Moon Palace*. New York: Penguin Books, 1990, 121–122.

22. Ibid., 123.

23. Ibid.

24. Ibid., 135.

25. Ibid., 134.

26. Ibid., 30.

Chapter 7

1. For example, Sabine Braun, "Audio Description from a Discourse Perspective: A Socially Relevant Framework for Research and Training," *Linguistica Antverpiensia* no. 6 (2007): 357–369. D. Fels, J. Udo, J. Diamond, and J. Diamond, "A Comparison of Alternative Narrative Approaches to Video Description for Animated Comedy," *Journal of Visual Impairment and Blindness*, 100, no. 5 (2006): 295.

2. Elena Di Giovanni, "Visual and Narrative Priorities of the Blind and Non-Blind: Eye Tracking and Audio Description," *Perspectives: Studies in Translatology*, 22, no. 1 (2014): 136–153.

3. For example see Julia Hoffman, "Disability Rights Between Legal Discourses and Policy Narratives: An Analysis of the European and Canadian Frameworks," *Disability Studies Quarterly*, 33, no. 3 (2013), http://dsq-sds.org/article/view/1778/3260.

4. Elaine Gerber, "Describing Tragedy: The Information Access Needs of Blind People in Emergency Related Circumstances," *Human Organization*, 68, no. 1 (2009): 73–81.

5. An exception to this generalization is this description of an arts residency program held at UC Irvine in 2012 where scholars and artists came together to sketch art projects with access features such as audio description incorporated into the design from the outset: Catherine J Kudlick, "Collision and Collusion: Artists, Academics, and Activists in Dialogue with the University of California and Critical Disability Studies," *Disability Studies Quarterly*, 34, no. 2 (2014), http://dsq-sds.org/article/view/4251/3609.

6. Rick Boggs, "How to Know What to Say," https://www.youtube.com/watch?v=JZlNVajYx9s.

7. The Described and Captioned Media Program, "Description Key," https://www.dcmp.org/descriptionkey/how_to_describe.html.

8. Joel Snyder, *The Visual Made Verbal: A Comprehensive Training Manual and Guide to the History and Applications of Audio Description*. Indianapolis, IN: Dog Ear, 2014, 60.

9. For example, David Bolt, *The Metanarrative of Blindness: A Re-reading of Twentieth Century Anglophone Literature*. Ann Arbor: University of Michigan Press, 2014.

10. Georgina Kleege, *Sight Unseen*. New Haven: Yale University Press, 1999.

11. Joel Snyder, ed., "Audio Description Guidelines and Best Practices: Work in Progress, Version 3.1, September 2010," American Council of the Blind's Audio Description Project, http://www.acb.org/adp/ad.html.

12. Mara Mills, "Listening to Images: Audio Description, the Translation Overlay, and Image Retrieval," *The Cine Files*, June 1, 2015, http://www.thecine-files.com/listening-to-images-audio-description-the-translation-overlay-and-image-retrieval/.

13. Chris Collins, "Hearing Pictures," *California Sunday Magazine*, November 2, 2014, https://stories.californiasunday.com/2014-11-02/rethinking-movies-for-the-blind/.

14. Georgina Kleege and Scott Wallin, "Audio Description as a Pedagogical Tool," *Disability Studies Quarterly*, 35, no. 2 (2015), http://dsq-sds.org/article/view/4622/3945.

Chapter 8

1. Elisabeth Salzhauer Axel, Virginia Hooper, Teresa Kardoulias, Sarah Stephenson Keyes, and Francesca Rosenberg, "Art Education for the Blind's Guidelines for Verbal Description," http://www.artbeyondsight.org/handbook/acs-guidelines.shtml. Accessed August 27, 2016.

2. Ibid.

3. The quotations that follow are all transcribed from MOMA's "Audio +" web page: http://www.moma.org/visit/plan/atthemuseum/momaaudio. Accessed August 27, 2016.

4. Georgia Krantz, "Leveling the Participatory Field: The Mind's Eye Program at the Guggenheim Museum," *Disability Studies Quarterly*, 33, no. 3 (2013), http://dsq-sds.org/article/view/3738. Accessed August 27, 2016.

5. Bridget O'Brien Hoyt, "Emphasizing Observation in a Gallery Program for Blind and Low-Vision Visitors: Art Beyond Sight at the Museum of Fine Arts, Houston," *Disability Studies Quarterly*, 33, no. 3 (2013), http://dsq-sds.org/article/view/3737/3278. Accessed August 27, 2016.

6. Krantz, "Leveling the Participatory Field."

7. Alice Wingwall, interview with the author, November 5, 2015.

8. David Johnson, e-mail with the author, November 20, 2015.

9. Ibid.

10. Carmen Papalia, "See for Yourself," *Arts and Disability, Ireland/ Curated Space*, http://www.adiarts.ie/curated-space/see-for-yourself. Accessed August 27, 2016.

11. David Johnson, e-mail with the author, December 13, 2015.

Chapter 9

1. Jean Sutherland Boggs, *Picasso & Things*. Cleveland, Ohio: Cleveland Museum of Art, 1992, 41.

2. Jacques Derrida, *Memoirs of the Blind: The Self-Portrait and Other Ruins*, trans. Pascale-Anne Brault and Michael Naas. Chicago and London: University of Chicago Press, 1993, 4–5.

3. *The Mystery of Picasso*, dir. and prod. by Henri-Georges Clouzot, 1956.

4. John M. Hull, *Touching the Rock: An Experience of Blindness*. New York: Vintage Books, 1992, 25.

5. "Sargy Mann, Artist—Obituary," *The Telegraph*, April 17, 2015, http://www.telegraph.co.uk/news/obituaries/11545135/Sargy-Mann-artist-obituary.html. Accessed August 28, 2016.

6. For a survey of depictions of blindness in Western visual art see Moshe Barasch, *Blindness: The History of a Mental Image in Western Thought*. New York: Routledge, 2001.

7. Interview with the author.

8. E-mail with the author, July 26, 2016.

9. The black-and-white reproduction does not do justice to Mann's work. To view this painting and others visit https://www.cadogancontemporary.com/artist/sargy-mann/.

10. For a thorough and compelling reading of this film see Michael Davidson, "Nostalgia for Light: Being Blind at the Museum," in *Concerto for the Left Hand: Disability and the Defamiliar Body*. Ann Arbor: University of Michigan Press, 2008, 146–167.

11. For a discussion of blindness and masculinity see Catherine J. Kudlick, "The Blind Man's Harley: White Canes and Gender Identity in Modern America Signs," *Journal of Women in Culture and Society*, 30, no. 2 (2005): 1589–1606.

12. At the exhibit "What Can a Body Do?" Curated by Amanda Cachia, Cantor Fitzgerald Gallery, Haverford College, 2012.

{ INDEX }

Note: Page references followed by a "*t*" indicate table; "*f*" indicate figure

The manufacturer's authorised representative in the EU for product safety is Oxford University Press España S.A. of El Parque Empresarial San Fernando de Henares, Avenida de Castilla, 2 - 28830 Madrid (www.oup.es/en or product.safety@oup.com). OUP España S.A. also acts as importer into Spain of products made by the manufacturer.

Printed and bound by CPI Group (UK) Ltd, Croydon, CR0 4YY

14/09/2026

02216295-0005

Active Assessment: Assessing Scientific Inquiry

Mentoring in Academia and Industry

Series Editor: J. Ellis Bell, University of Richmond, Virginia

---

Biology is evolving rapidly, with more and more discoveries arising from interaction with other disciplines such as chemistry, mathematics, and computer science. Undergraduate and Graduate biology education is having a hard time keeping up. To address this challenge, this bold and innovative series will assist science education programs at research universities, four-year colleges and community colleges across the country and by enriching science teaching and mentoring of both students and faculty in academia and for industry representatives. The series aims to promote the progress of scientific research and education by providing guidelines for improving academic and career building skills for a broad audience of students, teachers, mentors, researchers, industry, and more.

Volume 1 Education Outreach and Public Engagement
by Erin L. Dolan

Volume 2 Active Assessment: Assessing Scientific Inquiry
by David I. Hanauer, Graham F. Hatfull, Deborah Jacobs-Sera

David I. Hanauer · Graham F. Hatfull
Deborah Jacobs-Sera

Active Assessment: Assessing Scientific Inquiry

Springer

David I. Hanauer
Department of English
Indiana University of Pennsylvania
421 North Walk
Indiana, PA 15705
USA
hanauer@iup.edu

Graham F. Hatfull
Department of Biological Sciences
University of Pittsburgh
376 Crawford Hall
Pittsburgh, PA 15260
USA
gfh@pitt.edu

Deborah Jacobs-Sera
Department of Biological Sciences
University of Pittsburgh
376 Crawford Hall
Pittsburgh, PA 15260
USA
djs@pitt.edu

ISBN 978-0-387-89648-9 e-ISBN 978-0-387-89649-6
DOI 10.1007/978-0-387-89649-6

Library of Congress Control Number: 2009920530

Printed on acid-free paper

springer.com

We dedicate this book to the community of scientist-educators and to all – from both sides of the divide – who aspire to join them

Acknowledgments

We would like to extend thanks to our many colleagues at the University of Pittsburgh that have been integrally involved in the study of bacteriophage genomics. Dr. Roger Hendrix spearheaded the phage comparative genomics effort in the early 1990s, and it was from this foundation that the PHIRE program emerged. Roger has been a truly wonderful and inspiring colleague and collaborator through all aspects of the genome investigations and the PHIRE program. We also thank Dr. Jeffrey Lawrence who has been centrally involved in the phage genome projects since joining the University of Pittsburgh, and we are grateful for his frequently profound insights into microbial evolution as well as for the enormous investment of time and effort into the development of suitable bioinformatic tools and programs. Dr. Craig Peebles has aided in phage genome analysis in numerous ways especially in the identification of small tRNA genes and other features; he has also supervised many students in the PHIRE program.

We extend special thanks to Dr. Marisa Pedulla who was the PHIRE program coordinator when the program was initiated in 2002. As a dedicated scientist/educator, Marisa established a strong foundation for the PHIRE program and established many of the structures that ensured its continuing success including introducing David Hanauer to the PHIRE program team. The PHIRE program could not have been successful without Marisa's dedication to placing students at the heart of our phage discovery and genomic effort.

Dr. Bill Jacobs introduced GFH to the mycobacteriophage world in 1988 and has been a fantastic collaborator in every aspect of research and the PHIRE program. Bill has had undergraduate and high school phage hunters in his laboratory for many years and has been an inspiration for all of us working with mycobacteriophages.

We are fortunate to have a small genome center at the University of Pittsburgh that is dedicated to phage genomics, and over the years has had a wonderful team of research associates that have skillfully helped to sequence phage genomes and have tirelessly mentored students in genome sequence and analysis. We also thank Dr. Steve Cresawn who participated in all components of the PHIRE program, as well as designing and composing the Phamerator program for analyzing gene phamilies.

The PHIRE program and the work on this book were supported by a Professorship from the Howard Hughes Medical Institute. We are enormously grateful to the support that HHMI has provided, both financially and programmatically. Dr. Peter Bruns was helpful and supportive in all aspects of administration and execution of the PHIRE program and we are grateful for his leadership at HHMI. We also thank Maria Kozalka at HHMI for outstanding assistance, especially at the outset of the Professors programs and when we were establishing the PHIRE program. The HHMI Professors program provided a critical opportunity to meet and learn from many truly inspiring scientist/educators. There is not one of the professors that did not provide some special insight and perspective, but we would like to especially thank Drs. Jo Handeslman, Utpal Banerjee, and Scott Strobel for their insights and inspirations.

Our graduate students, postdoctoral researchers, research associates, and fellow faculty have joyfully participated in the grand PHIRE experiment. They have assisted in ways too numerous to mention, have helped mentor many students, and have shown remarkable tolerance for all the perturbations that can arise from having relatively inexperienced researchers in the laboratory milieu.

Contents

Chapter 1
Active Assessment

1.1 Scientists as Educators

Doing science is an exciting, fulfilling activity that contributes to the collected cultural knowledge of humanity. By doing science new knowledge is created and our understanding of the world around us is increased. Unfortunately, this sense of mission and personal feelings of excitement and fulfillment so characteristic of the active scientist are lost in most science education settings. This book, as with other publications from the authors of this book, evolved from the simple premise that active scientists should be involved in and develop serious educational programs designed around real scientific research questions. Science education is too serious a purpose that scientists can leave this to others to fulfill. The authors of this book hold a deep belief that the way to advance science education is through the development of in-laboratory science education programs that bring students into close contact with the experience and realities of authentic scientific inquiry. This book is designed to help active scientists to create authentic assessments that contribute to the educational process and provide meaningful data that can be used by the scientist-educator and student-scientist to enhance the educational process within the laboratory and thus enhance science. This book was written with the understanding that scientists may not feel comfortable with educational concepts and terminology and that this is one of the barriers to the creation of more laboratory-based, authentic science education programs. It is our hope that this book will provide a clear introduction to the approach to the assessment of scientific inquiry that we have developed and used in our own laboratory educational program and that this knowledge will ultimately lead to the creation and understanding of assessment in new laboratory-based scientific inquiry educational programs.

1.2 The Context and Aims of This Book

This book deals with a very specific educational context – the in-laboratory, scientific inquiry, educational program. The issue that this book addresses is the way

D.I. Hanauer et al., *Active Assessment: Assessing Scientific Inquiry*,
Mentoring in Academia and Industry 2, DOI 10.1007/978-0-387-89649-6_1,

to assess knowledge development and outcomes within this setting. This book has three main aims:

1. To provide scientist-educators working with in-laboratory scientific inquiry educational programs an approach to the development of a meaningful assessment program
2. To provide scientist-educators with a comprehensive understanding of issues of educational assessment and an overview of the work that has been done by science educators concerning the assessment of scientific inquiry
3. To provide scientist-educators with a case study and specific examples of one program that utilized the approach developed in this book to the assessment of scientific inquiry.

1.3 Relevant Historical Developments in Science Education

This book finds its source in three interrelated developments in science education. The first deals with the importance of enhancing students' understanding of the procedural knowledge of scientific activity. The most widely recognized statement of this type was the National Research Council's publication of their *National Science Education Standards* promoting scientific inquiry as a core element of scientific education (NRC, 1996). Over the years since this early publication, the same message of the centrality of scientific inquiry as an educational tool has been repeated in a variety of publications and national reports. Most importantly for undergraduate science education, in another NRC report prepared by the Committee for Undergraduate Biology Education to Prepare Research Scientists for the 21st Century and entitled *BIO2010: Transforming Undergraduate Education for Future Research Biologists*, an emphasis is placed on providing students with the experience, understanding, and skills required to conduct interdisciplinary scientific inquiries within the coming century.

The second educational development consists of the movement of science education out of the classroom and into the laboratory. This direction can be seen as the most direct implementation of the concept that science education should focus on scientific inquiry. As stated by Handelsman et al. (2004), "Scientists of all disciplines have developed inquiry-based labs that require students to develop hypotheses, design and conduct experiments, collect and interpret data, and write about results" (p. 521). Extending this argument Hatfull et al. (2006) and Hanauer et al. (2006) promote (and exemplify) the transformation of the professional research laboratory into an educational arena that brings students from a diversity of disciplines, ages, and interests into a laboratory in order to conduct authentic scientific inquiries. This requires the definition of in-lab research projects that are appropriate for a variety of incoming students with different knowledge bases but still culminate in authentic scientific discoveries (Hatfull et al., 2006; Hanauer et al., 2006).

The third educational development deals with the role of the science instructor. Under the heading of "scientific teaching," Handelsman and her colleagues in a number of initiatives and publications have promoted the concept that science teaching should be directed by the same principles that inform scientific research activity. Specifically as developed by Handelsman et al. (2007) scientific teaching should involve the same levels of "critical thinking, rigor, creativity and the spirit of experimentation" as those used by scientists in their research. The concept of scientific teaching integrates the activity of conducting scientific research with the activity of scientific teaching. Importantly, the concept of scientific teaching rests upon two core principles: the need for engaging educational experiences based on an understanding of scientific inquiry and the need for evidence that will allow the evaluation of all educational activities.

The outcome of these three developments in science education is the proposition that science education should focus on scientific inquiry, should optimally take place within a laboratory setting, and be directed by the principles of scientific teaching. An educational program of this sort should engage students in the process of scientific inquiry and allow scientist-instructors the ability to measure and evaluate the quality and content of the education their students are receiving. It is this last point that the current book addresses. The aim of this book is to provide scientist-educators with a set of conceptual tools that will allow them to create an assessment strategy and assessment tools that are appropriate for the assessment of an educational, scientific inquiry program situated within a laboratory setting. This book builds upon the basic ideas of scientific teaching by providing an approach to the development of assessment tools that can be used in a variety of settings and thus allow scientists to consider carefully the quality and learning outcomes of their teaching. It should be noted that the current book addresses assessment within the confines of the educational developments specified above, namely teaching scientific inquiry through in-laboratory experiences. This is a relatively complex educational context and accordingly specific approaches to this distinctive educational setting are developed in this book.

1.4 Active Assessment Defined

Active assessment is the process through which scientist-educators develop an assessment strategy and assessment tools that provide significant information that enhances the active learning experience of students involved in the scientific inquiry process. Active assessment is a process in that the scientist-educator is actively involved in the development of their own assessment tools. In other words, the scientist-educator is an active part of the process of understanding how her/his educational programs are assessed and is in no way a passive recipient of standardized, externally created assessment tools. In addition, active assessment is based on the idea that the students who are engaged in scientific inquiry within a laboratory setting experience the assessment process as integral to their scientific inquiry process and as a source of input that informs their work and understanding as scientists. The active assessment process requires the scientist-educator to be deeply involved in the design of an educational experience that provides serious feedback and makes the scientific inquiry process conceptually meaningful and scientifically valuable for both the instructor and student-researcher. The characteristics of active assessment can be summarized as follows:

1. Active assessment elicits significant information that can be used to assess the quality and content of the educational inquiry program.
2. Active assessment is embedded within the scientific inquiry process and reflects meaningful practice within the laboratory setting.
3. Active assessment is developed by the scientist-educator and reflects the core procedural and substantive understandings of the specific scientific inquiry process that is utilized within the laboratory setting.
4. Active assessment is meaningful to the student-researcher and provides significant feedback that contributes to the educational and scientific development of the student-researcher.

1.5 The Underpinning Principles of Active Assessment

The idea of active assessment as defined above is based on several basic principles of educational practice. The first characteristic – *Active assessment elicits significant information that can be used to assess the quality and content of the educational inquiry program* – is tied to the core concept of all assessment research that educational processes and outcomes can and should be measured. From the perspective of scientific teaching, decisions in relation to educational practice should be based on the presence of relevant and comprehensive data concerning the process and outcomes of learning. Active assessment as an approach to assessment is designed to provide quality-contextualized information that in a very direct way measures those aspects of the scientific inquiry program that represent moments of meaningful knowledge development in the student-researchers' projects. Evidence collected from the process of active assessment concerning students' knowledge can be used to evaluate the state of learning within the program by pinpointing areas in which development has (or has not) occurred. This information can be used to modify or enhance various components of the educational program. In other words, active assessment should provide the evidence through which the educational value of the scientific inquiry program can be measured.

The second characteristic – *Active assessment is embedded within the scientific inquiry process and reflects meaningful practice within the laboratory setting* – addresses the core understanding that scientific inquiry is a particularized activity and that learning science is best advanced through contextualized understanding. The basic educational principle exemplified within the in-laboratory scientific inquiry process is termed situated learning (Lave & Wenger, 1991). Situated learning proposes that meaningful learning takes place within authentic settings and as part of a process of participation within a community of practice. A series of researchers have posited the constructivist argument that learning is enhanced through participation in a contextualized, personally meaningful, problem-solving setting (Brown, Collins, & Duguid, 1989; Polman, 1999; Roth 1995; Wenger 1998; Williams & Hmelo, 1998). As argued by Lee and Songer (2003) authentic science practices within the cultural context of real scientific inquiry are important components of advancing scientific understanding. The movement of science education into the professional laboratory enhances the possibility that students get access to the personnel, tasks, and culture of scientific work. Active assessment extends this position on the importance of embedding learning within authentic contexts. As developed in this book, active assessment situates assessment within the framework and in relation to the authentic tasks and aspects of specific scientific inquiries. Rather than an imposed generalized approach, active assessment promotes contextualized assessment tasks tied to the specificity of the particular scientific inquiries. The assessment procedures closely reflect the actual work done in the laboratory and as such can provide evidence of understanding on the knowledge, concepts, and skills required to complete that particular scientific inquiry process. The embedded nature of the active assessment should make the procedures of assessment meaningful to the student-researchers as well as provide direct evidence of learning outcomes for the researcher-educator.

The third characteristic – *Active assessment is developed by the scientist-educator and reflects the core procedural and substantial understandings of the specific scientific inquiry process that is utilized within the laboratory setting* – addresses the central role the scientist-educators play in the development of both the educational program and its assessment procedures. The process of active assessment situates the scientist-educator in a central role in relation to the development of educational programs. Based on the principles developed within the framework of *Scientific Teaching*, the researcher-educator having developed an educational program should have interest in ways to measure knowledge acquired within that program. As described in the last point the types of task developed in the process of active assessment are closely related to the specific characteristics of the particular scientific inquiry process utilized as the basis for the educational program. The process of active assessment assumes that the specific scientific inquiry process is tied to the prime researchers' own scientific research agenda. Accordingly, the prime researcher is best qualified to know what is significant from both a substantial and procedural perspective. It is these understandings of the significance of particular types of knowledge within the scientific inquiry process that ultimately constitute the basic components of the active assessment process. In this sense the scientist-educator utilizes her/his developed understanding of science to make decisions concerning what is of significance for assessment.

The fourth characteristic – *Active assessment is meaningful to the student-researcher and provides significant feedback that contributes to the educational and scientific development of the student-researcher* – addresses the role of metacognition as an important aspect of learning. As described by Baird (1990) metacognition consists of the learner consciously recognizing aspects of their own learning and modifying or redirecting their educational actions in accordance with this understanding. Significant contextualized feedback can potentially play an important role in directing the students' attention toward areas where further understanding is required. On a different level, active assessment can play a role in making sure that the educational laboratory experience is not just a case of manipulating procedures but rather a truly conceptual process. White and Gunstone (1992) posit that the integration of the laboratory experience with metacognitive tasks enhances the learning of science. As conceptualized within this book, the aims of active assessment are formative, diagnostic, and summative. The student-researcher's usage of the assessment tools should provide information that is useful for the student in recognizing what has been learnt and what still needs to be learnt. The embedded, contextualized nature of the assessment process should ensure that the student gets specific feedback that is directly relevant to the scientific inquiry that is being followed. The outcomes of the assessment procedures need to become feedback to the student on the different aspects of the inquiry process that they are involved with. As a metacognitive process the feedback from the assessment procedures should direct the student to focus on areas that need to be addressed and thus allow learning to be individualized to the student's specific needs. Meaningful assessment that provides direct feedback to the student-researcher is a central aspect of the active assessment process.

1.6 On the Importance of Active Engagement

As can be seen in the definitions of active assessment provided above, active engagement and problem solving on the part of the scientist-educator and the student-researcher are core aspects of the approach to assessment that is developed in this book. This assertion concerning the importance of the active engagement of both researcher-educator and student-researcher within the active assessment process needs some clarification. In relation to the scientist-educator the emphasis on active engagement with the assessment process has two aspects to it. First, scientist-educators are coming under increasing pressure to become involved with educational processes. This pressure is directed by national educational bodies, funding agencies, university administers, department chairs, and most importantly from a deep-rooted sense that able students are choosing other professions rather than the sciences. The outcome of these forces is that the research scientist is being redefined, at least in part, as an educator and producer of quality science education programs. Understandably many research scientists do not feel comfortable with this role and may even feel that this is an imposition on the more significant aspects of their scientific work. In addition many research scientists do not feel that they are really qualified to make educational decisions in particular in relation to the assessment of learning outcomes.

The solution posed within this book is to redress the supposed distance between educational and research activity and to situate active assessment within the context of authentic scientific inquiry. The idea as developed with the work of Hatfull et al. (2006) and Hanauer et al. (2006) is to integrate the educational scientific inquiry process within the scientific research agenda of the professional laboratory. In the second half of this book, one such program The PHIRE program (Phage Hunting Integrating Research and Education) situated at the Bacteriophage Institute of Pittsburgh at the University of Pittsburgh will be described in detail. The idea behind the PHIRE program and other programs like it is that students are involved with authentic scientific inquiry as full partners in the process. Naturally, the specifics of the educational research project need to be carefully chosen and not every research project conducted in a professional laboratory is compatible with educational processes (see Hatfull et al., 2006 for a full discussion of this point).

Of utmost importance to this approach to science education is the idea that the prime educator is also the prime researcher and that these two roles are compatible. The educational component of the laboratory's research agenda is designed to serve the overall mission of the laboratory as a site of scientific knowledge construction. In an environment of this kind the scientist-educator's engagement is obvious. In the same way as the head of a laboratory is fully committed and actively engaged with the research agendas of the laboratory, the researcher-educator is engaged with the educational process of the student-researchers. All serve the same aim of constructing scientific knowledge. Active involvement with the process of assessment design in this framework is an extension of the same engagement. As will be outlined in the following chapters of this book, the process of developing an assessment procedure is directly tied to the prime researcher's understanding of the specific process of scientific inquiry that is being utilized in the educational program. In this sense, engagement in active assessment means really utilizing the prime researcher-educators' understanding of the scientific inquiry processes of her/his laboratory that have become part of an educational program.

The second aspect of the importance of scientist-educator engagement with active assessment could be defined as a quality of life issue. The development of an assessment procedure by the prime laboratory researcher can provide both a sense of control and achievement in relation to the educational component of the inquiry process. When done well, active assessment provides very close, real-time data on the quality of the students' knowledge, understanding, and work within the scientific inquiry process. Rather than thinking of assessment as an external process that is beyond the control of the prime researcher (and might influence future funding), as the designer of the assessment process, information concerning the development of student understanding is immediately accessible to the prime researcher-educator and, if necessary, changes to the program can be made to ensure that a quality education in the sciences is achieved. In addition, there is the potential for enormous satisfaction when evidence of student learning that is really meaningful is found. A by-product of this process of active assessment is the option for a second line of laboratory research. By becoming directly involved and engaged with the assessment process the scientist-educator develops a secondary research agenda that both allows the educational program to evolve and improve as well as offering a new source of publishable research. Within the PHIRE program mentioned above, research is published on both the scientific and educational research that is conducted within the laboratory.

The argument for student engagement in the educational process is supported by some quite clear research outcomes and current understandings of quality educational practice. Handelsman et al. (2007) in their discussion of active learning review several studies that support the position that active engagement in scientific education enhances the retention of scientific information from courses. Knight and Wood (2005) utilizing problem-solving activities, discussions of journal articles, and learning assistants demonstrated increased knowledge retention. Similar results for the benefits of active engagement for science education have been presented by Udovic et al. (2002), Hake (1998), Beichner et al. (1999), and Ebert-May et al. (2003). Handelsman et al. (2007) summarizes their discussion by stating "Consistent across these research studies are the findings that active engagement enhances learning and retention, and that active learning builds higher-order thinking skills" (p. 26). The concept of active assessment is the attempt to make the assessment process a direct part of generating active engagement on the part of student-researcher in relation to the educational process that they are involved in. The underpinning concepts of embedding active assessment within the cultural practices of the laboratory and making the assessment tasks authentic and meaningful are designed to enhance the engagement of the student in the learning process and to provide real feedback to allow the student to play an active role in their own learning.

1.7 The Design of This Book

The aim of this book is to provide scientist-educators with an approach to the assessment of educational programs situated within laboratory settings and involving scientific inquiries. The book is designed as two sections. The first section of the book develops the theoretical and practical concerns involved in the process of active assessment. The aim of this section is to ensure that the reader is grounded in the literature, concepts, and practical aspects that inform the approach developed within this book. The second section provides a case study that exemplifies the approach developed within this book. Chapter 1 introduces the concept of active assessment and some of the sources and reasons for this approach. Chapter 2 involves a discussion of the concept of scientific inquiry. The direction of this chapter is to redefine scientific inquiry in contextual–operational terms that form the basis of the type of authentic assessment proposed in this book to be a possibility. Chapter 3 offers an introduction to assessment by presenting and explicating the basic concepts of assessment. Chapter 4 develops a specific approach to the assessment of scientific inquiry. The chapter reviews research that has been conducted on the assessment of scientific inquiry and then develops an approach to assessment that places high value of authenticity. Chapter 5 operationalizes the ideas of authentic, active assessment and provides the reader with a conceptual framework that allows the development of an assessment program for educational scientific inquiry programs. The second section of this book provides a case study in which the ideas and frameworks presented in the first section are exemplified. Chapter 6 presents an introduction and overview of the educational scientific inquiry program (entitled the PHIRE – Phage Hunting Integrating Research and Education – program) in which the ideas for assessment presented in this book were developed and will be exemplified. Chapter 7 presents the specific assessment strategy that was developed for and utilized in this program. Chapter 8 presents a description of the specific tools developed for the PHIRE program assessment. Finally Chap. 9 is written from the perspective of the scientist-educator and presents the prime researcher's experience of utilizing the process of active assessment within his program.

Chapter 2
Conceptualizing Scientific Inquiry

2.1 Introduction

In order to develop a strategy for the assessment of scientific inquiry in a laboratory setting, a theoretical construct of the components of scientific inquiry needs to be developed. A basic principle of any assessment procedure is that the starting point of any project is the specification of the object that is to be assessed. In the case of active assessment the object to be assessed is scientific inquiry. Unfortunately, as discussed by Hofstein and Lunetta (2003) in their meta-analysis of 20 years of research concerning the use of the laboratory as a site for education, the term scientific inquiry has been described and defined in a variety of ways leading to the need for "greater precision and consistency" in the explanation of this term. The aim of the current chapter is to provide an understanding of some of the complexities within the educational context in defining scientific inquiry. The main problem that this chapter addresses is the definition of scientific inquiry as an object that can form the basis for the development of a program of assessment. The definition of scientific inquiry developed in this chapter posits a very significant role for the contextualized nature of scientific inquiry.

2.2 The Diversity of Scientific Inquiry

Since the widely referenced and acknowledged National Research Council (NRC, 1996) definition of *National Science Education Standards* there has been renewed recognition that the enhancement and propagation of scientific inquiry is one of the core elements of scientific education. The basic idea is that to learn science involves conducting activities that address the procedural and epistemological aspects of science. The National Science Education Standards (NRC, 1996) state that "scientific inquiry is at the heart of science and science learning" (p. 15). As conceptualized by the NRC, scientific inquiry includes a range of activities involved and related to the scientific process. Specifically the NRC defines inquiry in the following

D.I. Hanauer et al., *Active Assessment: Assessing Scientific Inquiry*,
Mentoring in Academia and Industry 2, DOI 10.1007/978-0-387-89649-6_2,

terms: "Inquiry is a multifaceted activity that involves making observations; posing questions; examining books and other sources of information to see what is already known; planning investigations; reviewing what is already known in light of experimental evidence; using tools to gather, analyze, and interpret data; proposing answers, explanations, and predictions; and communicating results. Inquiry requires identification of assumptions, use of critical and logical thinking, and consideration of alternative explanations" (1996, p. 23).

However, while there is broad agreement over the potential significance of scientific inquiry for science education, the definition of scientific inquiry has to a certain extent been quite elusive and on a practical level difficult to implement. Hodson (1996), in a historical overview and educational critique of the scientific inquiry movement, deconstructs the simplistic notion of scientific inquiry as a decontextualized set of abstract principles (such as those posed in the NRC definition) that can easily be transferred from one scientific context to another. Hodson (1996) points out that actual scientific inquiry is infused with specific theoretical knowledge and hence contextualized in very specific ways. As stated by Hodson, "The difficulty of an observational task depends crucially on what is being observed and what constitutes appropriate or significant observation. In other words, the task is governed by the nature of the concepts involved" (1996, p. 126). Meaningful scientific inquiry is contextualized within a specific and developed knowledge structure and not the abstract application of procedural knowledge.

A different direction of critique of the scientific inquiry movement comes from studies of in-school manifestations of scientific inquiry. Millar (1998) is skeptical about the ability of in-school laboratory experiments to provide alternative understandings of accepted substantive descriptions of scientific concepts. Millar (1998) describes this type of scientific inquiry as a rhetorical form designed to manipulate results in order to provide specific, historically defined answers. Nott and Smith (1995) show how teachers manipulate the actual classroom demonstrations so that they conform to the accepted position on how they are supposed to perform. Hanauer (2006) in a study of elementary school students reveals how under the heading of scientific inquiry a multimodal structure of oral, written, visual, and physical forms of communication direct students to required and predefined results. All these studies propose that scientific inquiry within the context of pedagogical discourse can become a persuasive communicative tool designed to convince students of the correctness of predefined scientific concepts rather than a tool of scientific discovery.

Several studies have analyzed the handbooks (manuals) that are used in schools to direct scientific inquiry laboratories. In an early study using a classification tool termed *The Laboratory Structure and Task Analysis Inventory* (Tamir & Lunetta, 1978; Lunetta & Tamir, 1979), Tamir and Lunetta (1981) coded three high school curricula in the disciplines of biology, physics, and chemistry. Their findings found that "almost all investigations were highly structured" and that "Seldom, if ever, are students asked to: (a) formulate a question to be investigated; (b) formulate an hypothesis to be tested; (c) predict experimental results; work according to their own design; (d) formulate new questions based on the investigation" (Tamir & Lunetta, 1981, p. 482). In addition these researchers point out that students are "often asked to perform a variety of manipulative and observational procedures and to interpret the results of their investigations" (Tamir and Lunetta, 1981, p. 482). In a later study using the same classification tool, Germann et al. (1996) studied nine biology laboratory manuals and found, once again, that biology laboratories are highly structured and that students were seldom provided with opportunities to "pose a question to be investigated; formulate a hypothesis to be tested; predict experimental results; design observation, measurement and experimental procedures; work according to their own design; or formulate a new question or apply an experimental technique based on the investigation they performed" (Germann, Haskins, & Auls, 1996, p. 493). The results of both these studies are strikingly similar and suggest that a wide range of in-school laboratory experiences emphasize physical manipulation over conceptualization and discovery.

A different approach to the definition of scientific inquiry was developed by Chinn and Malhotra (2002). In these researchers work, the epistemological and reasoning aspects of professional science were compared with school manifestations of scientific inquiry. Using the technique of examining school textbooks for hands-on activities, these researchers differentiate between three types of simple inquiry tasks: simple experiments (a single factor experimental design), simple observations (the careful observation and description of an object), and simple illustrations (following a specific procedure). These types of scientific inquiry were compared to authentic scientific inquiry in relation to the cognitive process involved and the epistemological aspects of the tasks. In relation to the cognitive processes of generating research question, designing studies, making observations, developing theories, and studying research reports, the differences between in-school scientific inquiry and authentic inquiry are pronounced. In relation to question generation and study design, in-school scientific inquiry is teacher-directed with students following directions, whereas, scientists function much more as independent problem solvers. In relation to making observations, explaining results, and developing theories, in-school scientific inquiry thought processes are directed toward straightforwardly addressing research questions without addressing the problems of observer bias, data transformation, experimental flaws, generalizability, theory development, conflicting data and inconsistencies, and more extensive literature. In authentic science the complications and ontological status of any scientific statement is a consistent concern.

In Chinn and Malhotra's (2002) study the epistemological underpinnings of in-school scientific inquiry activities are differentiated from authentic scientific inquiry in relation to the purposes, nature of reasoning, and social construction of knowledge. Specifically authentic scientific inquiry is directed at the construction of knowledge through a variety of forms of argumentation and in the context of a community of researchers. In-school scientific inquiry does not develop knowledge, is limited in its forms of argumentation, and is not related to the wider community of scientific researchers. Zachos et al. (2000) extends this differentiation through the distinction between what they term "personal" and "cultural" discoveries. The discoveries of scientists have a historical and cultural aspect in that they constitute moments at which new knowledge is created. In this sense they are cultural discoveries. Personal discoveries involve the development of new knowledge for the individual – a moment in which an understanding of phenomena is achieved – but not a move forward for the wider scientific community. In this sense they are personal discoveries. As seen in Chinn and Malhorta (2002), in-school scientific inquiry is designed to produce personal and not cultural discoveries.

As exemplified in the studies reviewed above, a major aspect of the confusion over the concept of scientific inquiry results from the fact that under the heading of scientific inquiry a wide range of different activities are being conducted. Wenning (2005; 2007) provides a useful heuristic through which this range of scientific inquiry activities can be addressed. Wenning (2005; 2007) develops a continuum of types of scientific inquiry that differentiates forms and educational uses of inquiry in relation to the degree of teacher control and required intellectual sophistication. Wenning (2005; 2007) presents the following levels and types of scientific inquiry:

1. *Discovery Learning*: This is the most basic form of scientific inquiry and consists of a teacher-controlled activity through which students are directed to make specific observations and reach predefined conclusions.
2. *Interactive Demonstrations*: This consists of a teacher-controlled manipulation of a scientific demonstration and the request for a prediction or the explanation of the phenomena. The teacher is in complete control of the demonstration, questions, and responses. The emphasis is on the teacher's manipulation of scientific equipment.
3. *Inquiry Lessons*: This consists of a teacher-controlled demonstration of an experimental procedure. This demonstration of an experiment is accompanied by a verbalization of the conceptual and physical aspects of the experimental design. The teacher also asks leading questions and models the thought processes involved in scientific inquiry.
4. *Guided Inquiry Labs*: This consists of a teacher-directed student inquiry. Students conduct a scientific inquiry that is directed by a question presented by the teacher and lab procedures defined and guided by the teacher. Students are directed to find the answer to a specific question through the usage of a provided set of procedures (Herron, 1971).
5. *Bounded Inquiry Labs*: This consists of a student scientific inquiry that is directed by a question that is identified and posed by the teacher. The students are expected to design the experiment and conduct the scientific inquiry (Herron, 1971).
6. *Free Inquiry Labs*: This consists of a scientific inquiry that is directed by a question identified and posed by the student and an inquiry process designed and conducted by the student.
7. *Pure Hypothetical Inquiry*: This form of inquiry involves students developing hypothetical explanations of laws and explanations of physical phenomena based on empirical outcomes. This type of inquiry emphasizes pure hypothetical reasoning.
8. *Applied Hypothetical Inquiry*: This form of inquiry consists of problem-based learning in which a specific real-world problem is presented to the student and

through a process of hypothesis formulation on the basis of factual knowledge solutions and explanations are posed. Posed solutions are supported through logical argumentation and informed reasoning.

Wenning's (2005; 2007) conceptual scheme of types of scientific inquiry, building upon Herron's (1971) earlier work, clarifies the problem with the definition of scientific inquiry. Scientific inquiry is an umbrella term for a range of educational and professional activities within the sciences. While the rhetoric has tended to conflate scientific inquiry with authentic professional science, the majority of studies that consider in-school activity suggest that there are significant conceptual, physical, and epistemological differences between professional and educational scientific inquiry.

2.3 The Characteristics of Authentic Scientific Inquiry

The discussion in the previous section has brought us forward in the sense that it is clear that scientific inquiry covers a range of types of activity that are very different from what is usually done within professional science. However, this discussion does not solve the main problem that this chapter addresses – the definition of scientific inquiry as an object that can form the basis for the development of a program of assessment. The context of scientific inquiry that this book addresses is different from the ones that were discussed in the previous section. This book describes an approach to the development of assessment procedures for in-laboratory, educational scientific inquiry programs designed around authentic scientific research questions, directed by a real research agenda of interest to the wider scientific community and coordinated by an active research scientist. This context presents from an educational perspective a new configuration of the components of scientific inquiry. Using the concepts developed in the previous section, the description of this form of scientific inquiry can be characterized as follows:

1. *Development of Personal and Cultural Knowledge*: A central aspect of the type of in-laboratory educational scientific inquiry programs addressed in this book is that they are directed by the presence of an active scientist with an authentic, scientifically valuable research agenda. In other words, the research that is being conducted by the student-researcher is designed to provide both personal and cultural knowledge. The scientific inquiry process may be educational in that it provides the student with the experience of learning how research is conducted, but ultimately the aim of this research is not limited to the realm of education but rather has the goal of the creation of new scientific knowledge that is publishable.
2. *Contextualized Scientific Knowledge*: The development of a research agenda and the ability to identify what research needs to be conducted and is of value for the wider scientific community require a comprehensive and sophisticated understanding of the scientific knowledge that exists within the specific discipline. By definition, research that is conducted with the aim of producing cultural knowledge is contextualized within a specific knowledge structure. Accordingly,

students studying within a framework of this kind are exposed to contextualized scientific inquiry practices relevant to a specific body of knowledge and are not involved in the application of abstract concepts of scientific inquiry. In addition, the assumption of a program of this sort is that the knowledge that will be produced will be presented in the settings and formats that characterize scientific communication such as research articles, research reports, posters, and conference presentations.

3. *The Progression Toward High-Order Problem Solving*: The cognitive aspect of an educational scientific inquiry program that is designed to produce publishable knowledge involves the movement toward argumentation and problem solving that is used within professional science. In other words, all the complexities of real research, such as the coordination of data and theory, the design of research, the resolution of problems that occur, and the discussion of anomalous results, are part of the educational program. As argued by Hatfull et al. (2006) for this to be practical the educational scientific inquiry program has to have an accessible entry point and progressively move to more complex structures. This creates a scientific inquiry program that starts from a research process that is guided and directed by knowledge, questions, and procedures from the instructor to a situation in which the student-researcher works independently in coordination and discussion with other members of the laboratory. In the terms developed by Herron (1971) and Wenning (2005) this involves the movement from a guided inquiry laboratory to a free inquiry laboratory. It is important to note that the last stages of the research project are open ended and cannot be predicted. They evolve as a result of informed decisions made as the situations arise. One ramification of this progression is that the student cannot stay on the level of physical manipulation of laboratory equipment but rather must acquire the substantive and procedural knowledge relevant to the discipline within which the specific scientific inquiry is being conducted.
4. *Social Interaction for Scientific Goals*: Professional science is characterized by extensive social interaction with other scientists. Science is not done alone but rather is the result of a community. In educational, scientific inquiry programs designed to produce cultural knowledge the wider community of scientists within the laboratory and beyond the laboratory will be addressed. In the early stages of the educational program the scientific inquiry process is guided and directed which involves extensive interaction with professional faculty in order to facilitate the development of relevant knowledge; at later stages of the process there is also extensive interaction with professional scientists but at this stage this consists of working out how the research agenda of the whole laboratory can be moved forward. Within programs of this type, student-researchers who create cultural knowledge are expected to interact with the other scientists through the professional lines of communication such as professional conferences.
5. *Scientific Inquiry as a Multi-stage and Multi-representational Process*: A professional scientific research agenda is characterized by the presence of multiple stages of research over an extended period of time. A scientific inquiry progresses through a series of laboratory stages which often involve the

manipulation of various properties of the physical world. At each stage different physical outcomes are found and recorded in writing and visual formats. As described by Latour and Woolgar (1986), actions taken within the laboratory become meaningful when they are transformed into representational inscriptions. In this sense a lot of science is visual and representational. Accordingly, a scientific research process can be described as a series of stages each characterized by the development of a specific representational outcome.

2.4 An Analytical Framework for the Definition of Scientific Inquiry

Based on these characteristics of the educational scientific inquiry program presented above, a two-part analytical frame can be proposed to define scientific inquiry. However, before the model is described it should be remembered that the basic principle of this model is that this model is fully contextualized within the framework of a professional laboratory involved in an educational scientific inquiry designed to produce cultural knowledge. Accordingly, it is assumed that the actual definition of a scientific inquiry that will form the basis for the development of an assessment program results from the specific application of the proposed analytical framework to the definition of the specific scientific inquiry process that forms the basis for the educational program. The proposed model has two analytical parts: it proposes a series of types of knowledge that are significant for any scientific inquiry process and it then proposes an organizational structure comprised of two intersecting axes for these knowledge types.

In a study that was designed to produce assessment tools, Hanauer (2007) analyzed the scientific process of a particular educational in-laboratory scientific inquiry program from a multimodal information processing perspective (Hanauer, 2006). As presented by Hanauer (2007) the analysis of this scientific inquiry process involved four different types of information: *physical knowledge*, *representational knowledge*, *cognitive knowledge*, and *presentational knowledge*. These different types of knowledge are assumed to work together in a multimodal-layered construct and were each considered to be knowledge that needs to be assessed when considering whether scientific inquiry knowledge is being acquired. These knowledge types were defined as follows:

- *Physical knowledge* consists of knowledge required to actually perform the laboratory tasks involved in scientific inquiry.
- *Representational knowledge* consists of the written and visual representations used within the laboratory.
- *Cognitive knowledge* consists of background disciplinary knowledge of scientific content and thinking abilities such as problem solving, decision making, and calculation.

- *Presentational knowledge* consists of the ability to summarize understandings from research, to conceptualize these in manner that is valuable for the scientific community, and present them in the formats that are used by the scientific community.

The approach taken here is that in order to understand and operationally define the process of scientific inquiry, in addition to an analysis of the stages of a scientific process, scientific inquiry needs to be analyzed in terms of the types of knowledge that are utilized as part of the inquiry process. This type of analysis produces a description of the scientific inquiry process and allows assessment materials to be developed on this basis. The types of knowledge proposed by Hanauer (2007) are modeled in Fig. 2.1.

As represented in Fig. 2.1, the process of scientific inquiry is a multimodal and multilayered phenomenon that integrates four different types of knowledge. Cognitive knowledge provides the background scientific information that is crucial to the actual understanding of the science involved in the scientific inquiry process. Cognitive knowledge also involves the ability to make informed decisions, interpret physical and visual results, and make calculations. This information source feeds into the physical activities that are actually conducted in the wet laboratory. The results of the laboratory process are in the form of visual and written representations that are stored in most cases within the framework of the laboratory notebook and as physical outputs from the laboratory work itself (such as plates or gels). To understand the visual representations that were produced, cognitive knowledge is

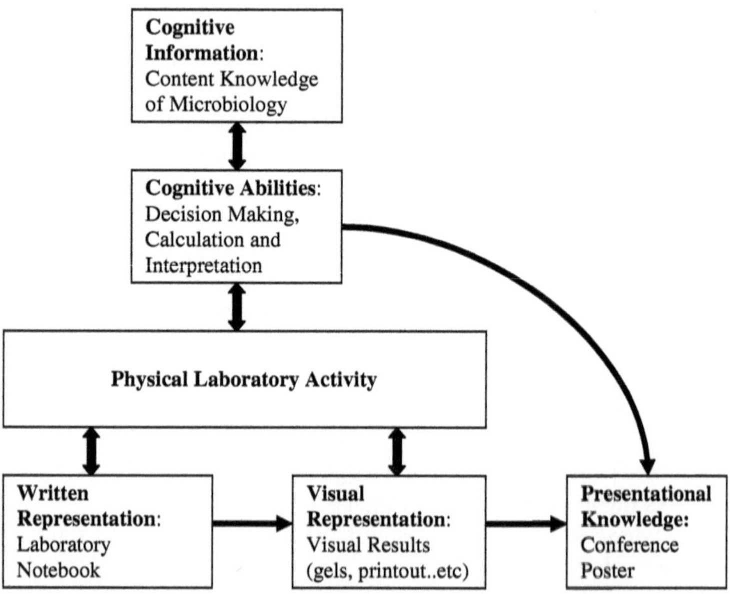

Fig. 2.1 A Schematic Representation of the Types of Knowledge Involved in a Scientific Inquiry Process

applied and decisions are made as to the future directions that need to be taken. Finally, presentational knowledge is to be considered the ability to produce a product that is useful for the wider scientific community to gain access to the research that was conducted. Presentational knowledge consists of the public presentation of conference posters (or perhaps written research papers or oral presentations) at professional conferences or within educational settings. The production of a poster integrates knowledge that comes from the notebook entries and other visual representations. The actual creation of a poster (or written/oral paper) involves the summarization and reconceptualization of the actual research that was conducted and the decision as to what makes this information important for the wider scientific community. As such to create a poster requires both the representational and cognitive knowledge sources used during the scientific inquiry. It should be noted that all the knowledge types presented above are of significance within the educational scientific inquiry program. It is the interaction between the different knowledge types that creates some of the complexity in assessing and understanding the scientific inquiry process.

The development of an assessment strategy for scientific inquiry requires a basic description of the components of scientific inquiry and the way these components are organized. The organizational approach used here specifies that scientific inquiry can be defined by two theoretical axes: the axis of knowledge source and the axis of stages of a specific scientific inquiry process. The basic idea behind this organizational structure is that scientific inquiry is a multi-stage process that involves the development of a series of in-lab outcomes (representations) over an extended period of time. Accordingly the definition of a scientific inquiry process consists of understanding the specific aspects of each knowledge source and how they develop over a period of time. Another way of understanding this model is to think of an extended scientific inquiry as a collection of much smaller scientific inquiries each of which produces a definable outcome and that collectively develop toward a research finding. For each specific stage, cognitive, physical, and representational knowledge is applied in order to reach the desired outcome, so that at different stages of the scientific inquiry different knowledge is required. Accordingly as the student progresses through the educational program knowledge will develop in relation to all the types of knowledge. From an assessment perspective, as will be discussed in later chapters, in the process of active assessment each of these axes requires a detailed analysis by the prime scientist-educator of the specific research project that is being utilized. Together the definition of knowledge for each of these two axes provides a detailed and operative description of a scientific process that can be used to generate a comprehensive assessment strategy. Figure 2.2 presents a schematic representation of the scientific inquiry process.

As an operational tool the two axes provide active researchers or observers of a scientific inquiry process a terminology and a conceptual heuristic with which to describe a scientific project in terms that are useful for assessment and educational design. The particular aspects and operational definitions of this framework are presented in Chap. 5. As seen in Fig. 2.2 the first axis divides a scientific inquiry process into representational "milestones." The idea is that a scientific process can

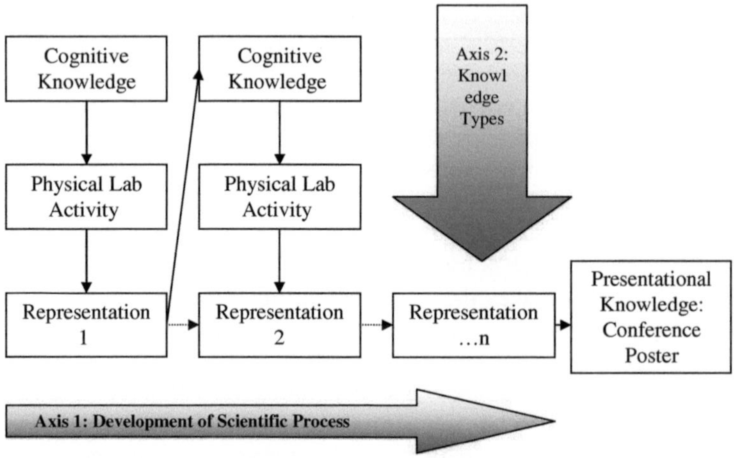

Fig. 2.2 A Schematic Representation of the Scientific Inquiry Process (*see* Color Insert)

be divided into stages according to the laboratory products that need to be produced. These products are termed representations in that they fulfill a representational role as the actual outcome of both a thinking process and physical laboratory activities. By analyzing the first axis a series of stages with specific outcomes can be defined and the overall process of scientific inquiry can be explicated. The second axis considers the types of knowledge that are required in order to produce the required laboratory representational "milestones". Every laboratory product results from the application of cognitive, representational, and physical knowledge sources. The analysis that needs to be done here is of exactly what knowledge is required to produce and comprehend each representation. This knowledge should be defined under the heading of cognitive, physical, and representational knowledge types. If both axes 1 and 2 are analyzed a detailed and operationally functional description of a specific scientific process should emerge. The detailed description of a specific scientific inquiry process is the basis upon which a comprehensive assessment program can be designed. In broad terms every assessment of an inquiry process would want to address the four knowledge sources of cognitive, physical, representational, and presentational knowledge and do so in relation to the different stages of the process itself.

2.5 Chapter Summary

The aim of this chapter was to provide an understanding of the concept of scientific inquiry that is applicable as a basis for the development of an assessment program. The following ideas and concepts were defined:

- The term scientific inquiry as manifest in different educational settings covers a wide range of diverse activities.
- The differences in types of scientific inquiry can be organized along a continuum according to the degree of teacher control and intellectual sophistication involved in each type of inquiry.
- Types of scientific inquiry can also be defined according to whether they produce cultural knowledge or personal knowledge.
- Authentic scientific inquiry is defined according to five characteristics: development of personal and cultural knowledge; contextualized scientific knowledge; the progression toward high-order problem solving; social interaction for scientific goals; and scientific inquiry as a multi-stage and multi-representational process.
- The definition of scientific inquiry that forms the basis for the development of an assessment program consists of a two-part analytical frame: the definition of knowledge types relevant to scientific inquiry and the definition of an organizational frame for these knowledge types.
- Four types of knowledge are significant for the definition of a specific scientific inquiry program: cognitive knowledge, physical knowledge, representational knowledge, and presentational knowledge. All four of these knowledge types are considered significant.
- These four types of knowledge are organized in a framework that consists of two intersecting axes: the axis of knowledge types and the axis of stages of a specific scientific inquiry. This framework describes scientific inquiry as multi-stage process that involves the development of a series of in-lab outcomes (representations) over an extended period of time.
- The definition of a scientific inquiry is contextualized within the framework of a specific research agenda in a particular scientific field that is directed by an active researcher.

Chapter 3
An Introduction to Assessment

3.1 Assessment and Science

Assessment like science is a practical, systematic, evidence-driven activity. Assessment like science produces knowledge that is used to make decisions about the nature and characteristics of the world. Simply put, assessment and science are conceptually compatible activities. It is therefore surprising that many scientists feel uncomfortable with the idea and practice of educational assessment within their educational activities. The aim of this chapter is to introduce some basic concepts and approaches to the development of assessment. As with other scientific activities, enhanced understanding of the underlying concepts and procedures that direct assessment should allow scientists an increased ability to understand their educational programs and practices. In addition, this should enhance the understanding of the specific approach to in-laboratory assessment that is developed in this book.

3.2 Assessment, Evaluation, and Testing

For many scientists one of the core points of confusion relates to the terminology of educational assessment. In this section, we will try and make some key distinctions clear. Zachos (2004) states that assessment "is the process of obtaining evidence to support inferences concerning the attainment of learning objectives" (p. 748). For Zachos, as for the authors of this book, assessment can be seen as a form of scientific inquiry process in which you collect data in order to understand student learning. Assessment in this sense is that process through which this information is attained and conclusions are reached through logical, reasoned extrapolation from collected data.

Assessment needs to be differentiated from the processes of evaluation and testing which are often used interchangeably. Evaluation refers to the process of using assessment data to judge the quality of a program or group of students. Testing refers to the tools and procedures used to elicit information that is part of the assessment

D.I. Hanauer et al., *Active Assessment: Assessing Scientific Inquiry*, Mentoring in Academia and Industry 2, DOI 10.1007/978-0-387-89649-6_3, process. This book deals with internal evaluation of in-laboratory science education programs and provides tools which can be used for evaluation purposes. However, it does not deal directly with the relationship of evaluation to external educational policy or funding. Testing is dealt with as part of the process of collecting data utilized in the assessment process. The main focus of our discussion is to provide a framework for the systematic development of an assessment strategy that will allow scientists involved in scientific inquiry teaching to assess the learning of their students.

3.3 Summative, Formative, and Diagnostic Assessment

Within the existing assessment literature a series of different aims for assessment have been defined. The National Research Committee on Classroom Assessment and the National Science Education Standards differentiate between formative and summative assessment aims. The core difference between summative and formative assessment is not the tool used to collect the data but rather the function of the conclusions from the data. Summative assessment is used for the aim of "offering a cumulative summary of achievement level" (NRC, 2001, p. 5). Formative assessment is used to "inform teaching and/or to influence learning" (NRC, 2001, p. 5). Within educational contexts summative assessment data are used to provide final grading or placement for a student taking a class. Formative assessment is used by the instructor as input in order to redirect and improve classroom teaching. In this sense formative assessment is used as a tool that informs instruction. The NRC (2001) propose that formative assessment is directed by the question "Where are you now" and that the answer to this question allows the teacher to design educational interventions that will help the student to achieve the end goals of the course. The concept directing this understanding of formative assessment involves a feedback loop between the formative assessment data that have been collected and the specific educational decisions made by the science instructor.

There is a third aim for assessment that is worth addressing. Diagnostic assessment aims to provide the instructor and the student with information concerning the current understanding and performance of the student. Diagnostic assessment has the function of identifying the student's specific strengths and weaknesses in relation to the information and procedures that are being learnt. The three aims of assessment discussed here and differentiated in relation to their functions can be summarized as follows:

- *Summative Assessment*: Aims to provide information for decisions concerning the final status of knowledge of the student
- *Formative Assessment*: Aims to provide information for decisions concerning the way to achieve the educational goals of the program
- *Diagnostic Assessment*: Aims to provide information for decisions on the current state of knowledge of the student.

These three aims for assessment should be seen as integrated and to a large extent utilizing the same data collection methods. Accordingly, an assessment strategy for an educational program usually involves all three of these assessment functions.

3.4 Distinctions in Elicitation Methods

There are a wide range of tools and procedures that can be used to elicit information useful for the assessment of student learning. A basic characteristic of all elicitation tasks is that they require students to respond to a particular prompt. The differences among elicitation tasks relate to

1. The modality of response and prompt (written, visual, physical, and/or oral)
2. The relationship of the task to authentic scientific practice (direct or indirect)
3. The discrete or integrative nature of the knowledge tested
4. The requirement to perform functions or provide knowledge in the response
5. Degree of provided structure

Elicitation tasks can be in any modality. It is common for elicitation tasks to have a written component in both the prompt and the response. But this is in no way a requirement. With a laboratory setting, for example, elicitation prompts could be verbal (for example, "show me how you use a micropipette") and the response may be physical (for example, actual usage by a student of a micropipette). This aspect of elicitation items is termed the modality of the task.

The task that is being tested could be directly drawn from the real task used within science or it could be a test of one abstract skill assumed to be significant within science. When an elicitation task is directly drawn from a real task used in science, it is considered to be an authentic task. Its authenticity is defined by the closeness of the elicitation task to the characteristics and components of the real scientific task. In some testing frameworks indirect elicitation tasks are used. An indirect task elicits information concerning a specific abstracted aspect of science. The indirect task is not modeled on a real task in science but rather is the result of an analysis of what is significant in this specific discipline and level of science.

As well known by any scientist, actually conducting scientific inquiries requires the integration of a range of skills and knowledge. Authentic elicitation tasks that are modeled on real science tend to integrate a variety of different skills and knowledge bases. Authentic elicitation tasks tend to be integrative tasks. Not all elicitation tasks are integrative. An elicitation task can address an individual part of a much larger knowledge structure. For example a student could be asked about her/his knowledge concerning the characteristics of the cell structure of a microorganism without being asked to integrate this knowledge with anything else. When the knowledge elicited from a student is done in a way that presents this knowledge as an independent item, this is termed a discrete item of knowledge. Typically, discrete elicitation tasks test one or other independent skill or content knowledge that is considered an important part of the educational aims of the course. Authentic tasks tend to be integrative and indirect tasks tend to consist of discrete items.

The prompt of an elicitation task can request that the student perform a task usually involving a form of problem solving. Tasks of this kind are termed performance tasks and the data elicited from a task of this kind is the ability of the student to do the task itself. Performance tasks address procedural knowledge of science. A prompt could also require the presentation of knowledge. Tasks of this kind are termed knowledge tasks and the data elicited from a task of this kind is the content of the knowledge presented. These tasks address substantive or content-based knowledge of science. There is a certain degree of knowledge and performance in every elicitation task. But there is difference in the intent of different types of elicitation tasks on this criterion. A performance task requires the student to actually do the task whereas a knowledge task request the presentation of knowledge.

A final characteristic of tasks refers to the varying degrees of provided structure. The structure of a task refers to the amount of guidance and direction that is provided to the student. For example, a scientific inquiry task could be open ended without any clarification of the specific tasks to be performed or it could consist of a series of prescribed directions that need to be performed. The former task would be considered to be relatively unstructured placing a large conceptual and planning responsibility on the student; whereas the latter task would be considered to be a highly structured task with detailed instructions.

For the purpose of assessment development, it can be helpful to differentiate between the specific manifestations of testing (such as multiple choice items) and the theoretical concepts that underpin these test types. Taken together the distinctions presented above in relation to elicitation tasks provide a way of classifying as well as generating elicitation methods. For example, consider a multiple choice test of substantive knowledge of a specific organism. A test of this kind would be written (modality), indirect (authenticity), discrete, knowledge-based, and structured. A test in which students are required to annotate a short sequence of DNA would be written, authentic, integrative, performance-based, and moderately structured.

3.5 Developing an Assessment Program

Tests of knowledge do not just happen. Like other forms of scientific inquiry, a basic principle of all educational assessment is that the construction of an assessment program is the result of careful and purposeful thinking. Doran et al. (2002) in their discussion of laboratory assessment specify eight stages that characterize the development of new assessments: State the Purpose, Select an Appropriate Task Format, Write or Modify the Task, Clarify Administrative Procedures, Develop a Scoring Rubric, Trial Test the Task, Revise the Task, and Analyze the Results. As specified by these researchers these stages function in a cyclical manner so that the development of appropriate assessment tasks is an on-going process of modification. These stages of development are defined as follows:

1. *State the Purpose*: The first stage of assessment development is conceptual. The initial stage of assessment development consists of defining the aims, functions, and types of knowledge to be assessed. For any assessment program there can be different aims for assessment including self-evaluation for improvement of the educational program, provision of data for external evaluation purposes, and the provision of feedback to students to enhance their educational process. The aims of program assessment should be tied to the actual aims of the educational program. If the program aims for generating knowledge of scientific facts then the assessment program should be assessing whether these facts have actually been retained by students. These real world aims are directly connected to the functions of assessment introduced in a previous section of this chapter. The concepts of summative, formative, and diagnostic assessment all define different potential functions of the assessment program. Having decided on the aims and function of the assessment program the types of knowledge to be assessed are addressed. Depending on the setting and aims of the educational program, assessment could address procedural knowledge or substantive, content knowledge of science. Furthermore the assessment designers at this stage need to consider the specific aspects of the types of knowledge that they wish to assess. Since the collection of assessment data is an extended process decisions have to be made as what will be chosen for assessment. It is assumed that all choices will address significant rather than trivial scientific knowledge.
2. *Select an Appropriate Format*: Having decided on the aims, functions, and specific knowledge that it is important to assess, the next stage of the planning process is to select an appropriate form of elicitation task for the assessment of this knowledge. As specified in a previous section of this chapter, types of elicitation task are defined according to five characteristics: modality, authenticity, discreteness, type of knowledge assessed (procedural or substantive), and degree of provided structure. The choice of specific elicitation task that will be used is directly connected to the decisions that have been made as to what is important to assess and what the functions of this data will be. For example, if the educational program aims to develop knowledge of a particular scientific concept, a written test of explicit knowledge may be suitable (the characteristics of written, indirect, discrete, and substantive). If an educational program aims to develop knowledge of a particular scientific procedure, the performance of the procedure within the laboratory and observation of the task may be suitable (the characteristics of physical, authentic, integrative, and procedural).
3. *Write or Modify the Task*: During this stage of the assessment development process, the planning that was conducted in the previous stages is translated into specific elicitation tasks that will be used for assessment purposes. Doran et al. (2002) state that issues of diversity need to be addressed at this stage. These include making the written tasks appropriate in style and language for different age groups, students with different language abilities, and students with a range of physical challenges. Before embarking on the actual writing and definition of an elicitation task it is worth considering the specific aims of the task that is being written. What knowledge does it address, is this knowledge significant,

and what type of knowledge is involved? The actual writing of an elicitation task involves making sure that what is required of the student does indeed address what the program wishes to assess. In some cases this can be straightforward as in the writing of an open-ended test question concerning factual scientific knowledge. In some cases, the development of an assessment task is more creative. It is well known within the context of testing that every elicitation task does indeed interfere with elicitation of student knowledge. Technically this is termed "task-effect" and consists of the negative contribution of the actual written tasks to the performance of the student on the task. As a result of the presence of task-effects, the writing of elicitation tasks needs careful consideration and piloting. The piloting and constant reevaluation of written tasks allows assessment developers to modify and change tasks when it is deemed necessary. In this sense the process of developing assessment tasks is an on-going task.

4. *Clarify Administrative Procedures*: Once a set of elicitation tasks has been written thought needs to be directed at the administrative and managerial aspects of the assessment process. The assessment process needs to be practical within the parameters of the educational process. Some of the practical aspects of assessment that need to be addressed are time constraints, safety procedures, ease of data collection, accessibility, and clarity. The completion of assessment procedures should be short, safe, accessible and clear to the students. While these aspects of an assessment process are obvious they are often forgotten as part of the planning of an assessment procedure. The importance of this stage is the idea that planning does not end with the development of the actual tools of elicitation but rather the actual process of administration of an assessment procedure requires consideration.
5. *Develop a Scoring Rubric*: The development of a scoring rubric consists of the exact specification of the way responses elicited from the student in relation to particular tasks will be understood by the assessment team. The development of an understanding of how the task will be completed by students is crucial for the construction of a meaningful assessment procedure. The scoring rubric should consist of sample answers, the assessment value attached to this type of answer, and the type of inference relating to the students' understanding that can be inferred from this response. In addition the scoring rubric should specify exactly the type and content of knowledge that is expected from the elicitation task. This collection of conceptual tool should allow assessment developers to define how specific answers will be understood and what they say about student learning.
6. *Trial Test the Task*: Piloting of a developed assessment procedure consists of an empirical study of the quality of the tools that have been produced. Before using the developed assessment procedure on an extensive basis with your target population, it is a good idea to evaluate the quality and characteristics of the assessment procedure by piloting the assessment procedure. The piloting of assessment materials should mimic the actual proposed usage of the tasks within the educational setting. As a piloting procedure the conclusions should be used for the evaluation of the tools and the assessment procedures themselves.

7. *Revise the Task*: The development of an assessment procedure is an on-going activity. Following the trail test of the developed assessment tasks, conclusions concerning the quality of the tasks need to be reached and any required changes need to be made. This process of revising the tasks should be considered after every administration of the assessment procedures. Through the interactive description of assessment development presented here and its associated revision of written tasks, it is assumed that assessment procedures will improve over time and become an ever more reliable method of assessment.
8. *Analyze the Results*: In principle, the analysis of the results of the assessment procedure is based on the rubric that was developed for this purpose. However, as a form of scientific inquiry, it is worth considering all results also for the ways in which they diverge from the expected responses defined by the rubric. This aspect of considering the unexpected can lead to new insights into the nature of student understanding (or misunderstanding), comprehensiveness of the rating rubric, and aspects of the task itself. While the main aim of result analysis is to provide information that can be used to assess the state of student learning and program outcomes, the analysis of the result should also be seen as having the option of providing new insights into the educational process that might not have been foreseen before administration of the assessment procedure.

3.6 Chapter Summary

The aim of this chapter was to develop basic concepts relating to the process of assessment. The following concepts and ideas were defined:

- Assessment is a form of scientific inquiry process in which you collect data in order to understand student learning.
- Assessment is differentiated from evaluation (the judgmental usage of assessment data) and testing (the procedure for collecting assessment data).
- The functions of assessment can be summative, formative, or diagnostic.
- Elicitation tasks can be defined according to five characteristics: modality, authenticity, discreteness, type of knowledge assessed, and degree of structure
- The process of developing an assessment procedure involves the stages of stating the purpose, selecting an appropriate task format, writing or modifying the task, clarifying administrative procedures, developing a scoring rubric, trial test of the task, revising the task, and analyzing the results.

Chapter 4
Assessing Scientific Inquiry

4.1 Introduction

The aim of the last chapter was to introduce some basic concepts and approaches to the development of assessment. In the current chapter, this discussion will be expanded so that it relates specifically to the issue of assessment that is addressed in this book – the assessment of scientific inquiry. This chapter reviews some of the proposals concerning scientific inquiry assessment and proposes its own approach to this issue. As discussed in previous chapters the approach taken to assessment in this book is one that places high significance on the contextual nature of scientific inquiry within an authentic research setting. Accordingly the chapter explores the concept of authentic performance assessment and discusses the importance of a deep understanding of the specific scientific inquiry process that is used in the educational program, as an initial stage in assessment development.

4.2 Approaches to the Assessment of Scientific Inquiry

The question of how to assess scientific inquiry has been addressed by several researchers and a series of assessment proposals have been presented. The differences among the approaches to assessment result from decisions concerning two issues: (1) the definition of the concept of scientific inquiry and (2) the type of elicitation method used. As described in the previous chapter the first stage in a process of developing an assessment program consists of the definition of the construct that one wishes to assess. As seen in the analysis of scientific inquiry in Chapter 2, a specific problem faced by anyone who wishes to create an assessment program for scientific inquiry is that scientific inquiry is a term that has a range of different meanings. To a certain extent the differences among the various approaches to the assessment of scientific inquiry result from the answer that each researcher provides to this question – what is scientific inquiry? A shared tendency among all the approaches to the scientific inquiry assessment is to define scientific

D.I. Hanauer et al., *Active Assessment: Assessing Scientific Inquiry*,
Mentoring in Academia and Industry 2, DOI 10.1007/978-0-387-89649-6_4,

Table 4.1 Approaches to the assessment of scientific inquiry

Source of approach	Definition of scientific inquiry	Methods of elicitation
Zachos (2004); Zachos et al. (2000)	*Core capabilities of scientific inquiry*: coordinating theories, underlying principles, precision, identifying error in measurement, and proportional reasoning	Written (open response), indirect, discrete, performance, and structured
Wenning (2007)	*Stages of scientific inquiry*: identify a problem, formulate a hypothesis, generate a prediction, design an experiment, conduct an experiment, collect (organize and analyze) data, apply statistical methods and reach conclusions, explain unexpected results, and report results	Written (multiple choice), indirect, discrete, knowledge-based, and structured
Bryce et al. (1983); Davis (1989); Welford et al. (1985)	*Practical skills*: planning, measurement, use of instruments and observation	Written, visual and physical, indirect, discrete, performance, and structured
Gott and Duggan (2002); Roberts and Gott (2003)	*Practical skills and concepts of evidence*: instruments (relationships, calibration, and error), reliability and validity of measurement, choice of instrument, sampling, design (variable structure, validity, choosing values, accuracy, precision, and tables), reliability and validity of design, data presentation, statistical treatment of data, patterns in data, and reliability and validity of investigation	Written, discrete, indirect, knowledge, and structured
Shavelson, Solano-Flores, and Araceli Ruiz Primo (1998); Solano-Flores and Shavelson (1997); Solano-Flores et al. (1999)	*Science performance assessment*: Four types of scientific inquiry – comparative, component investigation, classification, and observation	Physical and written, integrative, indirect, performance, and semi-structured
Lunsford and Melear (2004)	*Science as literacy act*: Scientific inquiry defined through the products of the portfolios, research reports, student demonstrations, student journals, and concept maps	Written and physical, integrative, direct, knowledge, and structured

inquiry in relation to a series of abstracted elements. The differences concern the type of abstraction that is proposed as significant and the way these abstracted categories of scientific inquiry are operationalized through a method of data elicitation. Table 4.1 summarizes the approaches to the assessment of scientific inquiry reviewed here and the nature of the differences in relation to the definition of scientific inquiry and methods of elicitation.

Zachos (2004) and Zachos et al. (2000), as a first stage toward the development of a scientific inquiry assessment program, conducted a study designed specifically to find those core capabilities that characterize scientific inquiry. The results of their study propose the following list of what Zachos (2000) terms critical "*scientific inquiry capabilities*:

- Coordinating theories with evidence,
- Search for an underlying principle,
- Concern for precision,
- Identifying sources of error in measurement, and
- Proportional reasoning." (p. 751)

In Zachos et al. (2000), these core capabilities were used as the conceptual basis for the design of a series of structured performance tasks. Three tasks – Floating and Sinking, Equilibrium on the Balance Beam and the Period of the Pendulum – were chosen from the research conducted by Inhelder and Piaget (1958) because they posed conceptual problems for students as they tried to construct and evaluate concepts of scientific phenomena. These tasks were considered to be useful for both developing and assessing scientific inquiry capabilities. However, Zachos (2004) suggests that the use of structured inquiry tasks and direct observation of performance is not feasible within educational systems in which the ratio of student-instructor is high and thus proposes that students be presented with the structured performance task and then asked to record "their responses on a special form" (p. 753). The responses would be assessed according to the core set of scientific inquiry capabilities that was defined by Zachos et al. (2000). In this sense the scientific inquiry capabilities are transformed into a set of performance indicators that are used to assess written responses to a structured inquiry task.

Wenning (2007), working within the context of physics education, designed a diagnostic multiple choice test of knowledge relevant for scientific inquiry. As specified by this test's creator, this test is not designed to "authentically assess student abilities to conduct scientific inquiry" (Wenning, 2007, p. 24). The test is designed to provide measures of students' development of knowledge concerning scientific inquiry and would be ideal for the pre- and post-testing of the development of such knowledge. As an initial stage of the test development process, Wenning (2005) conducted a literature review of academic materials that define scientific inquiry and proposed a list of stages that define the scientific inquiry process. This list was then reviewed by physics-teaching majors, scientists, and educators. The final list of stages was as follows:

- Identify a problem to be investigated.
- Formulate a hypothesis or model using induction from logic and evidence.
- Generate a prediction using deduction.
- Design an experimental procedure to test prediction.
- Conduct a scientific experiment, observation, or simulation to test the hypothesis or model.
- Collect meaningful data, organize, and analyze data accurately and precisely.

- Apply numerical and statistical methods to reach conclusions.
- Explain unexpected results.
- Use available technology to report, display, and defend results.

This list of the stages of scientific inquiry was used as a basis for the development of 40 multiple choice questions that cover the defined stages. Following repeated piloting, five questions were deleted and some questions changed and reworded leaving the final version of the test with 35 questions.

A different approach to the definition of scientific inquiry consisted of considering the practical, procedural aspects of scientific inquiry as central (Archenhold et al., 1988; Bryce et al., 1983; Davis, 1989; Welford et al., 1985). This type of approach sees issues such as measurement and instrument use as what needs to be taught and assessed within an educational inquiry program. The assessment of knowledge relating to practical skills could be in both a performance format in which students make readings of present instruments and a written format in which pictures of instruments are presented and students are required to provide a written response.

Gott and Duggan (2002) and Roberts and Gott (2003) working in the field of biology developed an approach to the assessment of scientific inquiry based on their concept of knowledge-based enquiry. According to Roberts and Gott (2003) knowledge-based enquiry is characterized by a focus on the understandings that result from a particular set of actions in a specific context of investigation. As such scientific inquiry involves an integration of a set of skills utilized within the laboratory and substantive knowledge addressing the same context. Specifically Gott and Duggan (2002) develop a set of concepts, termed concepts of evidence, that describe the types of understanding of action that they consider useful in characterizing scientific inquiry. This list consists of

- "Instruments: underlying relationships
- Instruments: calibration and error
- Reliability and validity of a single measurement
- The choice of an instrument for measuring datum
- Design: Variable structure
- Design: Validity, 'fair tests' and controls
- Design: Choosing values
- Design: Accuracy and precision
- Design: tables
- Reliability and validity of the design
- Data presentation
- Statistical treatment of measurements of data
- Patterns and relationships in data
- Reliability and validity of the data in the whole investigation" (Gott and Duggan, 2002, p. 117).

Roberts and Gott (2003), while careful not to associate the written test of concepts of evidence as an assessment of the performance of scientific inquiry, do suggest that their list of concepts of evidence can be used in a written format and provide useful information on the knowledge-based aspects of scientific inquiry.

Solano-Flores and Shavelson (1997) and Shavelson et al. (1998) have developed an approach to the assessment of scientific inquiry, termed science performance assessment (SPA), which is based on the presentation of structured performance tasks to students in conjunction with a clearly formulated scoring system. As stated by Shavelson et al. (1998) "SPA should put a student in a laboratory, pose a problem, and watch as the student devises procedures for carrying out an investigation, analyzes data, draws inferences by linking data to prior knowledge (e.g., relevant theory), and comes to a conclusion and a problem solution" (p. 171). These researchers divide the structured tasks that they create for assessment purposes into four different types:

- Comparative investigations (scientific inquiries that "compare two or more objects on some attribute while controlling other variables" (p. 172));
- Component-identification investigations (scientific inquiries that require the determination of the parts that make up the whole);
- Classification investigations (scientific inquiries that require the development of a classification scheme utilizing the attributes of a set of objects);
- Observation investigation (scientific inquiries that involve the recording of a systematic observation over a period of time).

A core aspect of these researchers' approach to assessment is the development of a reliable scoring system that addresses the central aspects of each inquiry type. For comparative investigation, the way the procedure is constructed and the accuracy of the problem are considered central. For a component-identification investigation confirming and disconfirming the presence of components is considered central. For a classification investigation usage of object attributes is considered central. For the observation investigation accuracy of results based on the observation and the development of explanatory models is central. The actual manifestation of science performance tasks consists of the construction of a specific task according to the guidelines of one of the research types, the performance of this task by the student, and the assessment of the task through the observation of the task in accordance with the guidelines of the scoring system.

In a later paper, Solano-Flores et al. (1999) widen their concept of science performance assessments by proposing a "shell" for the design of new performance assessments. These researchers define shells as "blueprints that provide directions for assessment developers to generate reliable, valid PAs [performance assessments] in a short time" (Solano-Flores et al., 1999, p. 294). The shell format builds upon the previous work conducted by this group of researchers and presented in Solano-Flores and Shavelson (1997) and Shavelson et al. (1998). Working within the scheme of the four inquiry types reviewed above, the shell divides the task into four student stages: planning, hands-on investigation, analysis, and interpretation and application. The shell also allows the manipulation of the task according to the type of equipment, the number of variables, the amount of conceptual information, the directions given, and the use of equipment. Through the manipulation of these factors the inquiry tasks can be conceptually simpler or more difficult. The manifestation of this approach is similar to that of the previous assessments conducted by these researchers. A task is presented to the student and this is assessed through assessment of student notebooks using the developed scoring system.

Using a more modest approach, Lunsford and Melear (2004) propose that the way to evaluate scientific inquiry is through a close consideration of the outcome of the scientific inquiry process. In their approach they avoid directly assessing the process of scientific inquiry and rather suggest that the final product of the inquiry can be used to infer what the student learnt and what was actually done in the project. Within this approach a variety of different outcomes could be assessed. They suggest the use of portfolios (observation notes, data, etc.), scientific research papers, laboratory practicals and student demonstrations, student journals, and concept maps. For each of these products a specific set of assessment criteria have been proposed. The criteria are based on the genre aspects of the form of writing and components that are found within each of these written products. For example a research report is evaluated for the presence of a research question; a hypothesis; a literature review; a methods section; data presentation in tables, charts, and graphs; usage of references; references in paper; a bibliography; good grammar; and punctuality.

This list of approaches is not intended as a comprehensive meta-analysis of all the work that has been done on the issue of assessment and scientific inquiry. But it does capture the conceptual directions that have been proposed in different educational settings. Broadly the approaches presented above can be differentiated into two groups: those methods which assess scientific inquiry as an abstracted form of knowledge that could inform a range of studies and those which require students to perform a structured scientific task. The latter group can be further differentiated between the assessment of practical knowledge of instruments and measures and those that require different levels of problem solving. A review of all these approaches to assessment and the way they define scientific inquiry presents an array of knowledge types that collectively seem to cover the nature of scientific inquiry. These types of knowledge and abilities can be divided according to the following scheme:

1. *Substantive Knowledge*: Knowledge of scientific concepts, facts, and processes; knowledge of the stages and components of a scientific inquiry
2. *Procedural Knowledge*: Knowledge of procedural aspects of how to conduct a scientific inquiry; knowledge of the equipment and materials within a scientific inquiry
3. *Problem Solving and Integrative Abilities*: The ability to solve problems, pose solutions, conceptualize results, and reach conclusions

Based on this review, scientific inquiry would seem to be a multifaceted activity that requires several different levels and types of knowledge that need to be used in an integrative and problem-solving manner.

All the ways of assessing reviewed here in varying degrees rely on indirect, inauthentic measures of scientific task performance. This results in a large extent from the mass education school age framework of the educational settings that they address. In-school scientific inquiry poses a series of problems such as large class sizes; the requirement to address national, state, and federal educational authorities; lack of equipment; difficulties in current scientific knowledge; classroom management issues; and the emphasis within schools on established knowledge that impede the use of authentic scientific inquiry organized around disciplinary significant research questions. For the authors of this book and the direction that is proposed here, authenticity is a serious issue.

Messick (1994), in a discussion of authentic assessment, points out that one of the problems in relation to validity of assessment measures is that of construct underrepresentation. As defined by Messick (1994) construct underrepresentation is a situation in which the authentic characteristics of tasks are not captured by the mode of assessment chosen. The multifaceted nature of scientific discourse, as well as the indirect, inauthentic way that it is assessed, poses the problem of construct underrepresentation in relation to the assessment of scientific inquiry. To have a valid assessment of scientific inquiry the different facets of authentic scientific inquiry need to be covered.

4.3 Authentic Assessment

A central aspect of authentic assessment is it situates the knowledge to be assessed within its social, physical, conceptual, and disciplinary contexts. As defined by Cumming and Maxwell (1999) authentic assessment considers real tasks in their context of performance and requires the person who is being assessed to apply expert problem-solving skills to the task on hand. Performance assessment focuses specifically on the completion of a specific task. What makes this approach authentic assessment is that the task requires the integration of disciplinary (contextually) specific knowledge in order to complete the task. Shavelson, Baxter, and Pine (1992) specify that performance testing requires students to perform concrete meaningful tasks that are assessed in relation to the types of reasoning and thinking that are applied to the task and not just the outcome. Stenmark (1991), in an early and rather open description, defines performance assessment as a procedure which involves "presenting a student with a task, project or investigation and then observing, interviewing, and looking at their products to assess what they actually know" (p. 13).

Herrington and Herrington (2006), summarizing the work of a series of researchers, offer the following set of characteristics that define the nature of authentic assessment:

1. Authentic assessment should involve an accurate recreation of the conditions under which the performance of the tasks would occur in its authentic setting (Reeves & Okey, 1996; Meyer, 1992; Wiggins, 1993).
2. Authentic assessment involves problem-solving skills and higher-order thinking (Reeves 2000; Newman & Wehlage, 1993)

3. Authentic assessment involves the production of new knowledge and not just the memorization and reproduction of established understandings (Newman & Archbald, 1992).
4. Authentic assessment involves complex tasks that involve student decision making and multiple steps (Wiggins, 1990; 1993; Linn, Baker, & Dunbar, 1991; Torrance, 1995; Reeves, 2000).
5. Authentic assessment is fully integrated with the activities that are the focus of the learning process (Reeves & Okey, 1996; Young, 1995).

As described above, authentic assessment implies a correspondence between the assessment task and the professional, real-world performance of the same task. From an assessment perspective, Gulikers (2006) provides an important criterion for evaluating the authenticity of an authentic assessment task when she states that "the authenticity of an assessment is defined by its resemblance to the real world" (p. 22). She defines this authentic, real-world task (termed the *criterion situation*) as the point of comparison for the assessment task. The degree of resemblance between these two manifestations of this task is the measure of the authenticity of the task. On this basis her definition of authentic assessment task is "*an assessment that requires students to use the same competencies, or combinations of knowledge, skills and attitudes that they need to apply in the criterion situation in professional life*" (p. 23). This definition of authentic assessment addresses a range of dimensions that function in relation to any real-world task. These include the nature of the task itself, the physical context of the task, the social setting and forms of professional interaction, the professional outcomes of this task, and the real-world criteria that are used within professional practice in relation to this task.

For the purposes of the approach to the assessment of scientific inquiry developed in this book, it is important to specify the ramifications of authentic assessment on the educational program. The first ramification deals with the concept of the construct validity of an assessment. Construct validity is defined as the degree to which an assessment task actually measures what it is supposed to measure. Since authentic assessment has a high degree of resemblance to the criterion situation and recreates the professional aspects of conducting the task under normal circumstances, authentic assessment tasks have very high levels of construct validity. Accordingly, the assessment of knowledge through an authentic assessment task should be a good predictor of the way the same task would be conducted within a professional setting. In other words, if one of the main aims of in-laboratory science instruction is to provide students with an experience of professional science and the instructor with some indicator of who has potential as a scientist, authentic assessment provides data on performance with an authentic laboratory task.

The second ramification is the inherent motivation and meaning that is found within authentic assessment tasks. Several researchers have specified that authentic assessment engages students and has a positive effect on student learning and motivation (Herrington & Herrington, 1998; McDowell, 1995; Sambell, McDowell, & Brown, 1997). As a result of the authentic contextualized nature of the performance of the task utilized for assessment, the procedure itself becomes part of the instructional design and provides diagnostic information that is directly applicable to the student's learning and development (Darling-Hammond & Falk, 1997). Authentic performance assessment has been recommended as particularly suitable for the development of scientific concepts and the enhancement of communicational skills required for problem solving in this context (Shymansky et al. 1997). This approach to assessment can legitimize the use of a wide variety of sources of information that provide evidence of both the process and outcomes of a student's learning process. Performance assessment really allows teachers to focus on students' higher-order thinking and reasoning. Finally and most importantly science students who were involved in performance assessment were found to have more metacognition of their reasoning processes and conceptualizations than students who underwent traditional testing procedures (Firestone Mayrowetz, & Fairman, 1998). In addition, authentic assessment which models professional activity is seen by students and instructors as a stage toward professional activity and not as an artificial measure of ability. As such, authentic assessment has the potential to be meaningful to the student on a personal level and provides the student with the option of really judging what the professional experience of science is like.

4.4 The Characteristics of Authentic Scientific Inquiry Assessment (ASIA)

As specified in the first chapter of this book, the context of interest for the current discussion of assessment is the in-laboratory scientific inquiry educational program. This educational setting is different from those that the previous approaches have addressed. However, from a conceptual perspective, the approach described here builds upon previous understandings of the ways to assess scientific inquiry. Specifically this approach builds upon the concepts of authentic assessment, the multifaceted nature of scientific inquiry, and the importance of carefully defining performance assessments.

The core characteristic of the approach described here is the importance it places upon authenticity in the educational program and the assessment of knowledge. For this reason the approach is best termed as authentic scientific inquiry assessment (ASIA).

As discussed in the previous section, authenticity in assessment is measured through the degree of comparison between the situation criterion (the real-world situation) and the assessment task. For an assessment task to be considered authentic it needs to have a high degree of equivalence with the tasks, the physical context, the social setting, forms of professional interaction, the professional outcomes of this task, and the real-world criteria that are used within professional practice in relation to this task. This form of assessment also requires students to use the same competencies or combinations of knowledge, skills, and attitudes that would be used in the professional setting.

The setting for assessment that the current discussion deals with is the in-laboratory, scientific inquiry, educational program directed by the presence of a research question that is significant within the wider scientific community. This specific educational setting allows high degrees of authenticity as it is situated in a laboratory and organized around real scientific research. The real issue for the development of an assessment program is to be able to accurately describe the nature of the educational, scientific activity and identify points of significance and value that constitute qualitative shifts in the understanding and practice of this scientific inquiry. In other words, the assessment procedures need to be able to accurately reflect the significant aspects of the scientific inquiry process that is at the heart of the educational program.

The answer that is at the center of the process of assessment development within the ASIA approach is the proposition that assessment development is preceded by empirical description of the scientific inquiry program. As seen in the approaches described in a previous section of this chapter, the definition of scientific inquiry was an early stage of most assessment development programs. The emphasis in ASIA is on the description of the knowledge, procedures, and representations that construct a specific scientific inquiry that is being used within the in-laboratory educational program. The assumption is that authentic scientific inquiry is a contextualized process that requires specialized knowledge. Accordingly, the starting point of assessment development is the empirical description of the specific aspects of this scientific inquiry.

The practicalities of an initial empirical description of a scientific inquiry that is relevant for assessment development pose a problem for most active scientist-educators. Accordingly the active assessment approach provides an analytical framework through which specific scientific inquiry programs can be analyzed in a manner that produces valuable distinctions. The next chapter provides a full description of this framework. From a conceptual assessment perspective, the approach used here involves a reversal of direction of the generative shell proposition for assessment development proposed by Solano-Flores et al. (1999). In the proposition of Solano-Flores et al. (1999) an analytic shell describing types of scientific inquiry tasks provided a framework for the production of new tasks following the same underpinning definitions. In the active assessment proposal, this analytic frame is used by scientist-educators to analyze the process of scientific inquiry that they are using in their laboratory. This analysis of scientific inquiry process produces a set of distinctions and categories of knowledge that can be used to define specific assessment tasks. The overall aim of this stage is to provide a theoretical framework for analyzing and characterizing the tasks that collectively define the scientific process that will be assessed. Since these assessment tasks are based on a process of empirical description conducted by the scientist-educator and drawn directly from the specific scientific inquiry utilized within the educational program, it is assumed that they will have a very high degree of authenticity.

An additional aspect of the ASIA proposal is the attempt for comprehensiveness in assessment. As seen in the previous section, scientific inquiry involves different types of knowledge and abilities. In order to capture the authentic aspects of the specific scientific inquiry used within the in-laboratory educational program it is assumed that assessment will need to be multifaceted, involve several different elicitation formats and be conducted at different times. In this sense, ASIA is a process that both follows and is integrated within the actual experience of scientific inquiry with the in-laboratory scientific experience.

The characteristics of ASIA can be summarized as follows:

1. *Authenticity Through Empirical Description*: A high degree of equivalence is required between the situation criterion and the assessment tasks resulting from an initial stage of assessment development that consists of the empirical description of the specific scientific inquiry process that is at the core of the scientific agenda of the laboratory and the educational process.
2. *Multimethod Approach*: Since scientific inquiry is considered to be multifaceted, in order to capture the different aspects of scientific inquiry an assessment program will need to involve different components using different elicitation methods.

4.5 Active Assessment Development

The active assessment development procedure consists of the following stages:

1. *Empirical Description of Scientific Inquiry*: The first stage of assessment development consists of in-depth qualitative research that explores the nature of the scientific process being investigated. The analysis of the process is conducted using a developed framework for the analysis of the process of scientific inquiry and the types of knowledge and abilities required in this inquiry process. The aim of this stage is to characterize the tasks that collectively define the scientific process that will be assessed.
2. *Definition of Educational Aims:* Following the empirical description of the scientific process that is utilized within the educational, scientific inquiry program, the educational aims of the program that the scientist-educator wants to assess need to be defined. A special aspect of the active assessment approach is the idea that the educational aims of program and the definition of significant scientific educational development are directly tied to the scientist-educators' understanding of the scientific inquiry process at the heart of the educational program. In other words, the definition of what is important to evaluate within the educational program results from the understanding and analysis of what is important within the scientific inquiry process itself. Specifically, in relation to active assessment, the scientist-educator will have to decide which of the various representational milestones (and associated cognitive and physical knowledge) is to be assessed. It is assumed that the whole process of assessment will address summative, formative, and diagnostic aims and will address representational, cognitive, physical, and presentational knowledge.

3. *Assessment Tool Development*: Once the scientific process has been characterized and the significant aspects of the process decided upon, the process of tool development can start. A core principle of this stage is the idea that the assessments need to be as authentic as possible and are directly tied to the analysis of the scientific inquiry process conducted as a first stage of active assessment. The development of specific assessment tools is the attempt to model directly the aspects of conducting the scientific inquiry itself. There are different ways of doing this, and tools of this kind could come in different elicitation formats. However, at every point it is important to understand that the tools should be directly tied and modeled on the analysis of the specific inquiry process that is being used in the educational program. The set of tools developed should comprehensively cover all the different types of knowledge used by professional researchers in conducting this type of scientific inquiry. In order for the assessment tools to be authentic they will need to integrate physical, representational, cognitive, and presentational knowledge.
4. *Scoring Rubric Development*: Having created a set of tools through which knowledge will be assessed in the educational program, a set of scoring rubrics need to be developed. As with the development of the tools themselves, a core aspect of the active assessment approach is that the scoring of the tasks is as authentic as possible. In other words, the criteria for success are drawn from the context of conducting the same tasks within the professional setting. The scoring rubrics should be defined according to the professional knowledge of the scientist-educator. As with all scoring rubrics, criteria for successful and problematic outcomes on these tasks need to be defined. The scoring rubrics provide the educational team and the student-researcher with both formative and diagnostic information that can enhance the educational program.
5. *Assessment Piloting*: As with any other assessment process, it is important to pilot the developed assessment tools. The process of piloting consists of using the developed tools with a smaller subset of the population and the constant reflective evaluation of the ability of the tools to assess the defined educational aims of the program. The stages of tool development, rubric development, and piloting are closely interrelated. A core assumption of active assessment is that piloting stage will evolve and change the tools that are used and the way they are scored. The outcome of this whole process should be an assessment strategy consisting of a series of piloted tools, which is authentic to the specific scientific process that is being taught, which is meaningful to the student and instructors, and which can be scored in a reliable, systematic manner.

4.6 Chapter Summary

The aim of this chapter was to review proposals concerning ways of assessing scientific inquiry and to propose a specific process for the assessment of scientific inquiry termed authentic scientific inquiry assessment (ASIA). The following ideas and concepts were defined:

1. A range of assessment procedures have been developed to assess scientific inquiry. These procedures differ in relation to the way they define scientific inquiry and the elicitation methods that they employ. These procedures rely on indirect, inauthentic measures of scientific inquiry.
2. A comprehensive analysis of the different definitions of scientific inquiry for assessment purposes defines scientific inquiry as multifaceted and involving substantive knowledge of scientific facts, concepts, and process, substantive knowledge of the stages and components of scientific inquiry, procedural knowledge of how to conduct a scientific inquiry, procedural knowledge of equipment and materials, and problem-solving abilities.
3. Authentic assessment creates assessment procedures that are closely modeled on real-world tasks and require the same conceptual, physical, and social abilities as the real-world task.
4. Authentic assessment enhances student engagement and motivation and limits questions of construct validity.
5. ASIA is an approach that is characterized through its definition of assessment tasks by a process of empirical description that enhances the authenticity of the assessment procedures and its emphasis on comprehensive multifaceted assessment of scientific inquiry.
6. The process of active assessment development consists of five stages: empirical description, definition of aims, tool development, rubric development, and assessment piloting.

Chapter 5
An Analytical Framework for the Development of Scientific Inquiry Assessment

5.1 Introduction

The aim of this chapter is to provide scientist-educators with a set of conceptual tools that can be used to develop an assessment program for in-lab, educational, scientific inquiry programs. This chapter operationalizes the concept of authentic scientific inquiry assessment (ASIA) within the active assessment approach. As argued in previous chapters, a core assumption of the active assessment approach is the idea that the prime researcher within a professional research laboratory is directly involved in the design of both the educational scientific inquiry program and the way this program is assessed. Accordingly, this chapter is designed to provide the scientist-educator with a terminology and conceptual methodology to fulfill this function.

5.2 Stages of Active Assessment Development

As described in the previous chapter, the process of developing an assessment program for scientific inquiry involves five stages: empirical description, definition of aims, tool development, rubric development, and assessment piloting. Figure 5.1 schematically represents the active assessment development process.

As discussed in the last chapter and schematically represented in Fig. 5.1, the core aspect of the active assessment approach to the development of authentic scientific inquiry assessment is the significance assigned to the empirical description of the scientific inquiry process. Active assessment aims to develop an overall assessment approach that is as authentic and as meaningful as possible. Accordingly the central task of assessment development is the explicit description of the scientific inquiry process that can form the basis of the assessment tasks. The authors of this book recognize that one of the problems that this poses to the scientist-educator is the actual conceptual organization of this knowledge in a format that can generate assessment tools. The sections that follow are designed to provide this conceptual framework through which the aims of active assessment can be achieved.

D.I. Hanauer et al., *Active Assessment: Assessing Scientific Inquiry*,
Mentoring in Academia and Industry 2, DOI 10.1007/978-0-387-89649-6_5,

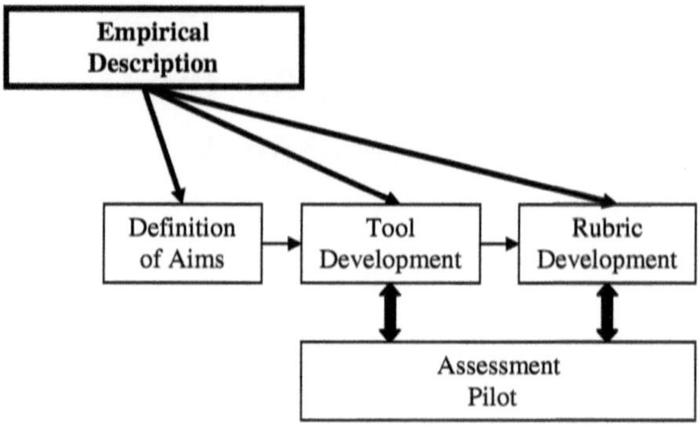

Fig. 5.1 A schematic representation of the active assessment development process

5.2.1 Stage 1: Empirical Description of Scientific Inquiry

The first stage of the active assessment process consists of the empirical description of the scientific inquiry process which constitutes the educational program. In some ways, the aim of this section, in helping professional scientists to define their scientific inquiry processes, is paradoxical. As professional scientists you are well aware of your own scientific inquiry processes and for your own professional activities you are not in need of any help from the authors of this book. However, in developing an assessment program, the conceptual framework developed here may be useful for its ability to create distinctions in the types of knowledge required and the ways these are integrated and organized across the scientific inquiry process. As will be described in the next section of this book, our experience within our microbiology laboratory has shown that this way of describing the scientific inquiry process is a useful way to generate a set of assessment tools and an overall strategy toward the assessment of our program.

The conceptual framework is constructed from the model of scientific inquiry proposed in Chap. 2 of this book and consists of a series of directed questions which should allow a clear description of a specific scientific inquiry process to emerge. As described in Chap. 2, the description of a specific scientific inquiry process consists of the analysis of two axes: Axis 1 consists of an analysis of the stages of development of the scientific inquiry process; Axis 2 consists of the types of knowledge required in order to complete the scientific inquiry process. As seen in Chap. 2 this is schematically represented in Fig. 5.2.

As seen in Fig. 5.2, the core assumption of this model is that professional scientific inquiry is an extended process and consists of a series of stages with concrete outcomes. Each of these stages and outcomes is seen as a form of "milestone" in the process of scientific inquiry and when accumulated these stages of the scientific inquiry process lead to potentially significant findings. Within the scientific inquiry process each of these stages or outcomes is seen through the presence of a particular form of visual representation. This representation might be as diverse as a

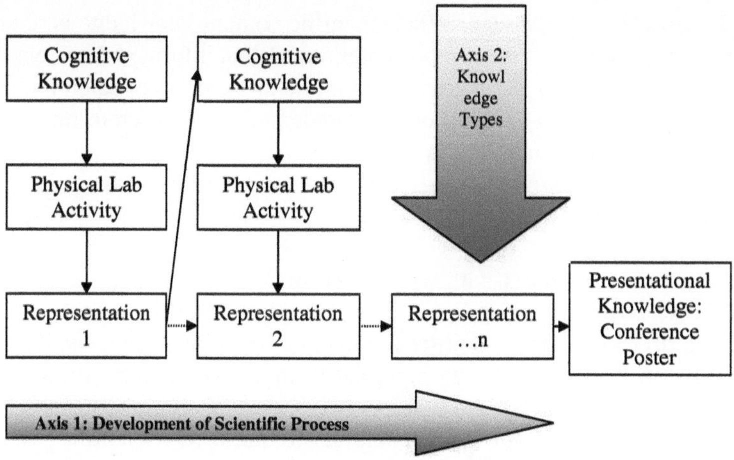

Fig. 5.2 A schematic representation of the scientific inquiry process (*see* Color Insert)

fluctuation on a computer readout or a plaque community on a dish. But there is some form of visual representation that marks the completion of a stage of the inquiry. Accordingly, these representations can be used to divide the scientific inquiry process into stages. For each of these stages specific physical manipulations will need to be done. In other words, the outcomes are dependent on some form of physical manipulation. For these manipulations and representational outcomes to be meaningful, the researcher needs to understand the relevant substantive knowledge and associated procedural understandings. Taken together, the cognitive, physical, and representational knowledge types organized along the developmental line of the scientific inquiry process should produce a description of the specific inquiry process used in the educational program.

The conceptual framework presented here consists of a series of questions asked and answered by the prime researcher and designer of the educational, scientific inquiry program. These questions are to be thought of as a form of reflective exercise in which the scientist-educator explores her/his own knowledge of the scientific inquiry process. It is assumed by the authors of this book that most scientists will be very well acquainted with their own research agendas and associated knowledge types. What this reflective exercise provides is a way of explicating, categorizing, and organizing this implicit knowledge base.

The first set of questions, designed according to the two axes of scientific inquiry, is planned to explicate the process itself and consists of the following:

1. *Axis 1: Representational Knowledge*: What types of representation are produced within the scientific inquiry process?
2. *Axis 2: Inquiry Process Development*: Is there a specific expected order for the production of these representations? What is that order (or potential orders)?
3. *Axis 1: Physical Knowledge:* What physical procedures are required to produce these representations?

4. *Axis 1: Cognitive Knowledge:* What scientific content knowledge is required to understand and interpret these representations? What informed decisions (or calculations) need to be made in order to continue this process of scientific inquiry? What does one need to know in order to understand the different representation produced within the scientific inquiry process?
5. *Axis 1: Presentational Knowledge:* In what ways and in what settings are the results of this scientific inquiry presented to the community of scientists?

The analytical process starts with a consideration of the specific representations found in the scientific inquiry process. The first question of this stage provides the basis for the division of the scientific inquiry process into stages. By focusing on concrete outcomes and their representational form a basis is created for the design of later assessment measures.

Having defined the specific representations found in this scientific process the second question deals with the way these representations organize the development of the scientific inquiry process. By focusing on the order of the representation the overall scientific inquiry process is divided into distinct stages according to the production of a specific outcome that is represented in a particular way. Through questions 1 and 2, the specific representations that are expected and the order in which they are expected create a timeline of the specific scientific inquiry that is being taught.

For some professional scientific inquiry programs, it is possible that the last stages of the inquiry cannot be determined at the beginning of the process, in that the scientific inquiry process is open ended (with every finding leading to yet another set of research questions). Accordingly, for some in-lab, educational, scientific inquiry programs it is assumed that only the first two-thirds of the program can be mapped out according to known representations.

Once the first two questions have been answered and a timeline of representations has been created, questions 3 and 4 address the physical and cognitive knowledge required to produce and understand each of these representations. The physical procedures that need to be assessed may include the working of equipment, ascetic practice, safety behaviors, and a wide range of laboratory work. For each representation, the physical actions which lead to this outcome need to be noted. In order to produce the specific representation, relevant scientific knowledge needs to be known. The prime researcher should consider what scientific knowledge needs to be known in order to understand what is happening that produces the required result from a scientific perspective. This will include factual knowledge of the processes and factors that influence any given outcome. In addition, the prime researcher should consider the problem-solving aspects associated with a particular stage of the scientific inquiry. What decisions need to be made? What are the range of options for interpreting the results found? What are the ways in which a particular representation can be understood? For most scientists the main problem with questions 3 and 4 is recognizing the depth of their contextualized scientific knowledge. Novice researchers will know far less than the expert and may often surprise researchers with questions that are truly basic. When considering the knowledge required in order to complete and understand a stage of a scientific inquiry, it is worth taking a very conservative approach to the amount of knowledge that students may have and to consider very basic as well as more sophisticated knowledge that contributes to the understanding of the process. The definition of physical and cognitive knowledge needs to be given for each of the representation along the timeline of the scientific inquiry process. The outcome of questions 1–4 should be a detailed description of a scientific inquiry process that includes physical, cognitive, and representational knowledge and is organized along a timeline of representations. The fifth question addresses provisional outcomes of the inquiry process and explores the ways in which scientific knowledge is commonly presented within the specific discipline.

5.2.2 Stage 2 – Definition of Aims

Having developed an explicit description of the scientific inquiry process, the second stage of active assessment development consists of deciding on the aims of assessment and the definition of significant scientific knowledge. During stage two, types of decision need to be made. The first decision addresses the relationship between the assessment and the objectives of the educational program. The second set of decisions addresses the definition of knowledge that is to be considered significant within the specific scientific inquiry process used in the educational program. Together these two sets of decisions define the purpose and content of the assessment program.

The first decision relates to the characteristics of the educational program itself. The prime scientist-educator needs to consider what the educational program is really trying to achieve from an educational perspective. The aims of the assessment program are tied directly to the overall objectives of the educational program. As such these aims need to be explicitly expressed so that the role of assessment in providing evidence that assess these aims can be defined. This stage of active assessment development is directed by the following two questions:

1. What are the aims of the educational program?
2. What are the aims and purposes of the assessment program?

In most scientific inquiry programs, the aims of assessment are summative, formative, and diagnostic. The aims of assessment are to provide evidence on the outcomes of learning (summative) and to improve instruction and facilitate student learning (formative and diagnostic). In science education, there may be specific aims such as the development of scientific literacy or acquaintance with a specific scientific discipline. The aims of the assessment program need to be explicitly and clearly written out. From a methodological perspective, these aims function as a set of research questions that direct the process of data collection in the form of assessment.

The second set of decisions deals with the content of scientific knowledge that is considered important for the specific scientific inquiry project that is utilized within the educational program. This stage is directly informed by the empirical description developed in the first stage of active assessment development and consists of deciding on the hierarchy of knowledge within the scientific inquiry process. A basic assumption of this stage is that the assessment process will address significant knowledge that is crucial for understanding this specific scientific inquiry. Accordingly, decisions need to be made as to what consists of significant knowledge within this specific scientific inquiry process. This aspect of active assessment is directed by the following questions:

1. Of the representations defined in this scientific process (see question 1 above), which of these representations could be considered a representational "milestone" in the development of this scientific process? (A limited set of crucial, milestone representations in the development of a scientific inquiry need to be chosen.)
2. What physical laboratory knowledge, cognitive scientific knowledge, cognitive interpretive and decision-making knowledge, and knowledge of visual representation are required to create and understand the milestone representations that have been chosen (see previous question)? (The required knowledge in each case needs to be explicated as fully as possible.)

The outcome of this analytical process is the decision that a subset of stages within the scientific inquiry process is of greater significance from a knowledge perspective than others in this specific scientific inquiry process. Each of the stages should be considered as a significant moment within the timeline of the scientific inquiry that can be used as a measure of the student-researchers' development of understanding of the scientific inquiry process.

5.2.3 Stage 3: Tool Development

The aim of this active assessment stage is the actual development of tools that can be used with student-researchers in order to assess knowledge development. As discussed in previous chapters, scientific inquiry is assumed to be multifaceted and as such a multimethod approach will be required to assess its different aspects. In addition, a core assumption of active assessment is the value placed on authenticity. There are several considerations that need to be addressed during the development of assessment tools:

- Comprehensively address representational, cognitive, physical, and presentational knowledge relevant to this specific scientific inquiry process
- Address significant knowledge within the scientific inquiry process
- Address the development of knowledge along the timeline of the scientific inquiry process
- Be as authentic as possible in designing the assessment tools

- Make sure that the assessment tools can actually provide evidence that is useful in addressing the aims and purposes of the assessment program

The development of assessment tools is a creative, problem-solving activity. The aims and scientific content of the assessment tools have been defined in previous stages. But these definitions need to be operationalized at this stage in the active assessment development process. To a certain extent, the process described here is simpler than those used by many other assessment development programs. As a rule of thumb, the direction taken in the active assessment approach is to use authentic aspects of the scientific inquiry process whenever possible. In other words, a large part of the tool development process is directed by the description of the scientific inquiry process (stage 1) and the decisions as to which aspects of this process are considered significant (stage 2). The development of assessment tools is relatively simple because it draws directly on the contextualized knowledge required for the completion of the scientific inquiry process itself and is based on the in-depth understanding of the scientist-educator of her/his own scientific inquiry process. In line with the concept of authentic performance-based assessment the actual assessment tools are actually tasks from within the scientific inquiry process that have been modeled. It is assumed that each of the significant milestones of the scientific process and the associated knowledge sources will be assessed. For some programs, this may mean actually observing the students' way of conducting the task; for others it may mean creating more indirect ways of eliciting the same knowledge. In this sense, assessment tasks can be modeled on the authentic tasks used in the scientific inquiry process. These may include completion of a laboratory process, the explanation of laboratory result, the writing and reading of a laboratory notebook, and the presentation of a poster. For active assessment, the idea is that actual authentic aspects of professional scientific inquiry be used as moments of student knowledge assessment.

When using authentic assessment tasks, it is important to make sure that all types of knowledge are assessed. In particular it is important that physical, cognitive, and representational knowledge are integrated in the evaluation of scientific inquiry. This will probably mean that the assessment tools will be of different types that use different methods of data elicitation. This multimethod approach should ensure that collectively the different types of knowledge comprehensively cover the different types of knowledge that are being assessed. This may manifest itself in an assessment program that consists of some performance of specific tasks, some indirect elicitation of cognitive knowledge, and some summarizing presentation task at the end of the scientific inquiry process. The tools of assessment need to be carefully designed and explicitly described and written.

5.2.4 Rubric Development

The aim of this stage is the development of scoring rubrics that can be used to rate the outcomes of student performance on the different assessment tools. In

Table 5.1 Summary of main aspects of active assessment development

Stage	Aim	Questions
1. Empirical Description	The aim of this stage is to develop an explicit description of the scientific inquiry process that is utilized within the educational program	*Axis 1: Representational Knowledge*: What types of representations are produced within the scientific inquiry process? *Axis 2: Inquiry Process Development*: Is there a specific expected order for the production of these representations? What is that order (or potential orders)? *Axis 1: Physical Knowledge:* What physical procedures are required to produce these representations? *Axis 1: Cognitive Knowledge:* What scientific content knowledge is required to understand and interpret these representations? What informed decisions (or calculations) need to be made in order to continue this process of scientific inquiry? What does one need to know in order to understand the different representation produced within the scientific inquiry process? *Axis 1: Presentational Knowledge:* In what ways and in what settings are the results of this scientific inquiry presented to the community of scientists?
2. Definition of Aims	The aim of this stage is to explicitly define the purpose of the assessment program and set priorities in relation to what is significant scientific knowledge in this specific scientific inquiry process	What are the aims of the educational program? What are the aims and purposes of the assessment program? Of the representations defined in this scientific process which of these representations could be considered a representational "milestone" in the development of this scientific process? (A limited set of crucial, milestone representations in the development of a scientific inquiry need to be chosen) What physical laboratory knowledge, cognitive scientific knowledge, cognitive interpretive and decision-making knowledge, and knowledge of visual representation are required in order to create and understand the milestone representations that have been chosen (see previous question)? (The required knowledge in each case needs to be explicated as fully as possible)

(continued)

Table 5.1 (continued)

Stage	Aim	Questions
3. Tool Development	The aim of this active assessment stage is the actual development of tools that can be used with student-researchers in order to assess knowledge development	The direction taken in the active assessment approach is to use authentic aspects of the scientific inquiry process whenever possible Tool development process is directed by the description of the scientific inquiry process (stage 1) and the decisions as to which aspects of this process are considered significant (stage 2) *Considerations:* (a) Comprehensively address representational, cognitive, physical, and presentational knowledge relevant to this specific scientific inquiry process (b) Address significant knowledge within the scientific inquiry process (c) Address the development of knowledge along the timeline of the scientific inquiry process (d) Be as authentic as possible in designing the assessment tools (e) Make sure that the assessment tools can actually provide evidence that is useful in addressing the aims and purposes of the assessment program
4. Rubric Development	The aim of this stage is the development of scoring rubrics that can be used to rate the outcomes of student performance on the different assessment tools	Scoring rubrics are based directly on the professional knowledge in conducting these tasks within the authentic setting
5. Assessment Piloting	The aim of this stage is to improve and validate the assessment procedures	To what degree do the assessment tools and the scoring rubrics provide evidence that can be used to assess the aims and purposes of the educational program?

accordance with the principles of authentic assessment it is assumed that the scoring rubrics are based directly on the professional knowledge in conducting these tasks within the authentic setting. In other words, the criteria for success are identical to the criteria used by professional scientists in conducting the same task. The scoring rubrics are a crucial part of the assessment program because the data elicited from the students is understood in relation to the standards of responses defined in the scoring rubric. Scoring rubrics usually divide responses into exemplary, acceptable, and unacceptable levels of response. The scoring rubrics need to be explicitly defined and written.

5.2.5 Assessment Piloting

The aim of this stage is to improve and validate the assessment procedures. All assessment tools and scoring rubrics need to be piloted. At the heart of the piloting program is the question

1. To what degree do the assessment tools and the scoring rubrics provide evidence that can be used to assess the aims and purposes of the educational program?

The process of piloting assessment tools requires the actual completion of the assessment tools by student-researchers and the scoring of these responses by different members of the educational team. It is a basic assumption of any piloting procedure that both the tasks and the scoring rubrics will be modified through the piloting process. In addition to the piloting of the materials with student-researchers, it is often useful to have professional scientists complete the assessment tasks as well and to look at the scoring rubrics. These professionals will ensure the authenticity of the materials developed and the relevance of these to the specific scientific inquiry process.

5.3 Chapter Summary

The aim of this chapter was to provide a conceptual framework for active assessment development. Table 5.1 summarizes the main aspects of this framework.

Chapter 6
The PHIRE Program

6.1 Introduction

The first section of this book (Chaps. 1–5) presents the theoretical basis for assessment of scientific inquiry and a practical framework for active assessment. This second section describes a case study and how the specific assessment strategies and tools were constructed and implemented. The first chapter of this second section presents a detailed description of the PHIRE program and establishes the context for authentic scientific inquiry and active assessment. The two subsequent chapters discuss the specific assessment strategies and the tools developed for active assessment within this program. The final chapter offers reflections from the perspective of the scientist-educator on the establishment of integrated research-education programs and the role of active assessment within this context. This case study is not presented with the expectation that it will be replicated elsewhere, but that it will provide a practical framework for establishing educational programs with fully integrated active assessment within the wide berth of sub-disciplines within the life sciences.

In this chapter we will provide a description of the PHIRE program and its development at the University of Pittsburgh. The acronym PHIRE is an abbreviation of the Phage Hunters Integrating Research and Education program and emerged several years after phage discovery activities begun in 2002 (further insights into the origins of the PHIRE program are provided in Chap. 9). The program name and acronym are rather informative. First, it places an immediate emphasis on the integration of scientific and educational missions, reflecting a core goal and motive for the program. Second, it introduces the concept of phage hunting, and while the general reader might know rather little about phages or the viruses of bacteria, it connotes the idea of searching and discovery. A key program theme is the idea of igniting enthusiasm in students through their involvement as research scientists, lighting a fire that will promote continued involvement in scientific research. It should also be noted that some of those involved in phage research often have a light-witted predilection to substitute "f" with "ph" at every opportunity!

A brief overview of the PHIRE program provides a context for a more detailed description. In this program, high-school and undergraduate students have the

D.I. Hanauer et al., *Active Assessment: Assessing Scientific Inquiry*, Mentoring in Academia and Industry 2, DOI 10.1007/978-0-387-89649-6_6, opportunity to engage in a research program focusing on their discovery of new bacterial viruses (bacteriophages, or phages), followed by purification and characterization of the new viruses that they discovered, with emphasis on determining the genomic DNA sequence. The new phage genome sequence is then annotated to show how the genetic information is organized and compared with other genomes to elucidate its evolutionary history. There are a variety of variations on this theme and these will be discussed later.

To fully understand the PHIRE program and why we believe it has some special attributes facilitating an integration of our research and scientific missions, we will first present some helpful background information about bacteriophages and the size and diversity of the phage population. These scientific concepts are central to the PHIRE program, and being familiar with them is important for fully comprehending the advantages that the PHIRE program has to offer.

6.2 What Are Phages?

Bacteriophages are viruses that infect bacterial hosts. They are commonly referred to as phages and share all the typical properties associated with viruses. They are not capable of duplication or growth by themselves and can only multiply once they have infected bacterial host cells. They are small and their morphological details can only be elucidated by examination in the electron microscope (one example is shown in Fig. 6.1). Phages come in many different shapes and sizes, but most are composed of two readily identifiable structures, the head (or capsid) and a tail. The tail can of be various types, the three most common being a short stubby tail, a long flexible non-contractile tail, and a contractile tail; the tail type is used for taxonomic grouping, with these types being known as the Podoviridae, Siphoviridae, and Myoviridae, respectively. To give a sense of scale, the diameter of the head is usually 50–100 nM, and the length of the tail (in the Siphoviridae and Myoviridae) is typically in the range 70–300 nM.

Chemically, bacteriophages are composed of two major macromolecules, proteins and nucleic acids, although some have associated lipids and carbohydrates. The visible structures are made of protein, but there are usually many different specific types of proteins, sometimes 20 or more. The quantity of each of the individual proteins is broad, ranging from fewer than half-a-dozen to several hundreds of others, all within a single viral particle. The genetic information is carried as nucleic acid, with the majority of viruses carrying double-stranded DNA (dsDNA), although there are examples of those containing single-stranded DNA (ssDNA) or RNA. The DNA genome is carried inside the head of the phage, typically in a linear form, and remains there until the process of infection occurs. When the tip of the tail associates with a specific receptor on the surface of the host bacterial cell, the genome exits the head, traverses through the tail, and is injected across the cell wall into the cytoplasm of the cell; the viral protein shell remains attached to the outside of the cell and plays no further role.

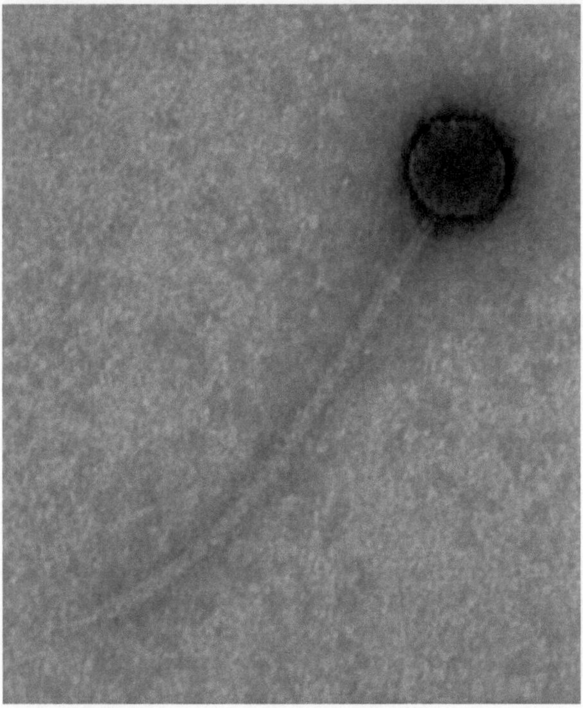

Fig. 6.1 Electron micrograph of mycobacteriophage Barnyard

Although phages are too small to see directly with a light microscope, they can be readily recognized and analyzed microbiologically. A common technique is called the "plaque assay," in which a phage sample and bacterial cells are spread across an agar surface in a Petri dish and incubated so that bacterial growth generates an opaque lawn across the surface; with most bacterial types this takes 12–24 h. Wherever a phage particle in the initial sample infects a host cell, it can reproduce to generate more copies of itself, typically 50–200, which are then released by disintegration (lysis) of the infected cell. These progeny – which are identical to the initial particle – can then repeat this process and continue to do so as long as the bacterial cells are growing. What is generated is a plaque, a small circular area in which the bacteria have been killed and the phage multiplied (Fig. 6.2). At the point when the bacteria cease to grow (12–24 h), there are typically 10^6–10^7 phage particles in a single plaque; all derivatives of the single particle that initiated that infection. This reproductive process requires the rapid and efficient production of many new copies of the phage genome and assembly of virion structures into which the DNA is packaged. The DNA replication process is accurate but not perfect, and thus all the progeny derived from a single particle will be extremely similar but not necessarily identical, with a small subset containing mutations making them just very slightly different to each other.

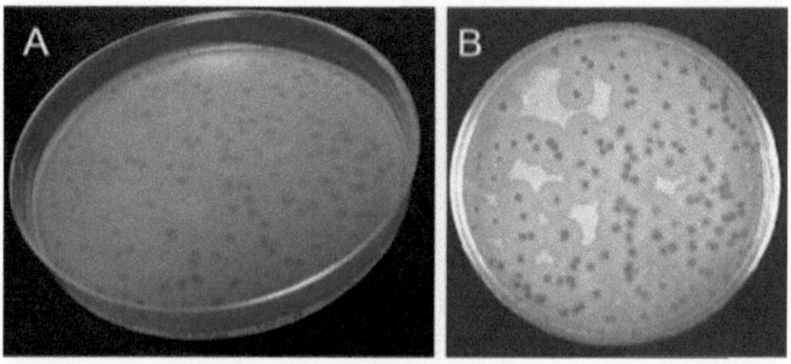

Fig. 6.2 Mycobacteriophage plaques on lawns of *M. smegmatis*. (**A**) Side angle view of a Petri dish containing a lawn of *M. smegmatis* containing mycobacteriophage plaques. (**B**) Top view of the same Petri dish, in which ~100 phage plaques are seen as small circles where the *M. smegmatis* cells constituting the opaque lawn have been killed

The plaque assay enables the simple recognition of a single viral particle in a sample, since one particle is sufficient for a plaque. Moreover, if there are many particles in a suspension, then through the process of purification by plating serial dilutions, it is possible to accurately separate and enumerate the phage particles in any sample. The number of particles is often referred to as its "titer," and when the titer is determined in this way it is usually expressed as the number of plaque-forming units (pfu) per volume of sample. For example, if 0.1 ml of a 10^{-6} dilution (which can be achieved by three serial 1 in 100 dilutions of the initial stock) provides 13 plaques on a particular host, then the titer of the stock can be described as 1.3×10^8 pfu/ml.

Preparation of bacteriophages stocks can be readily accomplished by mixing bacterial host cells and phage particles and allowing multiple rounds of phage growth and cell lysis to occur. Eventually all or most of the cells will be lysed, and after filtration the resulting sterile "lysate" can be stored and used for future experiments. There infections can be performed on solid agar medium in a Petri dish to generate a "plate lysate" or in liquid medium to generate a "liquid lysate." While either method can be used, some phages – including many of the mycobacteriophages – appear to grow better on solid medium than in liquid, thus generating higher phage titers. Either approach can generate stocks with very high titers (10^9–10^{11} pfu/ml), although there are many parameters that influence this, especially the number of phage particles that are initially added to the cells. Optimal phage production often depends on empirically determining this for any given phage.

6.3 Bacteriophages Are Ubiquitous and Host Specific

Bacteriophages were first discovered separately by Felix D'Herelle and Frederick Twort in the early 20th century employing the plaque assay as described above. It became clear that phages could be identified in many types of samples from many different environments, but that each phage type is specific to the bacteria they can infect. The collection of bacteria that any specific phage isolate can infect is referred to as its "host range," which can only be determined empirically by asking what bacterial hosts it is capable of forming plaques on. Some phage types have rather broad host ranges and may for example infect many different bacterial species within a given genus. Other phages have extremely narrow host ranges and may infect only a specific sub-type of one bacterial species. Phages have been isolated for the majority of bacterial species for which they have been specifically sought, and it is generally accepted that phages probably exist for the vast majority of bacteria in the biosphere. It is noteworthy that only a rather small portion of bacteria in the environment can actually be cultured in the laboratory, and it seems probable that all of the unculturable bacteria are also hosts for bacteriophages.

6.4 Bacteriophages: The Dark Matter of the Biological Universe

In the early 1990s, methods were developed enabling the simple determination of the number of nucleic acid containing items in an environmental sample using only a fluorescence microscope (Hennes & Suttle, 1995). When certain dyes are added (e.g., SYBR Green), bacterial cells and viruses absorb the dye, binding to the DNA and causing them to fluoresce. When seawater samples were examined (which are easy to collect), it was found that they typically contain 10^6–10^7 virus particles per milliliter, regardless of whether the samples were coastal, oceanic, surface, or deep (Wommack & Colwell, 2000); moreover, the ratio of viruses to bacteria (which are easily distinguishable as being larger than the viruses) was typically about 10:1. Similar numbers and ratios are estimated from terrestrial samples, and with a simple multiplication by the size of the oceans plus some factor for terrestrial areas, it can be calculated that there are about 10^{31} viral particles in the biosphere (Hendrix, 2002), of which the large majority are bacteriophages (i.e., they infect bacterial hosts). Since an independent calculation estimates that there are about 10^{30} bacterial cells in the biosphere (Whitman et al., 1998), this seems not unreasonable. However, the size of the phage population is truly stunning. The 10^{31} totality suggests that phages represent the numerical majority of all biological entities, i.e., there are more phage particles than all other forms of life taken together. If we assumed that each particle was on average 100 nm in length, then placing the entire population into a linear arrangement would generate an array that extends 200 million light years!

Recognizing the remarkable size of the phage population shows us how little we understand it. The total number of bacteriophages that have been described in the literature is perhaps a few thousand, and genomic analysis has been undertaken for just over 500 at the time of writing (September, 2008). We will provide further details into the comparative genomics of the phages in Sect. 6.7.8, but one simple conclusion is that they are genetically highly diverse; so these are not apparently 10^{31} particles that are minor variants of each other. In fact, the abundance of novel genes present in phage genomes suggests that the phage population represents the largest unexplored reservoir of genetic information in the natural world (Hatfull et al., 2006).

6.5 Goals of the PHIRE Program

Realizing the size and diversity of the phage population provides a foundation for understanding the goals of the PHIRE program. The program emerged as a means of introducing students to the scientific process, emphasizing the involvement of students that have little scientific training but are curious about science and the natural world in which we live. Involvement of students in a research project within an established research environment provides a forum for an education into both the process and content of science. We therefore wanted to integrate our research and educational missions in a context that broadly extends opportunities to a diverse student body – both high school and undergraduate – without bias except for their curiosity and desire to learn about science (Hanauer, 2007). The specific research projects needed to address authentic scientific questions could accommodate a significant number of students and most importantly be intertwined with the excitement of scientific discovery. The diversity of the phage population and the ability to isolate novel phages relatively easily thus offered an attractive framework for engaging students in scientific research.

6.6 The Power of Discovery

The number and diversity of the phage population provides a core underpinning for the PHIRE program. While we would not make the claim that phage hunting is uniquely suited for scientific discovery by beginner scientists, it does appear to be particularly well suited to it. The genetic diversity of phages is sufficiently high that new isolates recovered from the environment are highly likely to be novel and, in many instances, quite different genetically from any viruses previously discovered. Furthermore, the isolation of a new "plaque-forming unit" is fairly simple from a technical perspective and doesn't require specific training or special skills. It thus offers a simple entry point for anyone to begin the process of discovery, and students learn rather quickly that they can contribute to the scientific process. At the same time, it soon becomes apparent that the isolation and purification of a plaque-forming unit does not in itself provide any information about its novelty. Even if it is purified and examined by electron microscopy – an exciting moment of realization as to what the virus looks like – its genetic relationship to other phages is not known. It is only when the DNA has been extracted and the genome sequence determined that its relationship to known viruses is understood.

It is clear then that the process of phage discovery and genomic analysis is thoroughly imbued with scientific discovery. A "new" virus can be isolated and studied, but its novelty is understood only by pursing the process of characterization. The discovery – and the accompanying sense of project ownership – provides the impetus and drive to continue and to open the door to further discoveries unearthed by genomic characterization. Furthermore, the new genetic information derived is of broad importance to the larger scientific community and thus warrants publication in some form (Hatfull et al., 2006). It is an authentic piece of science.

6.7 PHIRE: A Ten-Step Program

Having established that the opportunities for scientific discovery by phage hunting and genomic analysis are suitable for integrating the research and educational missions, we will describe the component steps of a typical project within the PHIRE program. It will become apparent that there is a prescribed formula or shape to the projects, each of which differs primarily by the individual phages that students isolate. We discuss in further detail in Sect. 6.11 the relative merits of such parallel projects, but it provides a common platform in which we can identify ten individual steps, most of which follow each other in a logical and chronological order. We will assume that the reader may have only a rudimentary knowledge of molecular biology. A visualization of these steps is provided in Fig. 6.3.

6.7.1 *Step 1: Phage Isolation*

As noted above, a student joining the PHIRE program begins by isolating a bacteriophage from the environment. Step 1 involves the gathering of environmental samples – we typically encourage collection from soil or compost although students can be quite creative – in a 15 ml plastic tube. Back in the laboratory, samples are extracted with a simple buffer (phage buffer) and filtered to remove contaminating bacteria. A portion of this sample is then mixed with bacterial cells and thin agar

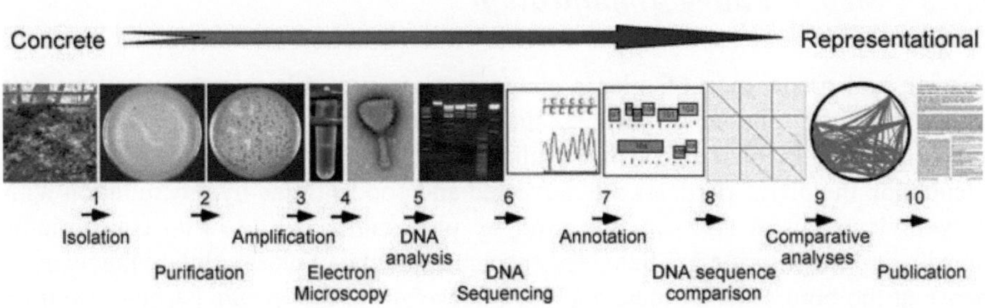

Fig. 6.3 The ten steps of the PHIRE program. Each of the ten steps in the PHIRE program are illustrated with the central arrow showing the transition from concrete to abstract comprehension from step 1 to step 10 (*see* Color Insert)

solution (top agar), and poured onto an agar base in a Petri dish. Once the top agar layer has solidified, the plate is incubated for 16–24 h and examined for the appearance of plaques on the bacterial lawn (see Fig. 6.2).

Most of our experience in phage hunting has been with using *Mycobacterium smegmatis* as a bacterial host although in principle any bacterial host can be used; we refer to phages that infect mycobacteria as mycobacteriophages. The proportion of samples containing identifiable plaques is relatively low (<10%) so that some students will be successful in their first set of samples, while others may have to continue to gather more samples before being successful. When plaques are observed, the numbers vary – often as few as just one but can be as many as hundreds. In the PHIRE program, close to 100% of students have succeeded in identifying at least one plaque. It should be noted that the samples probably contain large number of phage particles ($>10^6$) but most of which infect bacterial species other than *M. smegmatis*. We have not systematically monitored what bacteria are present in the samples that students collect, although this has rich potential for future program development.

6.7.2 Step 2: Phage Purification

Step 2 involves the purification of the phage sample to ensure that it is a homogenous sample. This is important since without a clonal population further characterization becomes overly complicated and since you then can't be sure of what you are really working with. The purification can be accomplished by "picking" the plaque by carefully stabbing it with a plastic pipette tip, transferring it to an aliquot of phage buffer, and re-plating dilutions to generate single plaques. With each plaque containing 10^6–10^7 particles, this can be fairly easily accomplished, provided that several dilutions are made to ensure that at least one gives a reasonable number of nicely isolated plaques. This is then repeated once or twice more to have confidence that a homogenous phage sample is achieved.

6.7.3 Step 3: Phage Amplification

Growth and preparation of a large phage stock is typically accomplished by first establishing the number of particles that will produce a maximum bacteriophage yield, followed by phage growth on solid medium using 30 large agar plates. After incubation the phage particles are harvested and concentrated by precipitation with polyethylene glycol and salt, followed by ultracentrifugation in an equilibrium-density cesium chloride gradient. This generates a tube of clear solution that is most dense at the bottom of the tube and least dense at the top; phage particles migrate to form a visible band of phage particles that have migrated to a predictable region (Fig. 6.4). Thus particles starting higher than this density will sink to the corresponding position, whereas those below will float upward. This concentrated layer

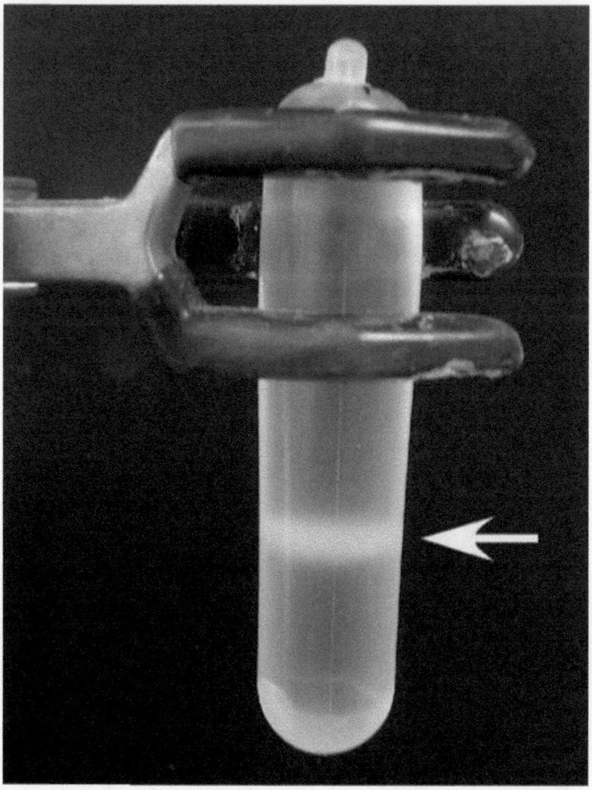

Fig. 6.4 Equilibrium density gradient purification of mycobacteriophage particles. A phage lysate harvested from 30 large Petri dishes was collected and centrifuged in a cesium chloride (CsCl) equilibrium density gradient for 16 h at 38,000 rpm. The starting CsCl density is 1.5 and during centrifugation a density gradient is established, with the bottom of tube more dense than the top. Phage particles migrate to a position corresponding to their own density and are visible as a bluish band (*arrow*). The total number of particles in the band is typically $\sim 10^{13}$

of biologically pure phage particles can be readily recovered with a syringe and needle. Phage samples in cesium chloride usually store well, although DNA extraction, electron microscopy, and other analyses require removal of the salt from the sample by dialysis.

6.7.4 Step 4: Electron Microscopy

Examination of the newly discovered phage by electron microscopy can be performed at any point after its purification, but it is an activity that students often look forward to and which may have significant impact on them. Up to this point, the idea of having a new phage in hand is something of an abstraction; they can deduce that there must be particles in the tube, because there is something there that kills bacterial cells and forms plaques. But the tube just has the appearance of a clear liquid.

Visualization of the virus particles changes and clarifies the nature of the phage (see Fig. 6.2). Students specifically comment on the impact of this visualization in their notebooks – it is as though a veil has lifted and the nature of the beast is revealed (Hanauer, 2007). A picture is worth a thousands words and provides a concrete description of an entity that could only be assumed to exist through an interpretation of its behavior. This is not only satisfying for the students, but raises their confidence in the interpretive aspects of science employed in the previous steps.

6.7.5 Step 5: Nucleic Acid Extraction and Restriction Analysis

Nucleic acid is extracted from the particles by chemical treatments that solubilize or destroy the integrity of the protein coat of the viruses. In our experience with the mycobacteriophages, all of the phages we have isolated contain DNA, although RNA phages (which require somewhat different procedures) are found with other hosts. Many different methods have been described in the literature, although we typically use a mixture of phenol and chloroform, which is immiscible with the phage buffer and thus easily removed. The DNA is soluble in the phage buffer and can be collected by precipitation with ethanol, washed, and resuspended in a suitable storage buffer.

Once the DNA is isolated it is helpful to determine the concentration of DNA and to perform a preliminary analysis by restriction digestion and gel electrophoresis. There are two alternative methods for determining the DNA concentration. First, the optical density at a wavelength of 260 nm can be measured in a spectrophotometer, and using the extinction coefficient of DNA (i.e., its absorption parameters) the concentration can be easily calculated. An alternative method is to examine a DNA sample by electrophoresis (see later) and compare the degree of staining with samples of known concentrations. The first is the most accurate but since other molecules (such as RNA and protein) can also absorb light at this wavelength, it is often useful to perform both methods and compare the results.

Useful and relatively simple insights about a genome can be gained from digesting the DNA with restriction enzymes and analyzing the results by agarose gel electrophoresis. Restriction enzymes are useful because they have the property of cutting the DNA at specific recognition sequences, usually a string of between four and six consecutive DNA bases (see Sect. 6.7.6); because any four-base sequence will occur more frequently than any (for example) six-base sequence, a four-cutter enzyme will cut more often and thus generate more DNA fragments than a six-cutter enzyme. Numerous different restriction enzymes are commercially available and their recognition sites are known.

Restriction digestion is easily performed by incubating a sample of DNA with a restriction enzyme and a simple buffer. Once the reaction is complete, the pattern of fragments generated can be determined by agarose gel electrophoresis, a process by which the DNA fragments can be separated according to their size. A gel matrix is generated by dissolving agarose (a gelatin-like substance) in a simple buffer by boiling and pouring the solution into a flat mold; a comb containing a series of teeth is then inserted toward one end of the mold and the agarose allowed to cool and set. The comb can then be removed to reveal a series of wells (small square holes) and the gel set in an electrophoresis apparatus to which buffer is added. The opposite ends of the apparatus contain electrodes that can be connected to a power supply that generates an electric current. DNA solutions, each containing different sized fragments, can then be inserted into each of the wells and the electric current applied. Since DNA is negatively charged, the fragments migrate within the electric field toward the positive electrode, but the smaller fragments snake through the agarose matrix faster than the larger ones and thus after about an hour or two of electrophoresis, the fragments are well separated. The approximate sizes of the fragments can be readily calculated by comparing their migration to those in a "standard" or a "marker", which contains a mixture of fragments of known sizes. An example of such an analysis is shown in Fig. 6.5.

For a preliminary analysis where the DNA sequence is not yet known, performing restriction analysis is most useful for comparing a genome with other genomes. One example is the circumstance in which several plaques are recovered on the initial isolation plate, and it is not clear whether they correspond to completely

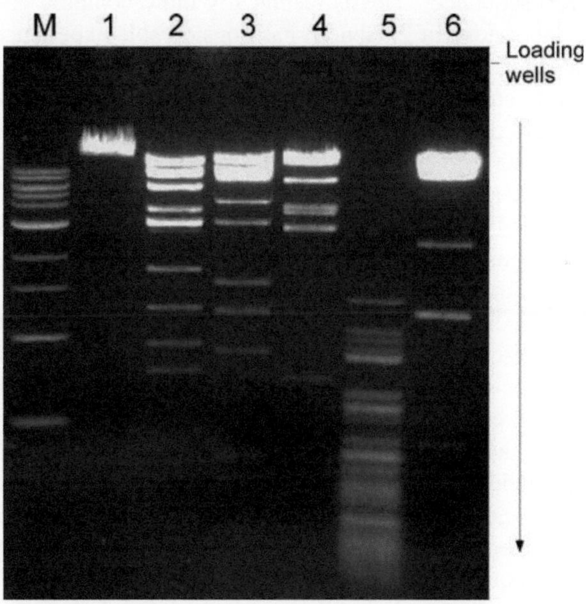

Fig. 6.5 Agarose gel electrophoresis of restriction-digested phage DNA. Approximately 0.5 μg of phage Mikdud DNA was digested with restriction enzymes and the resulting DNA fragments separated by agarose gel electrophoresis. The position of the loading wells and the direction of DNA migration are shown; smaller DNA fragments migrate hastily and are toward the bottom of the gel. Lanes contain marker DNA of known sizes (M), uncut phage DNA (lane 2), or phage DNA digested with *Bam*HI, *Cla*I, *Eco*RI, *Hae*III, *Hin*dIII (lanes 2–6 respectively)

different phages or whether they are related. Comparison of the restriction patterns will address this question, since if they are closely related then the restriction patterns will be similar.

A second but equally important utility of this analysis is for comparing the restriction pattern determined for a particular enzyme with that predicted once the complete genome sequence is determined. Because restriction enzymes cut at known specific sequences, the precise pattern can be predicted by computational analysis. Although there are some exceptions, for the most part a close correlation between the predicted and empirically determined digestion patterns is observed. The process of sequence determination involves breaking the genome into smaller pieces and then reassembling them like a jigsaw puzzle into the big picture of the complete genome sequence. Occasionally this assembly can go computationally awry, and this can be revealed through non-congruence of the predicted and empirically measured patterns.

6.7.6 Step 6: DNA Sequencing

To determine the genome sequence of the phages, we have primarily used methods that involve shotgun library construction followed by automated DNA sequencing using an ABI3730 sequencer. This is technically more complex than most of the prior steps. Our laboratory in Pittsburgh has considerable experience with this, so we closely guide students through the process. The standard process requires breaking of the DNA into smaller pieces (2–3 kbp) by hydrodynamic shearing, generating a library of plasmid clones in which each plasmid molecule contains a different and randomly selected segment of the phage genome, performing sequencing reactions in a thermocycler, and analyzing in the automated sequencer. The number of plasmid clones needed varies, but is typically 250–500 and depends on the size of the genome and the quality of the library. For the mycobacteriophages, the average genome length is about 70 kbp, but ranges from 40 to 150 kbp.

Each of the sequencing "runs" usually generates about 800 bp of sequence information. In brief, DNA is a polymer of repeated units, and genetic information is stored in the order, or sequence, of these units. There are typically just four types of units (nucleotides) containing four different bases – adenine, guanine, cytosine, and thymine, abbreviated as A, G, C, and T, respectively. In dsDNA, two strands of nucleic acid are held together through pairing of these bases, with the strict rule that A pairs with T and G pairs with C. The sequence of the bases is different on the two strands, but because of the base-pairing rules, if the sequence of one strand is known, then the sequence of the other strand can be predicted. Thus in a typical shotgun sequencing project each "run" gives a sequence of about 800 As, Gs, Cs, and Ts, and about 500–1,000 individual "runs" are needed (usually by determining the sequences from both ends of each plasmid clone). Since the phage pieces are randomly cloned and sequenced, the overlapping pieces can be computationally assembled together, such that a contiguous sequence of bases corresponding to the entire genome can be constructed.

Once the shotgun part of the project is completed, the sequence can usually be computationally assembled into one or a small number of "contigs" of continuous sequence information. Going from this point to a finally completed sequence can be tricky and requires the confirmation of weak areas in the sequence information, joining of the contigs, ensuring that information is acquired on both DNA strands throughout, and precise determination of the phage genome termini, if it contains defined ends.

In the past several years there have been dramatic advances in DNA sequencing technologies, especially with the pyrosequencing approaches as employed by the 454 sequencer (Roche Inc.) and the methods used by the Solexa genome analyzer (Illumina Inc.). These high-throughput methods can be applied to phage genome sequencing and should greatly simplify sequence acquisition especially if multiple genomes can be determined at the same time. The potential downside is the removal of much of the sequence determination methodology out of the hands of the student-researchers into a core facility. However, the gains in time should be considerable and 454 sequencing is anticipated to ensure that a higher proportion of students achieve complete genome sequencing and can move onto subsequent analyses.

6.7.7 Step 7: Genome Annotation

The raw DNA sequence information holds the informational code with instructions for how the phage grows and survives. Bioinformatic analysis involves the identification of genes and other features through computational analyses, using well-established sequence patterns to predict the overall genome organization. We have made use of the DNA Master program (J. Lawrence, University of Pittsburgh) to facilitate this process, enabling rapid and accurate predictions of gene locations. While this can be accomplished in just a few seconds of computer time, we recommend an up-close manual inspection by students of all of these data. This may take a good deal longer, but it is a powerful way to familiarize students with the nitty-gritty essence of molecular biology, for instance, how the two DNA strands relate to each other, the correspondence of DNA and amino acid sequence information, the difference between transcription and translation, and where genes start and stop. Usually this refinement of the initial crude annotation results in several revisions of gene parameters, identification of additional putative genes, and avoidance of genes improperly predicted by the automated methods. A screen shot of how the information appears to the student is shown in Fig. 6.6.

6.7.8 Step 8: Comparison of the DNA Sequence to Known Phage Genomes

With an annotated genome sequence available, the real fun begins, as the genome can be compared with other known genomes to explore the differences and similarities. There are fundamentally two levels of comparison that can be performed. First,

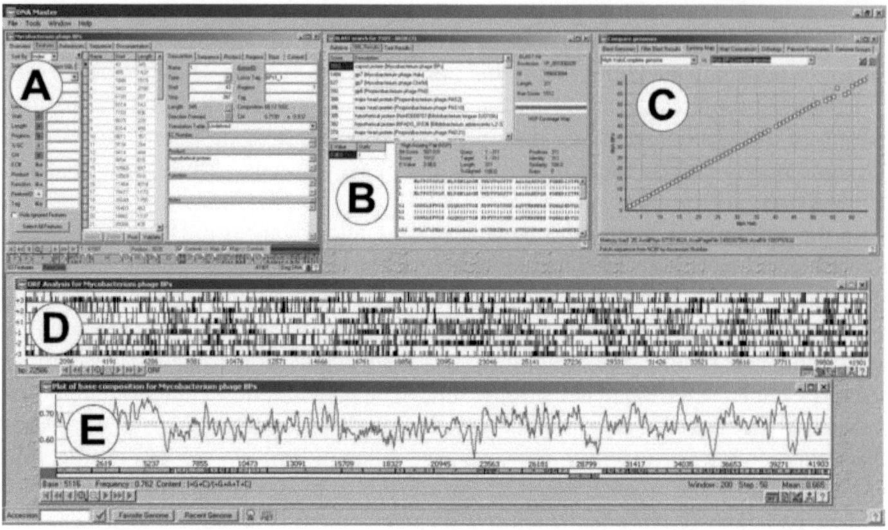

Fig. 6.6 DNAMaster: A program for phage genome annotation. Screen shots are shown from several representative windows of DNAMaster (**A–E**). (**A**) Window presenting features of mycobacteriophage BPs. The "Feature" tab is selected, showing a list of the genes with their coordinates. (**B**) The "Compare Genomes" window showing the results of a BlastP search of phage BPs gp7. (**C**) Comparison of phage BPs and phage Halo genomes, with each yellow box indicating the position of genes that are shared between the two genomes. (**D**) The "Frames" window showing the positions of stop and start codons in all six reading frames. The positions of identified opening reading frames are colored either *green* (forward direction) or *red* (reverse direction). (**E**) Plot of base composition showing the average GC% content across the BPs genome. These represent just a small subset of the available functions with DNAMaster (available as a free download from http://cobamide2.bio.pitt.edu) (*see* Color Insert)

the entire genome can be compared at the DNA sequence level with other known genomes. It is very rare to find substantial or significant DNA sequence similarity between phages that infect different bacterial hosts, and even phages infecting a common host can be totally different to each other. There are several readily available computer programs (such as Dotter or Gepard) for DNA sequence comparison. If several genomes are to be compared at the same time, the individual sequences can be concatenated and then compared. A typical example is shown in Fig. 6.7, in which dots are placed on the display where two sequences show similarity (specific parameters influencing the stringency of the comparison can be chosen). A diagonal line appears showing that each genome is the same as itself, but any lines off the diagonal reflect similarities between different phage genomes.

Comparison of the nucleotide sequences of 60 mycobacteriophage genomes reveals two fundamental facets of these phage genomes. The first is that even though these phages can all infect the same host (i.e., *M. smegmatis*) and are therefore in direct genetic communication with each other, there is a high degree of genetic diversity; they are all clearly not relatively minor versions of a common sequence. The second is that the relationships are not homogeneous, and there are groups

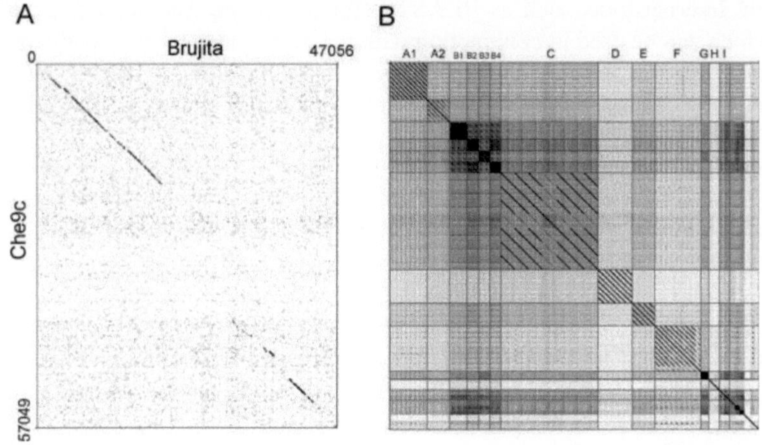

Fig. 6.7 Nucleotide sequence comparisons of phage genomes. (**A**) The nucleotide sequences of mycobacteriophages Che9c and Brujita were compared using the program Gepard, using a sliding window of ten nucleotides. Diagonal lines indicate that the genomes share significant nucleotide sequence similarity. (**B**) Nucleotide sequence comparison of all 60 sequenced mycobacteriophage genomes using Gepard as in (**A**). The names of the clusters are shown above

or clusters of genomes that appear to be more similar to each other, than to the other phages. Of the 60 phages, 55 can be clustered with at least one other comprising nine clusters (A–I). It should be noted though that the inclusion of a phage genome within a cluster is largely arbitrary, and the closeness of the relationships is determined by the appearance of the nucleotide comparison in plots such as that shown in Fig. 6.7. It should also be noted that some genomes can have nucleotide sequence similarity to more than the cluster, but spanning just a relatively small genome segment. This clustering is thus one of representational convenience, rather than one reflecting taxonomic differentiation (Hatfull et al., 2006). The appearance of clusters has changed dramatically as additional genomes have been added to the comparison and is expected to continue to do so. We predict that with greater coverage of the mycobacteriophage population the boundaries around these clusters will become fuzzy and may largely disappear in favor of a continuum of relationships.

6.7.9 Step 9: Comparative Genomic Analysis

The average size of bacteriophage genes is smaller than that of bacterial genes and is typically 600–700 bp (Hatfull et al., 2006; Pedulla et al., 2003); thus in a 70 kbp genome there are usually 100–110 genes. A key question is "what do these genes do?" Although this may require detailed experimental studies, much can be learned by comparing a new genome sequence to known phage genomes at the DNA sequence level and the amino acid sequence level. There are commonly available Internet tools such as BLASTP (for the amino acid sequence comparison), which can be used in conjunction with the tools and databases available at the National Center for Biotechnology Information (NCBI) site; the information gained by comparing predicted genes of a "new" genome to all known genes is extremely valuable.

When comparing a genome of – for example – a mycobacteriophage, there is a greater likelihood that the predicted gene products will have similarity (and thus descended from a common ancestor) to other mycobacteriophage gene products than to anything else in nature. However, we know now that the genome architecture of phages is typically mosaic, with different segments or modules of the genome having different evolutionary histories. This mosaicism can be best represented by examining in detail how each of the predicted genes relates to other mycobacteriophage genes. Steve Cresawn (James Madison University) has devised a program "Phamerator" that performs pairwise comparisons of all mycobacteriophage gene products and assorted then into phamilies (Phams) of related sequences. Phamerator can then display the genomes with each of the genes annotated in accord with its relatives (Fig. 6.9), providing an especially informative comparative genome representation demonstrating the mosaic relationships. The phamerator also produces individual bacteriophage genome maps (Fig. 6.8). Phamerator can also readily provide a representation of the relationships of each gene within a given phamily, which we refer to as "phamily circles" (Fig. 6.9). These phamily circles are essentially phylogenetic representations, but differ fundamentally from the more traditional diagrams of phylogenetic trees. One key advantage is that phamily circles enable

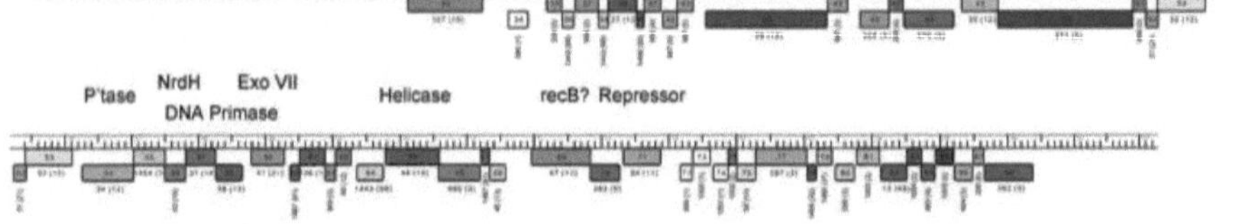

Fig. 6.8 Genome map of mycobacteriophage L5. The L5 genome is represented as a *horizontal bar* with markers spaced at 1 kbp intervals. Each of the predicted genes is shown as a colored box either above or below the genome; those above are transcribed rightward, and those below are transcribed leftward. The map was generated by the program Phamerator, which sorts the predicted genes into phamilies (Phams) as functions of their predicted amino acid sequence relatedness. The Pham number is shown above each gene with the number of Pham members in parentheses, and each gene is colored according to its Pham. Some of the predicted gene functions are noted (*see* Color Insert)

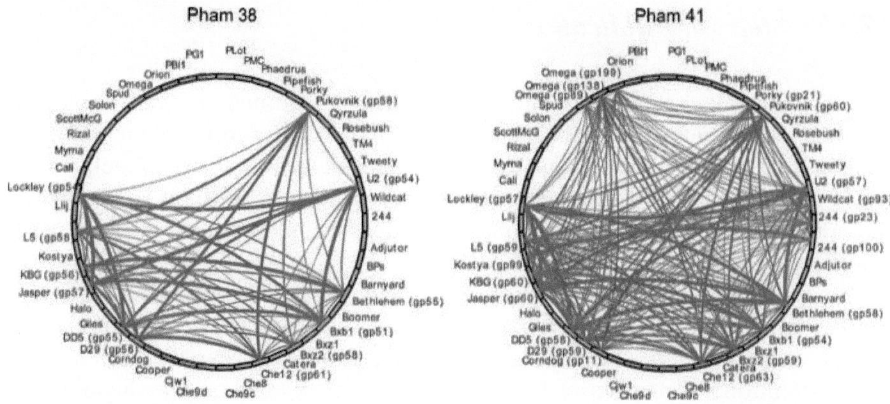

Fig. 6.9 Phamily circles. Phamily circles for Pham38 and Pham41 are shown. In the L5 genome (see Fig. 6.8), genes 58 and 59 are members of these two Phams, respectively, and the phamily circles suggest that they have distinct and different evolutionary histories. Each of the phages is listed around the circumference of each circle and an arc is drawn between members of each phamily with line thickness corresponding to strength of the relationship (*see* Color Insert)

the inclusion of all bacteriophage genomes in the comparison, even those that do not have a member of that particular phamily. Thus the phamily circles can be compared to reveal not only the strength of the relationships, but who participates in them.

This comparative genome analysis can get quite complicated, but it provides a wonderful forum for thinking about genome evolution and for understanding phylogenetic analysis. Performing these comparative analyses provides a really terrific opportunity for students to gain a first-hand experience in what evolution is and how it works. For example, if two adjacent genes in a genome are members of phamilies that have quite different phylogenies (see Fig. 6.9), then at some point in their evolution one or more recombination events must have occurred between them. A simple explanation for how this occurs is via an illegitimate – effectively random in regard to the specific DNA sequence – recombination event at some point in their history. When and how this occurs remains unclear, but the concept of genetic variation occurring in the absence of design or direction, followed by natural selection for the successful progeny, is a very nice illustration of the central tenets of Darwin's model for the origin of species. Interestingly, because bacteriophage genomes must also conform to fairly strict size constraints – i.e., there must be an appropriate length of DNA, because either too little or two much will not stably fit into the phage head – new variants could at least temporarily be selected other than on the basis of their function, in a non-Darwinian manner. Thus non-functional gene variants could survive within the phage population, but serve as substrates for subsequent recombination events giving rise to yet more new, possibly functional, variants. Genetic mosaicism thus represents a rather rich view of the process of biological evolution.

6.7.10 Step 10: Publication

An indication of the relevance of the genome sequence information is reflected in the importance of its publication. This is typically in one of two forms. First, all of the genomes that are completely sequenced and annotated are submitted for inclusion in one of the commonly available sequence databases (such as GenBank), from which they are accessible to the scientific community. This includes the authors of the work as well as all of the phage genome details.

The second form is the publication of the genome sequence information in the peer-reviewed scientific literature. When and how this occurs for each genome is dependent upon what has been learned from its isolation and characterization. Typically, submitting a manuscript for publication that contains only a single phage genome sequence requires either a stunning finding that warrants publication or considerable additional analysis and experimental dissection (see later). Much of what we have learned from phage genomics in the past few years has emerged from comparative analyses, and students who have contributed substantially to the work have been included as co-authors (Pedulla et al., 2003). In one such publication (Hatfull et al., 2006) a specific description is provided as to what each of the student-authors contributed.

6.8 Is That All?

It is helpful to understand that while learning about the genetic diversity of the bacteriophage population is important, the genomes and the genomic information also represent a resource and a good starting point for many other scientific inquiries. The reason why we have primarily focused on the viruses that infect mycobacterial hosts is not because we anticipate them to be systematically different to phages of other bacteria, but because the hosts are important and interesting in their own rights. *Mycobacterium tuberculosis* is a particularly special pathogen and kills nearly two million people each year across the globe (Raviglione, 2003). Approximately one-third of the entire world's population is infected with *M. tuberculosis* and the emergence of especially nasty drug-resistant strains further compounds the problem. In a 2006 study of an outbreak of extensively drug-resistant tuberculosis (XDR-TB) in Tugela Ferry, South Africa, 52 of the 53 patients died and the median time to death from collection of an initial sputum sample was 16 days (Gandhi et al., 2006). There is a desperate need for effective vaccines, new drugs, and rapid diagnostic tests for determining drug susceptibility. From the molecular microbiologist's perspective, these advances are likely to depend on having a strong understanding of the biology of *M. tuberculosis* and the availability of the genetic tools required for its facile genetic manipulation.

Because of the slow growth of *M. tuberculosis* (doubling time of 24 h) and its pathogenicity, the development of a system for genetic manipulation has been slow, compared with other bacteria. Bacteriophages provide a valuable resource for genetic development, since they are easy to grow and study due to their relatively small size and simplicity (Hatfull, 1994). They also provide a very valuable and efficient means of introducing DNA into their host cells, an attribute that has been exploited for targeted mutagenesis, transposon mutagenesis, and rapid diagnostic detection (Bardarov et al., 2002; 1997; Jacobs et al., 1993). Numerous specific genetic tools derived from mycobacteriophages have been developed, but the potential is huge and the surface has as yet been barely scratched (Hatfull, 2004). So for any new mycobacteriophage that has been isolated and genomically characterized, there are many potential projects that students can choose to engage in. These projects are more open ended and independent in nature, but students who have succeeded in the PHIRE program are well positioned to pursue them.

6.9 What's in a Name?

Scientific discovery is a powerful force. Within the context of the PHIRE program, discovering a new virus in the environment is an intrinsically exciting activity and is intimately associated with the concept of project ownership. Students recognize that isolating a new virus may be of importance to the community, but it is also important for them personally. If they do not decide to pursue its characterization and unlock its secrets, then who will? The discovery they have made is "money-in-the-bank," and further studies will result from the proud investment of their time and energy.

This sense of project ownership and discovery is further reinforced by the key step of naming the phage that they have discovered. Students are encouraged to use individual names rather than any more systematic scheme, with the justification that our genomic understanding of bacteriophages is that they cannot be readily arranged into hierarchical lineages because of the extensive amount of horizontal genetic exchange that dominates their evolution. The term "species" cannot be easily applied to bacteriophages, no matter what definition of the term is applied (Lawrence et al., 2002). So we use names that reflect this individualistic character. Examples of some of the mycobacteriophage names include Corndog, Barnyard, Giles, Pipefish, and Rosebush.

It is not uncommon for students to take some time in making the decision as to what to name their phages. A particularly illustrative example occurred when one of us (GFH) was giving a presentation of the PHIRE program and happened to have a program student in the audience. The student was asked to come to the podium (without prior prompting) and talk about his involvement in the PHIRE program. In response to the question "Why did it take so long to decide on the choice of a name for your phage," he thought for a while and then responded "Because it is so important!" This is a fairly common reaction, the idea that the phage they have isolated and characterized becomes a part of the scientific landscape and one that may be used by others for many years to come in various ways. Its name is therefore important, and not something to be taken too lightly. Enabling students with the authority to provide a name (we usually hold the power of veto, just in case) couples closely with the concept of project ownership, further cementing the association of the student with the phage.

6.10 Who's Qualified for the PHIRE Program?

The PHIRE program unusually combines the idea of being able to contribute to key scientific advances without the need for extensive and specific training or experience. In essence, this is a program that anyone – literally anyone – can participate in. As noted above, the techniques required in the initial stages are quite simple and can readily be performed in most high-school settings. There is also not really much that you need to know that would prevent someone from doing these initial steps. This should not be confused with the notion that there is no scientific content to the PHIRE program; clearly the opposite is true, but engagement and success in performing the experiments provides a platform to learn about the ecology, microbiology, genetics, evolution, and biochemistry that emerge within the program. Participants of the PHIRE program include undergraduates, high-school students, teachers, and even middle-school students. While not everyone will necessarily be fully engaged for all parts of the program or be inspired to complete all the steps described above, we have yet to find someone who is unqualified to start in the PHIRE program.

Perhaps this low barrier to participation seems unimportant or trivial, but it is a truly key element of PHIRE. Most importantly, all students have an equal opportunity for participation, and there is no need to employ biased and inappropriate conditions for selection. For example, when choosing students for participation we do not give undue weight to standardized test scores because of the limited validity of these tests for our educational program that is organized around the performance of actual scientific research. An expression of curiosity by students is usually a good indicator that they will benefit from the program, and we generally aim for as diverse a group of students as is reasonably possible. In essence, everyone is qualified for the PHIRE program, and it provides opportunities for students to find out if this is an endeavor in which they excel even if their past experiences may not necessarily have predicted it.

6.11 Parallel Projects: Pros and Cons

The fact that we are able to describe a ten-step project plan as part of a reflective process of program development and active assessment underscores another core PHIRE component. Essentially, while students enjoy the novelty of project ownership and discovery, the processes and techniques employed are essentially the same for each student. This can therefore be thought of as a massively parallel project structure and one that comes not only with some notable attributes but also with some detriments.

The detriments are reasonably obvious. If students are engaged in parallel projects then there is a compromise of the concept of doing truly independent open-ended research, where the outcome is not known and there are many decision points along the way. We regard this as an unfortunate compromise, but it also needs to be recognized that inclusion of any more than a very small number of students is difficult if each has a truly independent project. To conduct more open-ended projects students typically need a more sophisticated knowledge of the subject matter and usually require specific and close supervision. Unfortunately, the ratio of supervisors (graduate students and postdoctoral fellows) to student-researchers rarely supports more than a small handful of students performing open-ended projects in any medium-sized research laboratory.

There are, however, considerable attributes to having parallel projects. Most importantly, there is a well-defined set of approaches that will be used and these are established and thoroughly streamlined. But the supervision problem largely disappears, since more experienced PHIRE students are well positioned to assist more junior PHIRE students, having already mastered most of the early phases. This peer supervision also releases the constraints on the number of students in the program. In fact having a greater number of students is an administrative asset. It decentralizes the program operation and enhances communication between PHIRE participants. Thus, while acknowledging the compromises, there are really important practical advantages. Furthermore, students are nicely trained for moving onto more independent projects as they emerge from their PHIRE successes.

6.12 Mentees and Mentors: Opportunities and Responsibilities

Students entering the PHIRE program are usually assigned a specific mentor, another student who is already within the program. In most cases this will correspond to a more "senior" undergraduate mentoring a more "junior" undergraduate or an undergraduate mentoring a high-school student, although the apparent academic hierarchy is merely superficial. In several instances, for example, high-school students have mentored undergraduate students, provided that they are established in the program and been successful through the early phases.

This mentor–mentee system is important for program administration of the parallel projects as described above, but it has a more important underlying role. Students entering the program are the beneficiaries of the opportunities that they are provided with – opportunities to engage in authentic scientific discovery. As mentors, they learn that with these opportunities come the responsibilities associated with passing on what they have learned to others; mentor training can be readily facilitated through the Entering Mentoring program established by Jo Handelsman and colleagues (Handelsman et al., 2005). Mentoring is as central to the PHIRE program as it is possible. It is the "I" in PHIRE, the integrating of research and education, with the opportunities to do research, inseparably associated with the responsibilities of education. The PHIRE program thus strives not just to introduce students to the world of science – who scientists are, how science is done, and the scientific environment – but places them from the beginning as scientist/educators or educator/scientists. Where divisions between our research and educational missions throughout academia have caused evident damage, this emphasis is an especially positive attribute to the PHIRE program.

6.13 Scheduling and Flexibility

The PHIRE program is not a course, and the time that students invest in their project is mainly determined by them, just as graduate students or postdoctoral researchers do. Students may spend time in the program during the summer months, taking the advantage of large blocks of available time for research, or they may be engaged throughout the academic year. For undergraduate students, finding the time can be challenging, especially early in their programs since the first two years of college/university education can often be demanding with required and core course work. High-school students also have many demands on their time, but several have worked throughout the academic year on a PHIRE project, whenever time was available to them. Clearly, the project moves faster when more time is invested in it, but significant parts of the project can be performed within a flexile schedule, and there are few phases that require large extended periods of intense work that have to be done within a particular schedule at the expense of all other demands.

Once again, it is tempting to consider the suitability of PHIRE projects with flexible scheduling as a relatively minor program component, but it fits well with the other program components. In particular, in the absence of a pre-arranged rigid schedule, students must be self-motivated to engage in the research and schedule their time accordingly. With many students, this motivation is closely linked to the rewards of discovery and project ownership and a quick realization that the successes are often the direct result of the degree of commitment to the project. Without a rigid course-like structure, project ownership, discovery, and research successes are absolute requirements of the program.

6.14 Multiple Milestones of Success

While the PHIRE program involves quite a well-formulated path, we recognize that not all students will succeed with all stages. Students may not have time, some will progress slower or faster than others, various difficulties can be encountered along the way, and some students learn that this endeavor is something that they don't really have their heart in. Nonetheless, students achieving only part of the process can still enjoy some degree of success. They will with near-certainty have isolated a new phage, have been able to purify it, and prepare stocks. During this process they have learned about the laboratory environment and the scientific process, worked alongside other professional scientists, and absorbed a substantial amount of microbiology! In an environment within the United States in particular where there are significant concerns about the level of scientific literacy among the general public, these would seem not insignificant accomplishments.

6.15 Not All Failure Is Bad!

Perhaps it is obtuse to laud the attributes of failure, but there are surely some benefits. Being a successful practitioner of scientific research requires many skills, but one of the most important is problem solving – knowing how to recognize and address substantial experimental and technical challenges and how to circumvent or resolve them. Becoming familiar with these problem-solving issues and to address them is an important part of the experience in learning how to do science and provides a sense of empowerment to students when they learn how to solve problems for themselves. Furthermore, it is not uncommon to identify students who are interested and curious in doing research that have a history of extraordinary academic achievement, in which they have always excelled at the classroom challenges. It can be a very humbling experience for such students to find that it is they – rather than the academically "average" student next to them – that has yet to identify a phage.

While some of the steps in phage hunting and genomics are more technically challenging than others, the phage isolation procedure is a playing surface-leveling experience. Success is not something that can be easily controlled because the presence of phage particles for the host you are studying is not readily predictable (other than recognizing that phages tend to be found in the environment in the same places as their hosts). A lack of care in following the procedures, sloppy work, and poor attention to detail can all make the isolation more difficult, but academic preparation, knowledge of microbiology, and supreme self-confidence, all have little influence. Understanding what is within and what is beyond the control of the scientist is an important lesson for all students to learn.

6.16 Transitions: From Concrete Beginnings to Abstract Representation

When practicing science, it is easy to forget that most of what we do is to develop and debate abstract concepts. Learning about science is in large part the art of acquiring the language that is required and being able to understand and manipulate concepts that are often divorced from grounding in our everyday lives. Thus the relationship between abstract concepts and their concrete roots is a critical component in the learning of science.

An appealing aspect of the PHIRE program is that there is a built-in transition from the very concrete beginnings – digging up dirt and collecting it in a tube – to the thoroughly representational process of decoding thousands of letters and numbers of a genome sequence rolling over a computer screen (Hanauer et al., 2006). The transition is fairly gradual, as dirt collection leads to growth of bacterial cultures, followed by preparation and electron microscopy; this leads to DNA isolation and the much more abstract processes of DNA sequence determination and annotation.

6.17 Seven Attributes of the PHIRE Program

In this chapter we have hopefully established an understanding of the PHIRE program, its elements, and the reasons why we believe it has some successes associated with it. It is also helpful to note that it represents a very different perspective to how science is typically taught, especially in the K-12 setting. The K-12 culture – especially at the high-school level – is commonly a process of the communication of our known facts and concepts from the instructor to the students, and students who do well are those that perform well at listening, processing, retaining the information, and subsequently recalling it in the context of standardized and other tests. However, as discussed in Chap. 2, the process of scientific research operates on a different set of principles. It requires challenging our current understanding and utilizing inquiry-based operations to elucidate new knowledge. Doing so requires prioritizing ideas and concepts in order of importance and of thinking about those issues and topics that we don't comprehend. Finally, it requires an idea as to how new knowledge is obtained and indeed the basis upon which we assert that we know what it is that we know.

The concept behind the PHIRE program is that inquiry-based activities are the only way that students can learn science, as opposed to the facsimile that currently is adopted in most K-12 settings and sometimes at the undergraduate level, especially in the freshman and sophomore years. We recognize that, for all students, to take advantage of such experiences poses major challenges, but we also hope that these experiences with PHIRE and other inquiry-based programs will provide a focus on what needs to be done to make this happen. In this chapter we have discussed the scientific and education attributes of the PHIRE program, but in summary will list seven attributes here that are translatable items and could be used as building blocks to construct other such programs with strong integration of research and education (Hatfull et al., 2006).

6.17.1 Attribute 1: Technical Simplicity with Transition to Complexity

Phage isolation is technically simple, and while some techniques can be more demanding they occur later in the process. Even finding genes begins with the simple concept of pattern recognition.

6.17.2 Attribute 2: Conceptual Simplicity with Transition to Complexity

Some of the concepts that will be learned with the PHIRE program are quite complex, but they are acquired in an inquiry-based context and high academic achievement is not required for starting the program.

6.17.3 Attribute 3: Flexible Scheduling Compatibility

Students have many demands on their time besides doing scientific research, and flexible scheduling capability is important. This approach to scheduling provides a degree of control to the students over the progress of their project.

6.17.4 Attribute 4: Multiple Achievement Milestones

The only serious and significant "failure" within the PHIRE program is the inability to isolate a phage; however, this is rare (about 1% in our experience). All others enjoy some degree of achievement, even if not all steps are accomplished.

6.17.5 Attribute 5: Parallel Projects and Mentoring

There are numerous advantages to having a parallel project structure, of which the most important is an inherent suitability for students to mentor other students.

6.17.6 Attribute 6: Authentic Publishable Research

The science within the PHIRE program is important and interesting to a broader audience. There are therefore rich opportunities for publications in the peer-reviewed literature. Also, students readily recognize the difference between authentic research and an exercise, and the latter is often not well endowed with motivation.

6.17.7 Attribute 7: Project Ownership

The association of the discovery with the student is powerful, and naming the phage that they have discovered provides incentives for continued involvement and commitment to the project.

Chapter 7
The PHIRE Program Assessment Strategy

7.1 Introduction

This chapter describes the specific assessment strategy developed for the educational assessment of the PHIRE program. The PHIRE assessment strategy covers formative diagnostic and summative aims of an education in bacteriophage scientific inquiry. The strategy proposed in this chapter consists of the integration of five different types of tool that cover the four knowledge sources of physical, cognitive, representational, and presentational knowledge and is organized across the scientific inquiry timeline of bacteriophage isolation and genomic identification. The overall approach follows the guidelines of authentic scientific inquiry assessment and designs assessment procedures following an informed understanding of the specific scientific and educational process that is being assessed.

As specified within Chap. 5, the process of designing an assessment strategy and constructing assessment tools consists of a series of stages. As an initial starting point the scientific inquiry process at the heart of the educational program needs to be analyzed and described (see Chap. 6 for a description of the stages of this program); then a series of decisions concerning the aims of the program and which specific representations and their adjacent knowledge are considered to be significant need to be made; following this a strategy and a set of assessment tools can be designed. The design of this chapter follows a similar plan starting with an analysis of aims, a detailed analysis of the decision-making process at significant milestones of the phage-hunting process, and finally the proposition of an overall strategy for assessment of this scientific inquiry process. Further clarification and exemplification of the specific assessment tools used in the PHIRE program appears in the next chapter.

7.2 Aims of Undergraduate Phage Hunting

The aims of undergraduate science education within the PHIRE program have been articulated by the prime researcher and educator of the program, Prof. G. Hatfull. In his Executive Summary of the Phage Hunting Outreach Program (2006), he

D.I. Hanauer et al., *Active Assessment: Assessing Scientific Inquiry*,
Mentoring in Academia and Industry 2, DOI 10.1007/978-0-387-89649-6_7,

states that students should "learn how to do scientific research and how to discover nature's secrets." The educational program is designed to "elucidate the mechanism for viral evolution and to determine the extent of viral diversity through the isolation and characterization of novel bacteriophages." The program not only provides the framework within which each student can "isolate a new bacteriophage" but also has the wider aim of "demystifying the culture of scientific discovery" and provide each student with the scientific "understanding that will enhance whatever career path they ultimately pursue." Finally the program wishes to "correct commonly held misconceptions about scientific discovery – what it is and who does it – and to show these students that they can become the next generation of scientific explorers." In terms of assessment, the aims of this program for undergraduate phage hunters can be stated as follows:

1. *Summative Assessment: Development of Substantive Knowledge Concerning Bacteriophage*: As with any other undergraduate science program, the PHIRE program has the aim of developing substantive scientific knowledge in relation to the core scientific concepts that inform and direct the scientific inquiry process. In the case of the PHIRE program these core concepts relate to three basic issues: the nature and mechanisms of viral evolution, the physical and genetic characteristics of bacteriophages, and research into the potential applications of bacteriophages in associated fields such as medicine. Data collected from this form of assessment could be used to evaluate the substantive factual knowledge acquired by students involved in this program.
2. *Summative Assessment: Development of Procedural and Representational Knowledge Concerning the Microbiological Process of Isolating and Genomically Annotating and Analyzing a Novel Bacteriophage*: The undergraduate PHIRE program involves a specific scientific inquiry program and as such is designed to enhance student understandings of the scientific procedures and methods involved in the isolation and characterization of novel bacteriophages and the microbiological aspects of these organisms and their interactions with the environment. This knowledge base includes basic microbiological and bioinformatic epistemology and a clear understanding of the representational aspects of the phage-hunting process. The aim of the assessment procedure is to elicit assessment data that can be used to determine the levels of procedural and representational knowledge development achieved by the participants in this program. These data can be used to describe the outcomes of the educational program in relation to the specific aspects of the scientific inquiry process of the isolation and characterization of bacteriophages.
3. *Summative Assessment: Presentational Knowledge and Self-Perception Concerning the Bacteriophage Scientific Inquiry Process*: The PHIRE program aims to help students to develop a self-concept as a researcher and the professional knowledge associated with this role. This knowledge includes the ability to present research finding within formats that are authentic to the ways in which professional researchers presented their research. This form of knowledge is presentational and consists of genre of presenting information at professional

settings. The data collected from this assessment could be used to evaluate the outcomes of the student's scientific inquiry process and the ability of the student to clearly conceptualize and present these results in a professional manner.

4. *Formative and Diagnostic Assessment – Procedural, Substantive, and Representational Knowledge of the Microbiological Process of Isolating and Genomically Annotating Novel Bacteriophages*: The PHIRE program is an educational program designed to enhance scientific learning through undergraduate participation in an authentic scientific inquiry process. The PHIRE program aims to provide every student with the ability to master the procedural, substantive, and representational aspects of the phage-hunting process. Accordingly, formative and diagnostic assessment data are collected to ensure that quality feedback can be provided to the students so that the scientific inquiry process can be completed successfully. As opposed to other forms of educational practice a basic assumption of the PHIRE program is that there is real scientific value in the specific scientific inquiry processes conducted by each student. This educational program functions through a form of directed mentorship in which students conduct guided scientific inquiries, and in this context ways of collecting data that can be used to assess the knowledge of the student and provide direct and informed feedback are useful for enhancing the students' ability to complete a scientifically significant inquiry process. The basic aim of this assessment procedure is to provide scientist-educators with information to provide quality feedback to students involved in the inquiry process.

7.3 Detailed Analyses of Decision-Making Reasoning and Calculation in the Bacteriophage Isolation and Identification Process

As defined within Chap. 5, decisions need to be made as to what representational stages constitute milestones within the developing scientific inquiry process and can be used for assessment purposes. Once these representational stages have been chosen a full analysis of the adjacent knowledge sources needs to be conducted. In relation to the bacteriophage isolation and identification process there are several significant decisions that have to be made in order to complete the process. The following is the outline of significant decision making and calculation that are made according to the stage in the process:

a. *Step 1 – Phage Isolation*: Identification of plaques
b. *Step 2 – Phage Purification*: Generating a pure phage population
c. *Step 3 – Phage Amplification*: Calculation of lysate concentration: Selection of maximum bacteriophage yield

d. *Step 4 – DNA Comparison*: DNA restriction enzyme digestion and electrophoresis: Comparison of electrophoresis gel and decision as to value of continuation of process
e. *Step 5 – Genome Annotation and Analysis*: Gene Identification – Selection and identification of genes

Each of these decisions marks a point of transition in the whole process and as such is worth considering within the context of significant representational milestones that can be used for assessment of tool development. Below a detailed analysis of each of these decision-making processes is presented. The analysis presents the basic knowledge that is required to make the decision and describes the decision-making process using the formats of a schematic description and a logical inferential structure. The decision-making process for the first four decisions is within the environment of the wet laboratory and the last decision-making process is within the digital environment of a computer program.

7.3.1 Phage Isolation – Identification Through Infection

This conceptual reasoning process allows bacteriophages to be identified. The process is based on a basic understanding of microbiology – bacteriophages are viruses whose hosts are bacterial cells. Bacteriophages reproduce by exploiting the metabolism of the host bacteria. The bacteriophage delivers its genome into the cytoplasm of the bacterial host where it uses the cellular mechanisms of the host to reproduce. This typically results in the destruction of the original cell through the extensive reproduction of the bacteriophages and subsequent destruction of adjacent cells as the progeny of that first bacteriophage infects and destroys those bacteria. Accordingly, based on this characteristic of bacteriophages, a process of initial identification can be defined. If a sample potentially containing bacteriophages is placed in the controlled vicinity of a bacterial cell it will either infect or not infect the bacteria. If it does infect the bacteria, there is evidence of the presence of bacteriophages, which is revealed by the presence of a plaque, a circular zone of cell death causing a cleared zone in a bacterial lawn (see Fig. 6.2). If it does not infect the bacteria (i.e., no plaques are present), we assume that no bacteriophages specific to that bacterial host are present (and capable of infection under these controlled laboratory conditions). Schematically this process can be defined as follows:

Required Determination: Presence (+) of bacteriophages (or PFU, plaque-forming unit) in sample
Sample: 2 options: + presence of plaques (bacteriophages)
– absence of plaques (bacteriophages)
Empirical Test: Samples plated with bacteria
Results and Analysis: Infection (presence of plaques) = + bacteriophages
No infection (no plaques) = – bacteriophages

As a logical structure this can be represented as follows:

a. Bacteriophages infect bacteria
b. If plaques are present in a controlled environment, then bacteriophages are present
c. If plaques are not present, then bacteriophages are not present (or cannot be detected)

7.3.2 Phage Purification Through Selective Infection

This conceptual process allows a single bacteriophage to be selected from a sample which potentially includes several different bacteriophages. A basic assumption of this conceptual process is that during the process of infection, bacteriophages will create plaques that can be visually defined as "characteristic" of that bacteriophage. Accordingly, two different bacteriophages in the same sample may produce two visually different types of plaque morphotypes. If this occurs, then the aim is to generate a sample that contains only a single bacteriophage type. Thus at each stage of infection, when multiple different plaques are found, a choice is made as to which plaque will be chosen for further infection. This selection process gradually purifies the sample to the point at which all the plaques on the plate have the same visual characteristics. This situation is understood as the presence of a single bacteriophage type in that sample. Schematically this process can be represented as follows:

Required Determination: Presence of a single bacteriophage type in a sample
Sample: 3 options: – absence of bacteriophages
+ presence of a single bacteriophage type
++ presence of multiple bacteriophage types
Empirical Test: Repeated plating of samples with bacteria
Results and Analysis: Visual analysis of morphology of plaques

- Multiple plaques of different size, shape, and appearance = multiple bacteriophages (choose one plaque to repeat test)
- Multiple plaques of same size, shape, and appearance = single bacteriophage type (objective achieved, progress to next stage)
- No plaques = no bacteriophages

As a logical structure this can be represented as follows:

a. When infecting bacteria in a plated sample, each bacteriophage type creates a characteristic plaque according to its size, shape, and appearance.
b. If a plate has multiple plaques of different sizes, shapes, and appearances then different bacteriophages are present in the plate.
c. If a plate has multiple plaques of the same size, shape, and appearance then it is more likely that a single bacteriophage type is present.

7.3.3 Phage Amplification – Measuring Bacteriophage Concentration to Determine and Produce Maximum Bacteriophage Yield

The conceptual process involves working out the concentration of bacteriophage within a sample so that a decision on maximum phage yield levels for the production of large samples of bacteriophage can be made. This process involves the evaluation of a concentration (or amount) rather than a dichotomous present/absent judgment. The overall judgment as to the maximum phage yield level of bacteriophage concentration for amplification is done in three stages: first, the lysate is diluted at 10-fold intervals, plated, and titered (measured); second, the titer is manipulated to theoretically produce the maximum phage yield based on the assumption that 10,000 ± plaques will produce that yield, manifested as the desired "web pattern" in which just enough phage particles have been added to infect all – or nearly all – cells that are present; third, the assumed maximum phage yield calculations that will produce the web are tested at five close concentration levels to allow for variations among phage types. An empirical visual analysis of the web pattern on the plate determines the best concentration of phage to be used in the 30-plate infection.

Required Determination: Concentration (titer) of bacteriophage in a sample
Sample: 10 levels of dilution for bacteriophage sample
Empirical Test: 10 dilution levels plated
Results and Analysis: Visual analysis of the number of plaques at the most countable dilution and mathematical calculation to determine the titer (PFU/ml)

As a logical structure this can be represented as follows:

a. Each 10-fold dilution of sample produces a 10-fold decrease in the number of PFUs counted.
b. A plate of 20–200 PFUs is counted (this plate is used because it is considered the most countable plate).
c. The number of PFUs counted is used to calculate the titer according to the following equation: PFUs counted/amount of sample plated (μl) × Dilution Factor × 10^3 μ1/1ml = Titer PFU/ml.

Required Determination: Maximum phage yield concentration to be used for 30-plate infection, typically calculated to 10,000 PFU/ml
Sample: Using the titer, the maximum phage yield dilution is calculated, four additional dilutions are plated to empirically identify the desired web pattern:
Calculated maximum phage yield (MPY) concentration
One magnitude above MPY
Half of one magnitude above MPY
One magnitude below MPY
Half of one magnitude below MPY
Empirical Test: Five dilution levels of lysate plated

Results and Analysis: Visual analysis of plate plaque patterns

- Exhibits required (+) web pattern – determine this dilution level as optimal
- Exhibits a different pattern from the required (–) web pattern – determine that this dilution level is not optimal

As a logical structure this can be represented as follows:

a. A plate with maximum phage yield produces a distinctive pattern that can be recognized.
b. If the plate (each with different dilution levels) has the distinctive pattern of a MPY then that represents the best choice of dilution level for the production of large quantities of bacteriophage particles.
c. If the plate does not have the distinctive pattern then it is not a good choice for the production of large quantities of bacteriophage particles.

7.3.4 Electrophoresis

The conceptual process consists of determining the uniqueness of a bacteriophage DNA sample. This determination is made in relation to the procedures of DNA restriction enzyme digestion (RED) and electrophoresis (see Fig. 6.5). Restriction enzyme digestion of DNA is a process in which a restriction enzyme recognizes a specific sequence of bases and cuts the DNA at those specific sites. The segments generated are potentially of different lengths and each genome will produce a characteristic pattern of DNA fragments. These can be separated and analyzed by the process of electrophoresis in which samples containing mixtures of DNA fragments are loaded onto an agarose gel, to which an electric current is applied. DNA fragments migrate toward the negative pole with smaller fragments migrating faster through the gel matrix than larger ones. Within a given time frame all of the DNA fragments can be separated and their sizes measured by comparison to known size markers. In the determination of the uniqueness of a bacteriophage DNA sample, a series of five (or more) DNA enzyme digests are used individually, and the pattern generated compared with the patterns of previously characterized bacteriophages.

Required Determination: The uniqueness of the isolated bacteriophage
Sample: Two options: Unique pattern of DNA restriction fragments
Identical pattern of DNA restriction fragments
Empirical Test: Electrophoresis gels of restriction enzyme-digested DNA
Results and Analysis: Visual analysis of electrophoresis gels (the visual analysis involves an evaluation of the number, location, and intensity of the bands for each enzyme and the overall pattern of all of the digests, sometimes referred to as its "DNA fingerprint").
(–) Exhibits unique pattern of DNA restriction fragments
(+) Exhibits similarities to a DNA restriction pattern of another phage.

As a logical structure:

a. The electrophoresis of a DNA restriction enzyme digest produces a pattern that is made up of digested DNA segments ordered according to size (as seen according to the number, position, and intensity of the bands).
b. Each bacteriophage DNA will produce a characteristic pattern of digested DNA segments on an electrophoresis gel.
c. If the DNA restriction enzyme digest produces a pattern that is identical to another DNA restriction enzyme digest then the assumption is that this is a duplicate (or VERY similar) of a bacteriophage that has already been identified.
d. If the DNA restriction enzyme digest produces a pattern that is different from the other DNA restriction enzyme digest then the assumption is that this is a previously undiscovered bacteriophage.

   Required Determination: Evaluation of restriction enzyme digest pattern of a bacteriophage

   Sample: Electrophoresis of DNA restriction fragments of a bacteriophage DNA sample

   Empirical Test: Set up digests and run gel electrophoresis

   Results and Analysis: Comparison of the overall pattern of bands with the digests of other known phages determines the uniqueness of each bacteriophage.

7.3.5 Gene Determination (Annotation)

The gene determination process aims to identify genetic sequences that have high coding potential to be genes. This process is interpretive and utilizes a series of sources of information. The basic determination is in relation to the computer file output designating the complete genetic sequence of the bacteriophage DNA sample. The sources of information used in the determination are the DNA Master Program, the GeneMark program, the Glimmer program, the NCBI Gene Blast program, and general principles of bacteriophage genomic structure. The actual process of identifying and recording the identified genes is done in the DNA Master program. Following is a schematic description of each program and its output:

- *GeneMark Program*: Provides a prediction of gene locations according to DNA sequence characteristics that are in common to those of known genes. Visual analysis of a computer output containing a trace depicting the degree of coding potential in each of all six possible frames across the entire genome (Fig. 7.1). In addition to coding potential the output also includes the positions of potential gene start sites (as up ticks) and stop codons (down ticks). An open reading frame (ORF) – i.e., a region of DNA in which stop codons are absent – that contains a potential start site at the beginning, a stop codon at its end, and high coding potential throughout has high probability for corresponding to a gene.
- *Glimmer*: Provides a prediction of gene locations by analyzing the DNA sequence searching for characteristics that correspond closely to internal open

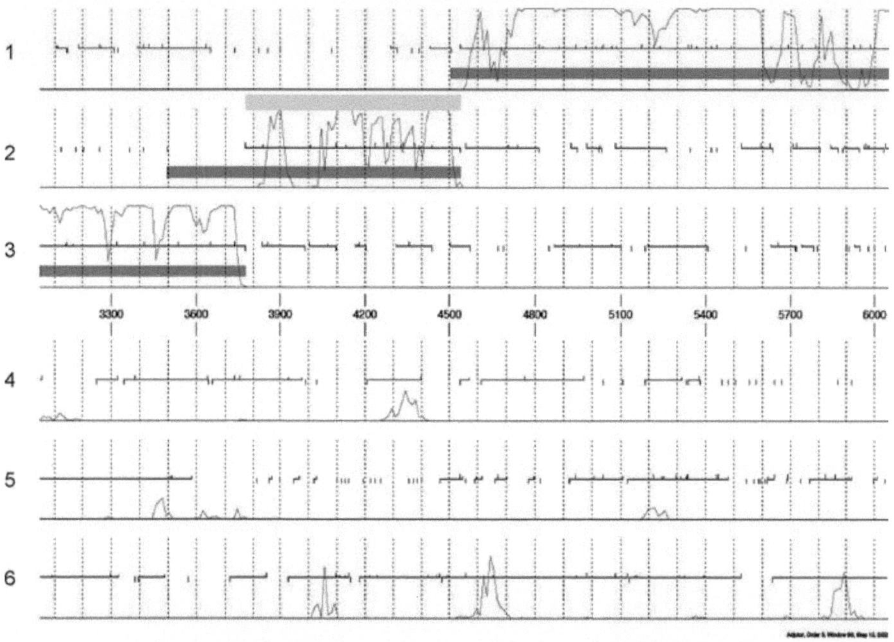

Fig. 7.1 Graphic Output of GeneMark Program. A segment of phage Adjutor genome sequence was analyzed using the program GeneMark, which generates a graph of the coding potential in each of the six possible open reading frames (ORFs) (labeled 1–6; frames 1–3 are expressed in the rightward direction, and 4–6 in the reverse direction). ORFs are identified as *horizontal lines* between translation stop codons (*down ticks*), and potential start codons are shown as *up ticks*. Coding potential is indicated by the line graph. The thick horizontal gray lines (still italicized) are considered areas of interest. One such gene is highlighted in *green* (*see* Color Insert)

reading frame features. The output is a computer file that depicts the coordinates of the start and stop of each gene (Fig. 7.2).

- *NCBI Gene BLASTing*: Compares the amino acid translation of a potential gene to a database of known protein sequences. The output is a computer file that identifies genes products that are statistically similar to those in other organisms (Fig. 7.3). The file provides a probability score for the quality of the relationship between the different gene products. If the BLASTed gene product has a BLAST score of acceptable significance, this provides further evidence for the gene identification.
- *DNA Master*: Compiles all data outputs together for evaluation by importing GeneMark and Glimmer data, providing a Shine–Dalgarno score to evaluate the potential for different start codons at the beginning of genes, and providing a six-frame translation for evaluation. It is in this DNAMaster program that all parameters and guidelines for the gene identification decision are synthesized into the best evaluation of genes in a genome (Fig. 7.4).

Microbial Genomes

GLIMMER (ver. 3.02; iterated) predictions:

orfID	start	end	frame	score
>Adjutor				
orf00001	43	309	+1	5.50
orf00002	421	1524	+1	11.60
orf00003	1568	1762	+2	7.44
orf00004	1772	1936	+2	19.55
orf00005	1946	2125	+2	2.27
orf00006	2136	3776	+3	9.08
orf00008	3773	4543	+2	7.48
orf00010	4540	6306	+1	13.68
orf00011	6328	7914	+1	15.10
orf00012	7925	8137	+2	8.51
orf00013	8134	8586	+1	6.27
orf00014	8555	8734	+2	9.56
orf00015	8822	9067	+2	1.62
orf00016	9235	9636	+1	6.98
orf00017	9669	10376	+3	10.88
orf00019	10392	10811	+3	10.24
orf00020	10848	12032	+3	12.62
orf00022	12029	12397	+2	12.81
orf00023	12400	12732	+1	7.05
orf00024	12729	13136	+3	7.45
orf00025	13129	13491	+1	8.23
orf00026	13488	13907	+3	5.12
orf00027	13944	14300	+3	8.89
orf00028	14312	14512	+2	4.14
orf00029	14541	15344	+3	9.78
orf00030	15426	16079	+3	10.30
orf00032	16102	16320	+1	8.00
orf00034	16322	21094	+2	10.80
orf00036	21084	22604	+3	14.22
orf00038	22601	24256	+2	12.44
orf00039	24256	26526	+1	13.24
orf00040	26526	28574	+3	11.64
orf00043	28574	29440	+2	4.49
orf00044	29450	29770	+2	11.76
orf00046	29773	30201	+1	4.90
orf00048	30210	31193	+3	10.50
orf00049	31190	31444	+2	7.17
orf00051	31715	32254	+2	2.39
orf00053	32238	32693	+3	6.68

Fig. 7.2 Glimmer Program Output. A segment of the phage Adjutor genome sequence was analyzed by Glimmer generating a list of potential ORFs, their start and stop codons, reading frame, and evaluative score. The *red box* designates one specific candidate gene (*see* Color Insert)

General Principles of Bacteriophage Genomics: Phage genomics is an emerging field. The data that guide the decision-making process of "correct" gene identification are fraught with incomplete information. Allowing Glimmer and GeneMark data to find the genes is relatively straightforward and reliable, but identifying the best start codon position involves subtle nuances requiring a trained human interpretive process. When choosing the "best" start codon, the following list of factors needs to be considered:

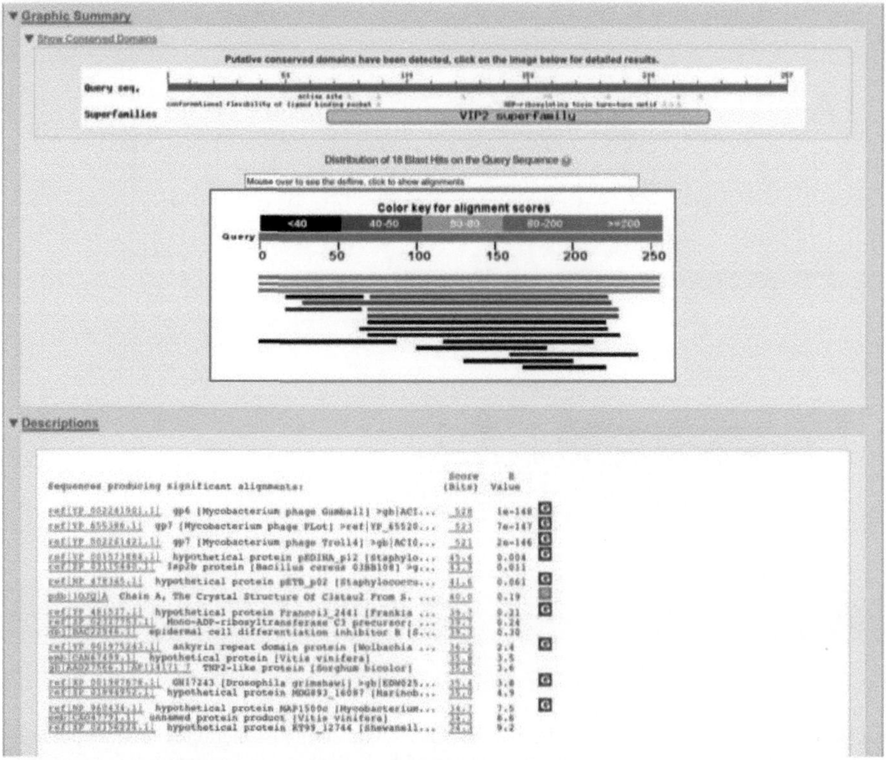

Fig. 7.3 Output of a BLASTP search using the BLAST server at NCBI. The amino acid sequence of a predicted phage protein was submitted as a search query to the server, which returned a summary of the search results; a screen shot of the results window is shown. At the *top*, a diagram shows the correspondence of a putative conserved domain identified in the search with a linear representation of the query sequence. Below that is a diagram of related sequences identified in the search, with the closest matches shown in *red*. The identities of the specific matches and their scores are shown in the *bottom panel* (*see* Color Insert)

- Phage genomes are tightly packed, so call the longest ORF.
- Genes are often found in groups in the forward or reverse directions.
- Genes do not extensively overlap. Overlap by a stop codon is common. However, if the overlap is greater than seven amino acids, then other data will be needed to provide additional support for that start site.
- Two genes are not called in the same space. Unless there is supporting data to the contrary, each segment of DNA only codes for one gene.
- Glimmer choice (start coordinate listed) is valuable.
- GeneMark choice (the beginning of the coding potential) is valuable.
- Shine–Dalgarno score (a feature of DNA Master) – the bigger the score, the better the potential start site.
- Shine–Dalgarno sequence – Translation initiation requires recognition of the correct location by binding of the ribosome to the mRNA. Specific sequences

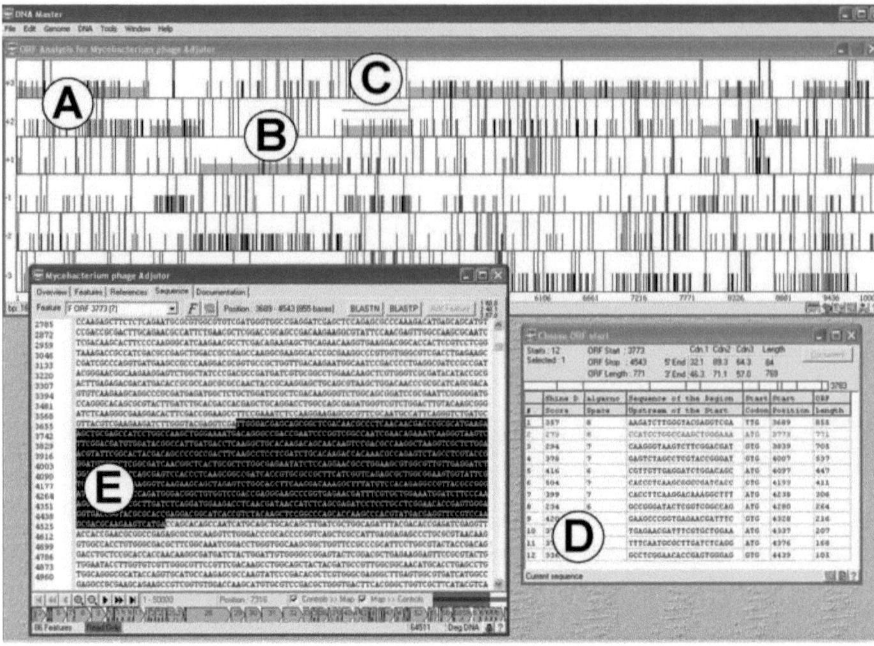

Fig. 7.4 Representations of genome analyses using DNA Master. (**A**) The output from the "Frames" routine in DNA Master showing six reading frames, with start (*short vertical lines*) and stop codons (*full height lines*) indicated. (**B**) ORFs with strong prediction for coding potential predicted by GeneMark and Glimmer are designated by a *thick green horizontal line*. (**C**) Clicking on a segment of a frame of interest produces a *thin green* line and also links to the "choose start" routine shown in (**D**) the ORF and start codon corresponding to the frame segment in (**C**) is in *red*. (4). (**E**) The genome segment highlighted in (**C**) is revealed as a selected segment (black background) in the "Sequence" panel of DNA Master and can be added to the annotation or copied as either a nucleotide or a translated amino acid sequence for BLAST analyses (*see* Color Insert)

(Shine–Dalgarno sequence) are recognized and bound by ribosomes. The consensus Shine–Dalgarno sequence in *Escherichia coli* is 5'-AGGAGGA spaced approximately seven bases upstream of the start codon but it is similar for many bacteria. For any given gene both the sequence and the spacing can vary.

- The three possible mycobacterial start codons have an overall distribution of 45% ATG, 45% GTG, and 10% TTG. Glimmer does not identify the TTG starts.
- Blast comparison – copy your call as a translation and submit a BLASTP request to NCBI BLAST. Does your predicted gene match other GenBank entries? If your gene is similar to a known gene but different start locations are chosen, it does not necessarily mean that yours is wrong.
- As the phage genome ORFS change direction, recognize that there probably needs to be intergenic space for promoters.
- Be cautious when identifying very small ORFS. The average length of phage genes is only 200 codons, but there are few smaller than 50 codons.
- Negative frame genes are somewhat more difficult, take time to get oriented.

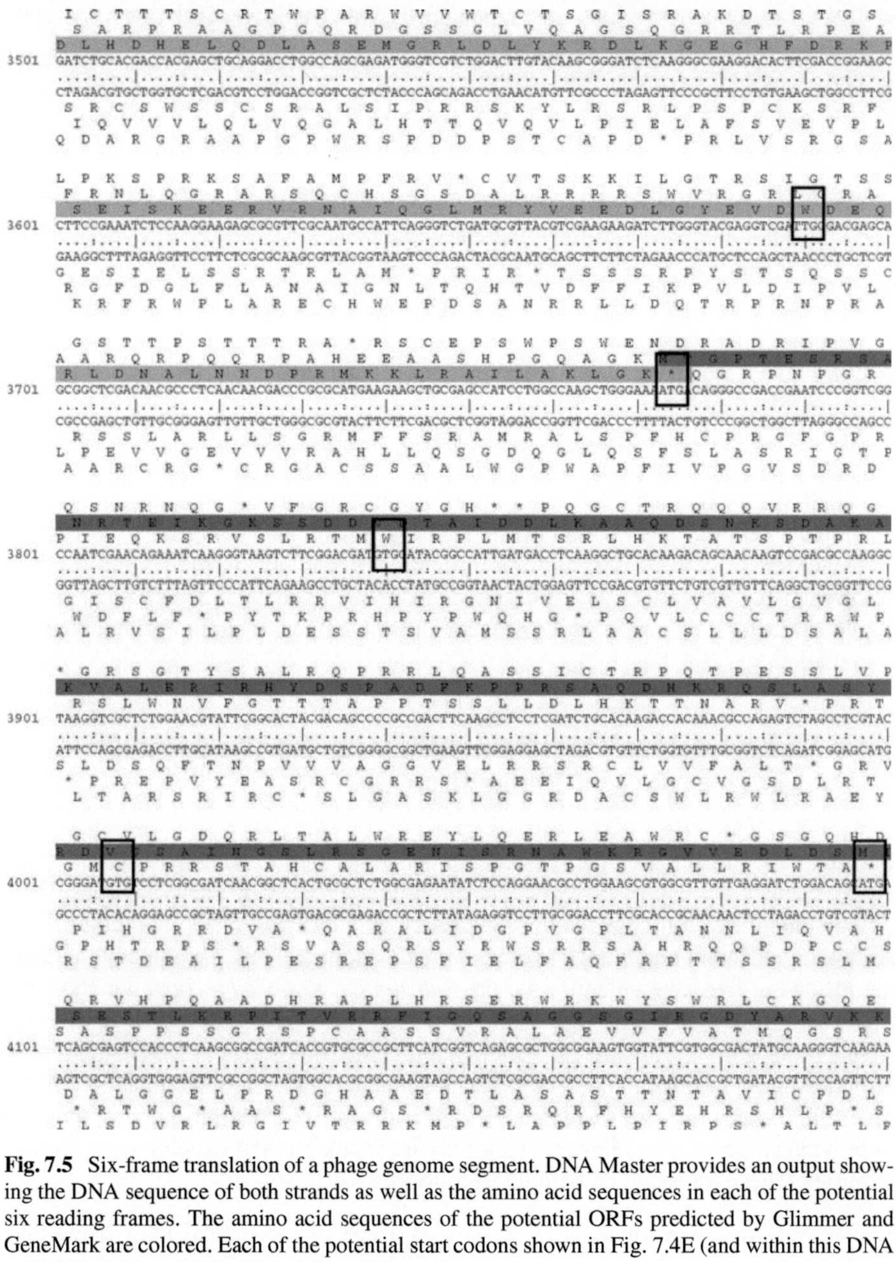

Fig. 7.5 Six-frame translation of a phage genome segment. DNA Master provides an output showing the DNA sequence of both strands as well as the amino acid sequences in each of the potential six reading frames. The amino acid sequences of the potential ORFs predicted by Glimmer and GeneMark are colored. Each of the potential start codons shown in Fig. 7.4E (and within this DNA segment) are shown *boxed* (*see* Color Insert)

- DNA Master stop codons are indicated by full frame vertical lines and start codons as 1/2 the height of the frame.
- Only DNA Master calls TTG starts.
- Check the gene calls at the right end of a circular genome to be sure there is not a gene that wraps around the end of the genome.

These information sources are weighted and evaluated differently in the determination of a gene. This decision-making reasoning process is interpretive (Figs. 7.4 and 7.5). Following is a schematic presenting of this process:

Required Determination: Identification of genetic sequences that have a high potential to be genes.
Sample: FASTA file – the complete genetic sequence for the bacteriophage genome in a common file format.
Results and Analysis: The process of identifying a gene within the complete genetic sequence is done in several steps. The recording of the analysis in its initial stages is conducted using a six-frame translation print out, GeneMark graphic output, and DNA Master. Using all of the programs (Glimmer, GeneMark, DNA Master) and the evaluations listed above, the potential genes of each bacteriophage genome are identified. This process is recorded in the DNA Master file and on the GeneMark and six-frame translation printouts using a marker.

7.4 An Educational Assessment Strategy for the Scientific Inquiry Process of Phage Hunting

In order to fulfill the aims of the assessment program and address in a contextualized manner the nature of the scientific inquiry process of bacteriophage isolation and identification, a series of assessment tools utilizing different methods and addressing different knowledge sources were developed. In all, the strategy includes the following five assessment tools: the *Substantive Knowledge Test*, the *Physical Checklist*, the *Visual Literacy Test*, the *Notebook Assessment Tool*, and the *Knowledge Presentation Performance Test*. Taken together this series of assessment tools provides in-depth information on the achievements of the students involved in the scientific inquiry process of phage hunting and also information that can be used to provide students with relevant and timely feedback on their developing scientific inquiries. These tools can be defined as follows:

1. *The Substantive Knowledge Test*: This is a test of the factual knowledge that develops as a result of the specific scientific inquiry experience of working in a microbiology laboratory. This test has the format of a written test designed to elicit factual scientific knowledge. The test can have the format of a multiple-choice or open-ended question format and is parallel to other tests developed within the university courses that relate to substantive knowledge. This test is divided into two sections, one conducted in the middle of the program and one

at the end of the program and is a final summative test of substantive knowledge development. This test involves professional content knowledge relating to bacteriophage. The knowledge assessed by this tool is significant in that it provides information on the factual knowledge of microbiology that has been achieved during this educational scientific inquiry experience.

2. *The Physical Checklist*: Working in a laboratory is a basic aspect of most scientific inquiries. Within the phage-hunting program a significant amount of the student's work is actually conducted in the microbiology laboratory. Accordingly the development of a tool that assesses basic working knowledge of a laboratory is a desirable aim. This tool addresses the basic physical knowledge that is required to function within the wet laboratory. The tool is designed for the novice workers in the microbiological laboratory and addresses basic techniques that have wide-based application in many of the different protocols used in the stages and steps of the bacteriophage isolation and identification process. An analysis of the physical knowledge utilized in the various stages of the phage-hunting process revealed five physical techniques that were repeated and considered basic to many of the procedures conducted in the microbiology laboratory. The five techniques are Use of a Pipette Gun; Use of a Micropipettor; Centrifuge Use; Aseptic Technique; and Plating Technique. The assessment tool has the format of a checklist specifying the required usage of each of these techniques and differentiating between different aspects of the technique. This assessment tool is used in an on-going manner and in relation to the students' real work in the phage-hunting program. In other words, the student is not artificially tested; rather, as the student works, the instructor-mentor closely observes the student's work and "checks-off" on the checklist the quality of the student's functioning with the different techniques. This happens in relation to every relevant usage of these specific techniques and as such is a rolling procedure in which a series of dated evaluations of physical technique are conducted. The physical checklist is designed as a diagnostic and summative assessment tool. As a diagnostic and formative tool, the checklist provides mentors with specific information on the functioning of the students. If any problems are found, the instructor comments on these and provides instructional feedback in relation to the specific step or stage of the phage-hunting process that the student is conducting. As a summative assessment tool, the checklist shows levels of mastery of these different basic microbiological laboratory techniques and is to be considered the development of procedural scientific knowledge. The knowledge assessed in this tool is significant on three levels: (1) it directly influences the quality of the microbiological research conducted by the student; (2) it provides a basis of physical knowledge concerning microbiological research that allows results to be interpreted and comprehended; and (3) it provides a basis for exploring developments in self-understanding as a researcher.

3. *The Visual Literacy Test*: A central aspect of the microbiological process of phage hunting consists of the ability of the researcher to conduct a visual analysis of various representations used in the microbiology laboratory. To understand and interpret these representations, different knowledge sources need to be

addressed. The interpretation of a visual representation requires the integration of substantive microbiological knowledge and procedural knowledge of the cognitive, representational, and epistemological aspects of microbiological research. Accordingly a test that is based on the interpretation of authentic visual representations used in the phage-hunting process elicits information that can be used to assess the development of the cognitive and representational knowledge that is specific to the phage-hunting process. In addition this test elicits information that can be used to assess the understanding of the microbiology of organisms that are researched and the specific process of scientific inquiry utilized in the phage-hunting program. For the PHIRE program five specific stages were chosen and the visual components of these reasoning processes were analyzed. Five specific visual analysis tasks were chosen for the construction of this test: Phage Isolation: Identification of plaque; Phage Purification: Generating a pure phage population; Phage Amplification: Calculation of lysate concentration (titer), Selection of maximum bacteriophages yield; DNA Comparison: DNA Restriction Enzyme and Electrophoresis: Evaluation of uniqueness of isolated bacteriophage; and Genome Annotation and Analysis: Gene identification. These five tasks cover the length of the phage-hunting process and are directed toward points in the process in which informed decisions need to be made. The format of the visual analysis test consists of a series of specific visual representation and questions designed for each task. The visual analysis test is administered by the student-mentor at the completion of each stage in the phage-hunting process to which it is relevant. As such it comes after the student-researcher has conducted her/his own research and can provide information on the understanding that has been acquired in relation to that stage. Since the visual analysis tasks cover the whole of the phage-hunting program, by considering the complete set of visual analysis tasks a picture of knowledge development in relation to the internal aspects of the phage-hunting program can be constructed. As with the physical checklist, the visual analysis test provides data that can be used for diagnostic and outcomes assessment. The administration of the test by the instructor is an opportunity for an interpretive discussion with the student concerning different ways of understanding the visual representations and can be an opportunity to provide direct feedback and instruction (if necessary) concerning the understanding of the process. The knowledge assessed by this tool is significant on three levels: (1) it provides information that can be used to assess the on-going cognitive development of microbiological understanding concerning the phage hunting program; (2) it provides information on the accumulated cognitive understanding of phage hunting and bacteriophage as an organism; and (3) it provides a basis for exploring developments in self-understanding as a researcher.

4. *The Notebook Assessment Tool*: The process of conducting a scientific inquiry within a professional research laboratory is a lengthy process that involves a range of physical, cognitive, and representational skills. The role of the laboratory notebook is defined as a scientific report that documents the on-going

scientific activities and thought processes of the researcher. Previous research (Hanauer, 2007) suggests that the notebooks as used by student-researchers may not be fully attuned to the professional understandings of the role of notebooks in the laboratory. The main conclusion from this situation is the need for further clarification with students as to how to use these literacy products as part of the scientific inquiry process. However, as proposed here, the laboratory notebook has the potential as a highly significant assessment tool if appropriate instruction and feedback are provided. As an authentic assessment tool, the scientific notebook indeed provides the instructor with the option of fully following both the educational and the scientific process of phage hunting and also provides an on-going log of all activities and the understanding of these activities. The assessment of the notebook is an on-going activity of the instructor and part of the regular educational process. The knowledge assessed by this tool is significant in that it provides an opportunity to observe the on-going development of the scientific inquiry process and for the instructor to provide timely instruction and feedback on this process.

5. *The Knowledge Presentation Performance Test*: This test involves the assessment of the student's ability to synthesize, contextualize, and theorize the results of the scientific inquiry process and present these within an acceptable scientific format. Observation within the laboratory has shown that the most frequent form of scientific inquiry presentation used consists of the conference poster format and accordingly the current assessment proposal suggests that a similar format be used as an assessment tool. As an assessment tool, the presentation of the outcomes of a scientific inquiry process in the form of a conference poster has two main sections: assessment of the conceptualization of the scientific content and assessment of genre form of the poster. As an assessment tool, rubrics for both of these elements have been developed. The knowledge presentation performance test is conducted at the end of the course in a physical format that is very similar to actual conference presentations. The showing of the posters can be public and offers a professional atmosphere that encourages the students' sense of authenticity. The knowledge assessed by this tool is significant in that it assesses the students' real understandings of the outcomes of their scientific and educational endeavors.

7.5 Weighting and Timing

The assessment strategy presented in this chapter involves the construction of a composite score from five different assessment procedures that are collected at different times during the course of scientific inquiry. The assumption of the authors of this book is that these information sources do not have equal weighting in relation to their relative importance to the educational process. The weighting of

Table 7.1 Assessment Measures, Knowledge Types, Timing, and Weighting of Assessment Measures

Assessment procedure	Knowledge assessed	Assessment timing	Weighting
The Substantive Knowledge Test	Summative assessment of substantive factual knowledge	Middle and end of program	20%
The Physical Checklist	Diagnostic, formative, and outcome assessment of physical activities in the wet laboratory	On-going first half of phage-hunting process	5%
The Visual Literacy Test	Diagnostic, formative, and summative assessment of cognitive and representational aspects of the phage-hunting process	On-going through the program. The five visual analysis tasks cover the length of the phage-hunting processes	25%
The Notebook Assessment Tool	Diagnostic and formative information relating to substantive, procedural, cognitive, and representational knowledge of the phage-hunting process	On-going throughout the program	25%
The Knowledge Presentation Performance Test	Summative assessment of presentational knowledge	End of program	25%
			100%

different assessment tools relates to the conceptual understanding of the educational significance of the various components for the scientific inquiry process. Table 7.1 summarizes the roles of the different assessment measures, the timing of the assessment, and the suggested weighting for each item.

Chapter 8
PHIRE Assessment Tools

8.1 Introduction

This chapter provides further clarification and exemplification of the specific assessment tools developed and used within the PHIRE program to evaluate student educational progress. As described in Chap. 7, the overall assessment strategy was based on a contextualized, multimethod approach and consists of five different tools: the substantive knowledge test, the physical checklist, the visual literacy test, the notebook assessment tool, and the knowledge presentation performance test. In the sections that follow each of these assessment tools is described individually.

8.2 The Substantive Knowledge Test

The substantive knowledge test is a tool that assesses the development of factual scientific knowledge as an outcome of the process of scientific inquiry. The substantive knowledge test is the most traditional of the methods used in the current set of assessment tools. The substantive knowledge test used within the PHIRE program consisted of a multiple choice question and open-ended question format and addressed factual knowledge of bacteriophage. As an initial stage, the prime researcher and his team regarded the type of knowledge that they thought could be considered significant as an outcome of the specific scientific inquiry conducted within the PHIRE program. Particular emphasis was placed on factual knowledge that informed the process of scientific inquiry and related to the nature of the organism and the specific processes of scientific inquiry. A list of questions covering the different stages of the PHIRE program and addressing very basic as well as more complex degrees of knowledge was developed. Below are three example questions relating to the early stages of the PHIRE program:

1. What is a bacteriophage?

    a. A bacteriophage is a virus that infects bacterial cells
    b. A bacteriophage is a bacterial cell

D.I. Hanauer et al., *Active Assessment: Assessing Scientific Inquiry*,
Mentoring in Academia and Industry 2, DOI 10.1007/978-0-387-89649-6_8,

c. A bacteriophage is a virus that directly causes disease in humans
d. A bacteriophage is the cause of tuberculosis

2. A bacteriophage can

a. Not metabolize or replicate its own DNA without a host cell
b. Reproduce independently
c. Intake and digest energy from other viruses
d. Needs a food source to survive

3. $CaCl_2$ is added to media and buffer used for phages and *M. smegmatis*. Why is Ca^{2+} needed?

a. Ca^{2+} is needed in the metabolic pathways for bacterial growth as well as for phage to bind to cell surfaces
b. Ca^{2+} is needed to stabilize and preserve the solution of phage
c. Ca^{2+} is needed to prevent phages from lysogenizing
d. Ca^{2+} is needed to maintain the structure of phage capsid

8.3 The Physical Checklist

The physical checklist is a tool that assesses basic working knowledge of a laboratory. In the case of the PHIRE program, working with novice undergraduate students with little or no experience of microbiology, the decision was made to focus on core microbiological techniques. This assessment tool is relatively simple to construct as it directly reflects correct usage of equipment within the setting of the professional laboratory and in many cases this has already been described in a protocol handbook used within the laboratory. The idea behind the use of this assessment tool is also quite simple. Rather than setting up an artificial context for tool usage, the idea is that actual work conducted by the student-researcher during the process of scientific inquiry is observed by the scientist-educator and assessed. The physical checklist is an aid in allowing the scientist-educator to assess and record in a systematic way the physical, procedural knowledge of the student-researcher. In this sense the physical checklist is a performance test that is conducted as the students actually conduct their scientific inquiry.

As an assessment tool that is practical to use, several quite simple procedures need to be followed in order to transform the existing knowledge concerning physical work within the laboratory into an assessment tool. The first simple action that needs to be taken is to decide on the specific physical laboratory actions that are important to assess as part of the scientific inquiry process. Naturally this will change in relation to each scientific inquiry process and level of student-researcher. Once this list of actions, procedures, and equipment that needs to be addressed from an assessment perspective has been generated, the second and most important transformation is to delineate, in a checklist format, what correct usage of a piece of equipment or a specific procedure actually consists of. The detailed explanation of the checklist, set out as a user-friendly table, is designed to provide the assessor with a basic set of ideas of what is important to consider in relation to the student's physical work in the laboratory and is ultimately the instrument that is used to record the students progress and understanding of the physical environment and actions within the laboratory. Once the checklist has been developed decisions need to be made as to when to assess each of the procedures described on the checklist. This decision is directed through the empirical analysis of the physical knowledge required for each of the representational milestone stages of the scientific inquiry process. To most prime researchers, this will be an obvious decision.

To exemplify the nature and form of the checklist, below is an example of the checklist developed for the basic microbiological technique of plating.

Physical technique	Subcategory	Correct usage	Perceived problems	Notes
Plating technique	Overall usage			
	Holds pipette gun at 45 degree angle			
	Control bubbles when dispensing media			
	Spreads liquid evenly			
	Correct labeling			
	Allows plates to cool			
	Incubates plates according to protocol			
	Uses warm top agar			
	Appropriate use of micropipette or pipette gun			

8.4 The Visual Literacy Test

The visual literacy test is a tool that is designed to assess the contextualized and integrated understanding of the specific scientific inquiry process that is at the heart of the educational program. As set out in the first sections of this book, the process of scientific inquiry can be set out as a series of representations with associated cognitive knowledge and physical actions. The aim of the visual literacy test is to use these milestone representations as significant points of assessment and to consider what it is that the student actually understands about this scientific process. This method of assessing scientific inquiry knowledge is designed to differentiate between those students who have good control over the mechanical components of the laboratory (as assessed in the physical checklist tool presented above) and the actual conceptual understanding of the process of scientific inquiry. Accordingly, this test integrates a visual analysis of representations in the microbiology laboratory with both cognitive and representational knowledge.

This test, more than any of the tools described in this chapter, is directly based on the empirical description of the specific scientific inquiry process that is used in the educational program. In the last chapter, it was specified that five representational milestones were identified for the PHIRE program: Step 1 – Phage Isolation:

Identification of plaques; Step 2 – Phage Purification: Generating a pure phage population; Step 3 – Phage Amplification and Purification: Calculation of lysate concentration: Selection of maximum bacteriophages yield; Step 5 – DNA Comparison: DNA Restriction Enzyme and Electrophoresis: Comparison of electrophoresis gel and decision as to value of continuation of process; Step 7 – Genome Annotation and Analysis: Gene Calling – Selection and identification of genes. A specific test was designed for each of these stages with the assumption that student-researchers would be tested following the completion of the in-lab work. A detailed analysis of the cognitive and representational aspects of each of these stages was conducted. In order to aid in the development of an integrated assessment tool, a basic knowledge and cognitive abilities template was designed based on the analysis of the specific representations. For the four wet-lab tasks, this template consists of

1. Knowledge of an organism's characteristics
2. Understanding of the manipulated environment
3. An ability to selectively focus on specific visual information in the representation
4. The ability to infer the state of the organism from the visual analysis through an argument structure
5. The ability to make an informed decision on future action that is required

This basic knowledge and set of abilities provide the structure of information that needs to be assessed in relation to these tasks and was reflected in the questions for the visual analysis task.

The last task – Gene Identification – is different from the first four tasks in that its decision-making structure uses symbolic core characteristics and is an interpretive, knowledge integration task. This template specifies basic knowledge and abilities that are required for making a decision in this setting:

1. Knowledge of the characteristics of an organism
2. Knowledge of the translation of the organism's characteristics into symbolic form
3. Understanding of the workings and outputs of the different computer programs
4. Understanding of the nature of the basic analysis conducted by the different computer programs which led to the specific output that is produced
5. The ability to weigh and integrate different information sources in making an informed decision.

This basic knowledge and set of abilities provide the structure of information that needs to be assessed in relation to the gene identification task.

The form of the visual literacy test is an open-ended question format dealing with the visual analysis of presented laboratory representations in the form of digital photographs. The representations were drawn from work actually conducted in the laboratory and the questions were designed according to the question template above. The result is a test which includes a visual representation and a set of associated questions. For example consider the following page from the test of the Phage Isolation stage (Fig. 8.1).

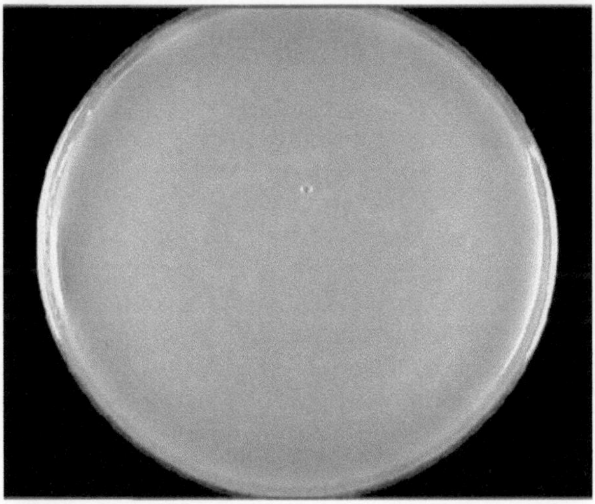

Fig. 8.1 Sample picture used for visual literacy test one

Visual Literacy Test One: Identification of Bacteriophage

Look carefully at the picture of Figure 8.1 and answer the four questions listed below. Questions:

1. Are there any bacteriophages on this plate?
2. How do you know if a bacteriophage is present on a plate? Specify exactly what evidence from the plate you are using to make this decision.
3. The plate in the picture is covered with bacterial cells. Why is this important and how does it help you to identify the presence or absence of bacteriophages?
4. What is the next stage of working with this specific plate?

As can be seen in this example, a digital photograph of an authentic outcome has been presented and is the basis for the set of questions that is being asked. The questions address the understanding of the representation and are designed around the analysis of the cognitive and factual knowledge required to actually understand and conduct this specific scientific inquiry. Naturally, a specific response rubric was developed for each of the visual analysis tests following the piloting of the materials.

8.5 The Notebook Assessment Tool

Scientific notebooks have enormous potential as educational and assessment tools of the process of scientific inquiry. This potential is based on two central ideas: (1) the scientific notebook is an authentic part of professional scientific inquiry; (2) the scientific notebook provides an in-depth, up-to-date description of the procedures, outcomes, and thoughts concerning the process of scientific inquiry conducted by the student (Hargrove & Nesbit, 2003). The notebook assessment tool is designed to collect data on the whole of the scientific inquiry process conducted by the student. Specifically, the aims of the laboratory notebook assessment procedure are

1. To elicit assessment data that can be used to determine the levels of procedural and representational knowledge development achieved by the participants in this program.
2. To provide diagnostic information that can be used to enhance each student's understanding of the substantive, procedural, and representational aspects of the bacteriophage hunting process and formative information to the scientist-educator so that changes can be made to the educational plan if necessary.
3. To provide summative data on the specific aspects of the scientific microbiological inquiry process of the isolation and characterization of bacteriophage

It is should be noted that the use of laboratory notebooks as part of the educational assessment process does not guarantee the collection of useful summative, diagnostic, and formative data. Hanauer (2007) and Ruiz-Primo, Li, and Shavelson (2002) note that within the notebooks they studied, the recording of the procedures and results were problematic leading to a situation of difficulties in replicating or directly following what the students were doing or how they understood their studies. In addition, in many cases the results were not written in a way that would allow conclusions based on evidence or patterns of significance to emerge. The notebooks did not reach their full scientific and educational potential as a full record of the scientific and thinking aspects of scientific work.

One of the central issues in utilizing laboratory notebooks as assessment tools concerns the role of the instructor. The instructor's role in properly introducing the laboratory notebook as a scientific literacy practice and providing on-going feedback on the quality of the science and the description of the entries is pivotal in making the laboratory notebook a valuable scientific and educational tool. The role of the instructor can be divided into three time periods: (1) at the very beginning of the program, the introduction of laboratory notebook writing; (2) throughout the program, the provision of feedback in relation to the quality of the science and notebook entries in describing the scientific process; and (3) at the end of the program, the assessment of the completed laboratory notebook. The full protocol for the usage of the notebook as a scientific and educational tool is provided below in relation to these three time periods.

8.5.1 Program Beginnings and Notebook Introduction

At the very beginning of the scientific inquiry program the presence and usage of laboratory notebooks needs to be introduced. This introduction is crucial in that it defines the aims and usage of this specific literacy practice. In our assessment procedure we used the following handout for this purpose.

Principles of Notebook Writing

1. ***The Principle of Autonomous Replication***: The main scientific principle directing the writing of laboratory notebooks is that the scientific inquiry that is described in the notebook can be followed and understood autonomously by an outside reader without the need to search for additional information from other sources. In other words, *the notebook stands as an autonomous, comprehensive, and explicit description of the scientific inquiry that was conducted and the results that were achieved.* A basic test of the quality of the notebook is that, if necessary, the outside reader could replicate the whole study and reach the same results.
2. ***Full Presentation of the Scientific Argument***: In order for the outside reader to be able to fully follow the specific details of the scientific inquiry process, the entries made in the notebook need to construct a full scientific argument in relation to each set of specific procedures and results that are presented. The scientific argument consists of the following entries that need to be included and presented in this specific order:

   - *Aims and Purposes of the Proposed Procedure*: Before presenting any specific scientific procedure, *the aims of the proposed methodology need to be explicitly stated in the notebook.* This might be as simple a statement as "I need to clean my samples from excess dirt so that I can later be able to plate them." Or in some cases the description of the aim of the procedure may include the specification of a quite complex problem that needs an experimental design to differentiate between different options. In other words, the student-research needs to explicitly answer the question as to why any specific procedure is being conducted. The presentation of the reasons why a procedure was conducted allows an autonomous outsider reader to follow the thoughts of the student-researcher in conducting this procedure and the decision-making processes that were involved.
   - *The Accurate and Comprehensive Reporting of a Scientific Procedure*: A basic aspect of any notebook is the full, explicit and accurate reporting of the procedures that were conducted. In principle a full description of every action taken in relation to the scientific procedure is required. In some cases the student may be following a well-known protocol and every step is followed in exactly the way it is described in the protocol. In this case reference can be made to the protocol. It is important to *remember that an outside reader must be able to follow exactly what was done in the scientific inquiry without the presence of the writer and just by reading the description of the procedure followed.* In some cases the description of the scientific procedure followed may include visual elements such as hand-drawn pictures. Whether the description is visual or verbal it is important that it is comprehensive, accurate, and explicit. The student-researcher needs to answer the question – How was the scientific inquiry completed? An explicit answer to this question provides a full description of the procedure.

- *Accurate Reporting of Results*: The accurate reporting of the results found within the scientific inquiry process and as an outcome of the specific procedures described in the notebook is a core aspect of the laboratory notebook. *The description of the results needs to be as accurate and as comprehensive as possible*. In many cases within the wet laboratory, this may include digital photographs or other visual representations of the actual results themselves. All visual material must be properly labeled and of a high quality. In some cases you may need to provide a mathematical description of the results that a specific procedure or experiment achieved. These results need to be detailed and present a full picture of what was found. The basic principle here is that the outside reader can fully comprehend what the actual results of the procedure were. With this entry, the student-researcher needs to answer the question – *what was the outcome of the application of this specific procedure?* An explicit answer to this question will provide a full description of the results that were found.
- *Interpreting Data and Reaching Conclusions:* Having presented an accurate and full description of the results, it is necessary to explain what the results mean. The results need to be interpreted and conclusions for the continuation of the scientific inquiry process discussed. The interpretation of the results leads directly to the specification of an aim for the next stage of the scientific inquiry process. It is particularly important to report on the presence of any unexpected findings and problems that arise. The interpretation presents the student-researchers understanding of what the results show and what this tells her/him about the scientific inquiry process they are involved with. Basically the student is trying to answer two different types of question: *What do the results mean? and What do I need to do now?* The first question relates to the results themselves and the second question connects to the continuation of the scientific inquiry process. Table 8.2 is a schematic representation of the types of notebook entry that constitute the scientific argument and the relationships among them.

8.5.2 On-Going Laboratory Notebook Usage and the Provision of Feedback

Good laboratory notebook writing practices will develop if the scientist-educator reads the notebooks and actively provides feedback to the student-researcher on the quality of the notebook from a scientific and educational perspective. This is particularly important in the first third of the scientific inquiry process as this is the time at which long-term scientific writing behaviors can be encouraged and normalized. During this initial period, the notebook is reviewed at on a weekly (perhaps bi-weekly) basis and explicit face-to-face instruction provided to the student. In order to facilitate this process we developed the rubric for laboratory notebook assessment presented below (Tables 8.1 and 8.2):

Table 8.1 Rubric for assessment of laboratory notebooks (scientific argument)

Notebook entry categories	Inadequate	Adequate	Comments
Statement of purpose of procedure			
Description of procedure			
Verbal presentation of results			
Visual presentation of results			
Interpretation of results			
Presentation of thoughts, problems, and deliberations			
Overall evaluation of reporting of experimental procedure			

As can be seen the rubric relates to the elements of the scientific argument that are present within the laboratory notebook. Particular attention is directed at the full contextualization of the procedures and results that are presented. Previous research has shown that students do not usually enter these into their notebooks.

8.5.3 Final Assessment of Laboratory Notebooks (End of Program)

As weighted within the current assessment strategy, the laboratory notebook constitutes 25% of the final assessment of the student. As a component in the final assessment the notebook needs to be assessed for its value as a scientific document and for its ability to provide the instructor with information on the student's demonstrated knowledge of substantive, procedural, and representational aspects of the process of bacteriophage isolation and genomic annotation. At the end of the program, the laboratory notebook is used as a scientific and educational document that allows the assessment of the outcomes of the scientific inquiry process that the student-researcher was involved with. To simplify this educational assessment process a series of specific questions that the researcher-instructor can ask following the reading of the laboratory notebook were developed. These questions are designed to direct the instructor's attention to specific issues in the assessment of the notebooks. The final assessment of the laboratory notebook is based on the instructors answer to the following questions:

1. Does the notebook provide you with sufficient information that would allow you to replicate the study if necessary? Does it allow you to fully understand the results that are presented and the specific procedures that led to these outcomes? (*Validity as a scientific document*)
2. Does the notebook provide you with sufficient information that allows you to follow and clearly understand all the different stages of the presented scientific inquiry? (*Validity as a scientific document*)

Table 8.2 Rubric for assessment of laboratory notebooks (scientific argument): instructor key

Notebook entry categories	Inadequate	Adequate
Statement of purpose of procedure	Does not provide or provides in a limited fashion a statement of the purpose and aims of the procedure that is to be followed	Provides a clear reason and explanation of the procedure to be followed. The reason given is accurate within the context of the type of scientific inquiry that is being conducted
Description of procedure	The description of the procedure does not allow the reader to understand exactly what was done by the researcher. The description of the procedure is very limited and partial	The description provides a clear and detailed description of the procedure followed so that the reader can understand and be able to replicate exactly what was done by the researcher
Verbal presentation of results	The reader has difficulty in understanding what the results are and how they relate to the procedure. This may result from a very limited or very partial presentation of results or the lack of clear connection between results and procedures described	The verbal presentation of results provides information that allows the reader to fully comprehend the results that were found. In some cases the verbal results may be an annotation attached to a visual presentation. But taken together the reader understands exactly what results were achieved from the conducted procedure
Visual presentation of results	The photographs, pictures, drawings, or graphs: are not of a quality that allows results to be understood; are not properly labeled; only partial results have been attached	The photographs, pictures, drawings, or graphs are presented in manner that allows the viewer to fully comprehend the results that were achieved. The visuals are properly labeled and presented in a visually clear and coherent manner. The visuals are of a good quality that allows a detailed examination

(continued)

Table 8.2 (continued)

Interpretation of results	There is a very limited (if any) presentation of the researchers' interpretation of the results and what new steps need to be taken to continue the process of scientific inquiry	The researcher writes out her/his interpretation of what the results mean and how they reflect the scientific procedure followed. In addition, the researcher explicates what new steps need to be taken following this interpretation of results
Presentation of thoughts, problems, and deliberations	There are very few (if any) comments relating to the research thought processes, problems, or deliberations. The researcher may be using the notebook to make personal comments which are not relevant to the scientific inquiry process itself	Throughout the description of the scientific inquiry process, the researcher explicates in written form the problems, deliberations, and thoughts that arise in relation to the scientific process itself. This series of entries allows the reader of the notebook to follow the thought processes of the researcher while conducting this scientific inquiry. These comments may include emotive presentation dealing with the results of procedures and the excitement of discovery or frustration of the unexpected
Overall evaluation of reporting of experimental procedure	Following the reading of the notebook entries the reader was not able to reconstruct the exact procedures, results, understandings, and thought processes used by the researcher in conducting their scientific inquiry. The reader was involved in an extensive process of inference and guessing in order to fill in the missing information. Signs of confusion as to what scientific process was conducted, what was found, or what it meant to the researcher are signs that the notebook description is lacking	Following the reading of the notebook entries the reader was able to fully reconstruct the whole process of scientific inquiry including the reasons for the procedure, the exact procedures that were followed, the details of the results, and the researcher's understandings of what was found. The scientific study described in the notebook is fully replicable from the description that is provided

3. Based on the evidence presented in this notebook, is it your evaluation that the student-researcher has a good understanding of the procedural and representational aspects of the bacteriophage isolation and genomic annotation? (*validity as a scientific document*)

8.6 The Knowledge Presentation Performance Test

The knowledge presentation performance test involves an authentic summative assessment of the scientific inquiry process that the student-researcher conducted. The knowledge presentation performance test is basically the public presentation of a conference poster constructed and designed by the student. Discussion with the scientist-educator is considered a central part of the presentation process and the point at which the assessment data are collected. A professionally produced conference poster presents information in a coherent, concise, and relevant manner and allows the instructor to asses the student's ability to synthesize, contextualize, and theorize the results of the scientific inquiry process and present these within an acceptable scientific format. The aims of the knowledge presentation performance test are

1. To elicit assessment data that can be used to determine the scientific outcomes and value of the student's research
2. To elicit summative assessment data concerning the student's understanding of the substantive scientific aspects of their scientific inquiry process
3. To elicit assessment data on the student's ability to synthesize, contextualize, and theorize the results of their scientific inquiry process
4. To elicit assessment data on the student's ability to present their research in accordance with the guidelines of professional scientific presentation

Conference posters have enormous potential as both educational and assessment tools. The advantage of the conference poster is that this is a real genre that students can actually produce and use to summarize their research. However, for this to work within the context of an educational program and as an assessment tool, the researcher-educator has a crucial role to play in creating an authentic context for the presentation and discussion of research. As with any research project, the conference poster comes only after significant data have been collected and is a form of conceptualization and summary of findings and outcomes. Accordingly, the knowledge presentation performance test is used at the very end of the undergraduate scientific inquiry process. Discussion of the conference poster is conducted during the last quarter of the scientific inquiry process. Basically there are two stages to be considered in the usage of the conference poster as an assessment tool: the development stage and the presentation stage. The full protocol for the usage of the conference poster as a scientific and educational tool is provided below in relation to these two stages.

8.6.1 Conference Poster Development

The development of a conference poster is a reflective and summative process that transforms the raw material of the scientific inquiry described in the laboratory notebook and the associated visual representations into a focused presentation of a significant scientific outcome. This process of transformation is highly valuable from an educational perspective in that this is one possible point at which the student can really consider what she/he has found out and relate this to understandings within the wider scientific discipline. The process of developing a conference poster incorporates this educational aspect of personal reflection on the scientific inquiry process. Hanauer (2007) defines five stages of poster development: development of poster genre knowledge; reflection on notebook and visual data; production of a written theme or core discovery of the inquiry process; construction of a conference poster; and construction of an accompanying oral explanation. In our assessment process we used these stages to design the educational process of conference poster development. These stages are as follows:

1. *Development of Conference Poster Genre Knowledge*: As a first stage of knowledge development the instructor presented the ASM (American Society of Microbiology) criteria for conference poster presentations. The initial introduction specified the elements that needed to be in the poster including an abstract, background, methods, results, conclusions, future directions, and references. This was followed by the analysis of real conference posters from professional meetings.
2. *Reflection and Discussion of Notebook and Visual Data*: Time was allotted for the student to carefully consider her/his notebooks and associated scientific inquiry data. Of particular importance was the consideration of the different visual representations that she/he has collected as part of her/his inquiry process. The student was directed to carefully consider all of her/his data and decide what she/he thought is important to present at a professional conference. At this stage, consultation with the scientist-educator and other peers could be valuable in helping the student to understand the value of her or his research project.
3. *Production of a Written Narrative*: Following discussion with the instructor students were required to produce a brief abstract of the main directions of the conference poster. The students were instructed that the brief abstract presents the main findings of the scientific inquiry that the student conducted. The student chose those visual representations which were most relevant in the presentation of these specific findings. It is important that the student fully contextualize the findings with the framework of a scientific argument that provides the reader with access to the background, methods, results, and conclusions concerning the study. This written abstract is presented to the instructor and subsequently discussed.
4. *Development of Conference Poster*: The process of actually developing the conference poster involves making good design decisions based on the abstract that has been written and discussed with the instructor. It is important to specify and

reinforce the sections that need to be present with the conference poster and that the visual representations have to be carefully chosen to provide the most relevant visuals for the poster format. Basically the conference needs to have a title, the name of the researcher, an abstract, background, method, results, conclusions, future research directions, and references. In addition the results sections need to present the appropriate visual representations for the specific findings to be presented. The student needs to consider the appropriate organization of the poster so that it flows correctly and provides the viewer with all required information. The use of poster computer programs such as Canvas is to be encouraged as it allows cut and paste options and the ability to try out different presentation styles. It is important to specify that the poster needs to be professionally presented.

5. *Development of the Accompanying Oral Statement*: Once the poster has been printed out the student was instructed to develop a succinct 5 min description and explanation of the poster. The description includes a statement about the main findings of the inquiry, the methods used to reach these findings, and the significance of the study. A good way of conceptualizing this process for the student is to think of the oral presentation as "taking your viewer on a guided tour of the poster and its associated scientific inquiry process." The oral presentation is written out and practiced by the student so that it is fluent.

8.6.2 Conference Poster Presentation

In order for the conference poster to function as an authentic scientific process, the instructor needs to construct a setting in which the conference posters are presented. It would be best if this was not during class time and included other members of the faculty and student bodies. The conference poster session can be simply the designation of a room and time for the presentation of the conference posters. This can be publicized so that there is access to this research by a variety of university members. Once a setting has been found students are told that the knowledge presentation performance test will be conducted during this open poster presentation session. The assessment of the conference posters consists of three components: assessment of the scientific inquiry; assessment of student understandings; and assessment of presentation abilities.

Assessment of Scientific Inquiry: In order to assess the value of the scientific inquiry process conducted by the student-researcher, the instructor considers whether the information collected and presented by the student has real scientific value within the scientific discipline. On a very basic level, the value of a scientific inquiry can be that it provides new data, new methods, or new insights. For example, it is assumed that the contribution of the majority of the student posters dealing with phage hunting would be on the level of new data concerning unique bacteriophages. The question the assessor needs to ask is

1. Does the data presented in the student conference poster really involve a development in scientific knowledge?

This question is at the core of all scientific inquiry and accordingly is significant in the evaluation of the final product of this specific scientific inquiry process – the conference poster.

Assessment of Students' Understandings: As part of the knowledge presentation performance test the student will be required to develop a poster, an oral statement concerning the poster, and provide interactive responses to instructor questions concerning her/his presentation. Having carefully viewed the poster, heard the oral presentation, and interacted with the student concerning the poster, the assessor considers the following questions:

2. Do the conference poster and the oral presentation fully contextualize the scientific findings that they present?
3. Having viewed the conference poster and heard the oral presentation are you convinced that the student fully understands the results that they have presented and the specific methodological procedures that were used to produce these results?
4. Does the student understand the importance and scientific value of the findings?
5. Having viewed the conference poster and having heard the oral presentation are you convinced that the students have a good understanding of the scientific inquiry process that is presented on the poster.

Assessment of Presentation Abilities: In addition to the scientific value of the inquiry and the student's scientific understanding of their specific inquiry process, the assessor can assess the quality of the conference poster and oral presentation. The quality of the poster addresses both the esthetic and informative aspects of the poster and oral presentation. The instructor can ask herself/himself the following questions:

6. Does the conference poster present information in a coherent, concise, and relevant manner?
7. Is the accompanying oral presentation coherent, concise, and informative?
8. Do the poster and the accompanying oral presentation synthesize, contextualize, and theorize the results of the scientific inquiry process and present these in formats that are acceptable to a scientific audience?
9. Is the poster esthetically pleasing and professionally produced?
10. Is the oral presentation fluent and articulate?

The final assessment of the conference poster takes into account all the information addressed in the 10 questions presented above. This is a composite score that addresses the quality of the scientific inquiry, the students understanding of this process, and the ability of the student to present this information in a format relevant to professional science.

Chapter 9
Reflections from an Active Scientist-Educator

9.1 Introduction

In the previous three chapters we have presented and discussed the PHIRE program as a case study for the development of strategies and tools for assessment. In this final chapter, one of us (GFH) will share his perspectives from the vantage point as head of a research laboratory that developed the PHIRE program and – together with my co-authors – developed the assessment procedures associated with it. A basic assumption of all our educational work is that real science is and should be at the heart of any science education program. For us science education and the actual development of valuable scientific knowledge should be integrated. The premise I will discuss in this chapter is straightforward: that there are a multitude of exciting opportunities to develop structured educational programs taking advantage of the research environment and incorporating active assessment procedures. The creation of new science-based, education programs would move both science and education forward. However, many of these opportunities remain unfilled, and while there may be many reasons for this, the barrier doesn't need to be nearly as high as it appears to be. My experience with the PHIRE program and the assessment tools we have developed offer some useful guidelines that I hope will be helpful to other scientist-educators as they contemplate developing their own programs.

Although the PHIRE program has many attributes that we like – and are described in Chap. 6 – it is certainly not unique. It is a component within a broader effort to fully embrace scientific inquiry with our educational missions, and there have been many other successful efforts toward this goal. Science education in the United States is in a peculiar position; on the one hand, K-12 science education is reported as underachieving greatly, but on the other hand, the United States continues to dominate the world of scientific discovery and publication in the peer-reviewed scientific literature. How can this be? While the roots of this paradox may be complex, programs such as PHIRE have the potential to change the game, extending positive advances to both the research and educational enterprises.

I have presented and discussed the PHIRE program in several different forums over the past couple of years and some common questions often arise. How do you find the space? How do you find the time? How do you pay for this? How do you

D.I. Hanauer et al., *Active Assessment: Assessing Scientific Inquiry*,
Mentoring in Academia and Industry 2, DOI 10.1007/978-0-387-89649-6_9,

select students for the PHIRE program? Doesn't this detract from your research productivity? What does your institution think of this? Will the PHIRE program work for me? How are the students and program assessed? I will try to address these and other questions here that may help to lower the barriers for other scientist-educators to explore exciting new programs and projects in science and education in their laboratories and classrooms.

9.2 Two for the Price of One: Integrating the Missions

I do not consider PHIRE an education program. At first glance, a program that provides laboratory opportunities to high school students might seem to naturally fit into that classification. But it could be better described as a research program that is particularly well-tailored as an introduction to scientific research. This "introduction" is aimed at undergraduate students, high school teachers, and other novice scientists (journalists, public officials, etc.), in addition to high school students. Perhaps such programs are not appropriate for all life science laboratories, but I'm sure there are many that are. Furthermore, within many research laboratories – including my own – only a subset of the experimental approaches may be suited to this introductory category. The critical issue though is that the project should be commensurate with the on-going research directions and not at odds with them. This is good news for scientist-educators thinking about establishing such programs, since it is likely to be a great deal easier initiating a project situated within the strength of their research expertise, rather than trying to start something new solely from the perspective of educational advantage. The context of the research laboratory, and the professional research conducted therein, is therefore of paramount importance, a theme that penetrates much of the book.

An excellent starting point for the development of an educational scientific inquiry program and its associated active assessment components is for the scientist/educator to conduct a brief self-review of the short-, medium-, and long-term research goals and professional scientific activities. It may also be helpful to review the population of students that you might target and the space available in – or close to – the research lab. Having done this, a series of potential projects could be considered, evaluating them for their suitability as an introductory nature – i.e., those that do not require a lot of prior scientific knowledge, prior research experience, or technical skill. In my experience, these projects are very different from the types of projects that most principle investigators are used to formulating for postdoctoral researchers and graduate students. They are also different to the types of projects that are often suggested to individual independent undergraduate researchers, whose projects are often scaled down versions that might be proposed to a beginning graduate student. Programs such as PHIRE aim to engage 8–12 students at any one time and suitable projects are likely to encompass many of the project attributes discussed in Chap. 6, such as project ownership, parallel project structures, peer mentoring, and progression from concrete beginnings to abstract processing.

If scientist-educators can devise a project that meets their research goals, many of the other essential elements, including active assessment, may well fall into place. Coming up with the right project is the key then to integrating the educational and research missions, with good prospects for advancing both missions. An interesting aspect is that once a project is established then the assessment goals and practices become much clearer. As described in this book, the process of active assessment is tied directly to an analysis of the knowledge, visual representations, laboratory procedures, and conceptual understandings that comprise the specific types of scientific inquiry utilized within the research laboratory and offer a contextualized approach to assessment. For us, both the educational and assessment aspects of the scientific inquiry program should evolve from the core scientific activity of the prime researcher and the laboratory setting. It is also important to note that as happened in our case, the educational projects can take on a life of their own, presenting new research directions that either the scientist-educator or a collaborator specifically interested in educational and learning issues can advance. Thus, a new line of research emerges from within the laboratory setting, one that ultimately enhances interest in science and the specific research agendas of particular laboratories.

9.3 Some Practical Concerns

One of our aims of this book is to promote the usage of in-laboratory science education programs. From my perspective as a scientist and scientist-educator, I know that the practical issue of setting up a program of this type may often seem formidable and there are indeed numerous practical issues that arise when considering the establishment of research-educational programs such as PHIRE. To ease this thinking process, I would like to share some of my thoughts on the practical issues of space, time, and money.

9.3.1 Space: The Final Frontier

Identifying appropriate laboratory space can be one of the toughest of these issues to satisfactorily address. I have been fortunate to have access to a small laboratory that is adjacent to the rest of my lab space and is physically adjoined to it. This has turned out to be ideal, since it is close enough that the PHIRE students are integrated into many normal operations of the laboratory and the use of common equipment, are sufficiently displaced so as not to “take over” the other functions of the laboratory, and work as a cohort in which they can readily work together and interact. In general, the amount of space is perhaps less critical than its location relative to other research activities. One bench at the end of a laboratory or a small lab displaced further away might also work, and given that space is often a prized commodity the investigator has to get whatever she/he can acquire. In general, when it comes to requesting space from a higher authority in the institution such as a Dean or a Department Chair, the scientist-educator has a distinct advantage, since the educational missions are often more closely aligned with the broader goals of the institution, and undergraduate research has become a strong selling point as universities and colleges compete for talented undergraduate students. Thus requesting space for an organized undergraduate research program may well be more effective than asking for more pure research space, which typically results in a discussion of how many research dollars are being brought in to support the research.

9.3.2 *Money and Time*

Running a program such as PHIRE is certainly not free and the shape and nature of the program are likely to depend on what financial support can be mustered. There are two main components. Perhaps the most critical is the need for funds to employ a program coordinator who can provide the direction and responsibility for overall implementation of the program. The coordinator is critical, since she/he can assist in choosing students for the program, organizing and mediating group meetings, addressing research problems, and all aspects of coordination. There are many nitty-gritty issues in implementation that the coordinator can and should be responsible for, and if all of these fall to the investigator, then the program may be difficult to sustain. This is central to the issue of time management of the researcher-educator, as running a program like PHIRE could become so time-consuming that it detracts from other duties and responsibilities. Obviously, the specific arrangements will depend on the size of the program and the number of students, but assistance with program coordination is not negotiable. The good news is that with a fully integrated education-research program there is a broad range of sources that can be explored for financial support, including research grants, local foundations, education-based federal grants, and the home institution. This is another example in which the educational components advance the research goals and vice versa.

The second main funding issue is that of student stipends. This is primarily an issue when students are working in the summer term, since most of them cannot afford to forego the opportunity to earn the money that they need to continue their education. Depending on the number of students, this can of course become quite costly, although once again, there can be quite substantial research advances in this time period, provided that a suitable project is in place. The same sources of funds can be explored as described above. If the program runs primarily through the academic term and if external funding is not available, then students could enroll in such a program for credit toward their degree.

9.4 Why Bother with Assessment?

A well-formulated project that is well suited to inexperienced students can be expected to have considerable educational advantages, and in some senses the more inexperienced the students are, the greater the education benefits that can accrue. But how do you know if any educational benefits are occurring at all and what is happening to students' understanding of the project and science in general beyond the simple accomplishment of assigned technical manipulations. Most scientist-educators are well positioned to assess whether the research goals are being met, but perhaps less so than when it comes to determining whether the educational goals are being achieved. Broadly and as set out in the principles of scientific teaching (Handelsman, Miller, & Pfund, 2007) the educational elements should be considered similarly to research elements, as experiments that are conducted whose results need to be evaluated. Active assessment, as described in this book, provides a conceptual framework and a method for collecting data that can be used to directly assess the value of the program in relation to educational outcomes. Rather than an external and abstracted approach to the assessment of knowledge, in this book we propose high emphasis on authentic, contextualized assessment directed by the prime researcher's extensive understanding of the scientific inquiry that is at the heart of the educational program. This approach to assessment should allow the prime researcher to collect data that allow both the assessment of the educational outcomes and controlling the actual quality of the research that is conducted in the laboratory, an issue that is always of prime concern for any scientist working with undergraduate researchers. On a different level, any information obtained that demonstrates the effectiveness of the education (or reveals program aspects that function less well) can not only be used to enhance and enrich the program, but also present a compelling argument when requesting support for program continuation. As described throughout this book, assessment of research-education projects does not have to be onerous provided that the assessment process is situated within the context of both the educational and research missions. I have found it to be an asset to my understanding of what my student-researchers are actually doing and learning in my laboratory.

There has been a substantial amount of research aimed at assessing the educational value of research experiences, and there is broad and general agreement that research is educationally valuable for undergraduate students (Handelsman, Miller, & Pfund, 2007). In general, the question as to whether undergraduate research is educationally advantageous seems to be well-resolved in the affirmative (Lopatto, 2004; 2007). Rather than attempting to revisit this large and important question, the key areas of assessment for the scientist-educator are those directly related to the context in which your specific program is conducted. In other words, consider assessment in the terms developed within this book as a way of really understanding undergraduate research conducted within your laboratory and as part of the process of the development of scientific knowledge. The previous two chapters give a clear description of how we have developed and implemented active assessment tools in the context of the PHIRE program.

9.5 Program Attributes Revisited

In order to further enhance the process of developing research-based scientific inquiry programs, I would like to revisit some of the attributes that I think are central to this type of educational program. In Chap. 6 we discussed a set of attributes that we had identified in the PHIRE program that we propose as guidelines in the development of new projects. One of these is the idea of *project ownership*, an element that is of importance since it fuels the self-motivation and independence that facilitate full engagement of students in their projects. A notable example is the program developed by Scott Strobel at Yale University in which students gain project ownership through the isolation and characterization of novel endophytes with interesting and unexpected properties (Strobel & Strobel 2007). A second and related key attribute is that students should be *performing authentic academic research*. On the whole, students can readily distinguish a laboratory exercise from an authentic research investigation, and the latter has considerable impact on activating the needed self-motivation. An excellent example is the program established by Utpal Banerjee at UCLA in which a substantial group of undergraduate students authored a peer-reviewed publication (Call et al., 2007; Chen et al., 2005). Lastly, *parallel project structures* offer tremendous attributes in that the commonality of techniques and the inherent compatibility with peer- and near peer-mentoring systems build coherence within the project, provide a common ground for students to discuss their projects, and facilitate a variety of assessment strategies.

9.6 Summary and Conclusions

My involvement in the PHIRE program has been a real joy. Observing students gaining enormous satisfaction from their research achievements and sharing with them the joys of publishing their data has been a particular pleasure. The use of active assessment strategies contextually adjusted to the research laboratory is a powerful way to learn what it is that students are learning and how the program can be refined to better achieve its research and education goals. Assessment of the type we propose is not construed as an extraneous intrusion into the education and research of student-researchers. As we have tried to show throughout this book, the type of assessment we developed that was situated within and attuned to a specific scientific inquiry process that we use in our laboratory directly enhances both our understanding of the educational benefits of our program and the quality of the student research that we produce. In this sense active assessment fulfills the aims of both good educational practice and quality control of undergraduate research.

At present, the research laboratory as an integrated environment for achieving educational goals is greatly underused. It is my and my collaborators hope that this book, with its explication of the basis for active assessment coupled with the PHIRE case study, will inspire numerous other scientist-educators to devise innovative programs that engage high school and undergraduate students in authentic scientific research. Our aim in writing this book was to make assessment relevant and accessible to a range of potential science educators. We believe that bringing students into the laboratory and assessing them closely in relation to specific scientific inquiry processes is the way forward. This is an approach that sees science as a specific, humanly valuable activity. We have experienced the excitement that students feel when they are involved in real science and active assessment has allowed us to carefully assess what this learning actually means in conceptual, physical, and representational terms. We know that the students who graduate from our program are well versed in what conducting microbiological science means. Our hope is that this book will help scientists to become scientist-educators dedicated to the enhancement of science and science education through the processes of integrated science-based, education programs evaluated using active assessment procedures. Ultimately our belief is that real science inquiry processes and the development of valuable scientific knowledge must be at the center of educational and assessment practices in the sciences. If done properly this could result in a revolution in the way science education is conducted around the world. Just imagine 100,000 laboratory-based science education programs producing scientific knowledge utilizing even just 10 undergraduate student-researchers. This would change the face of how science is understood and developed around the world.

References

Archenhold, F., Bell, J. D., Johnson, S., & Welford, G. (1988). *Science at Age 15: A Review of APU Survey Findings*. London: HMSO.

Baird, J. (1990). Metacognition, purposeful enquiry and conceptual change. In E. Hegarty-Hazel (Ed.), *The Student Laboratory and the Science Curriculum* (pp. 183–200). London: Routledge.

Bardarov, S., Pavelka, M. S., Jr, Sambandamurthy, V., Larsen, M., Tufariello, J., Chan, J., et al. (2002). Specialized transduction: an efficient method for generating marked and unmarked targeted gene disruptions in Mycobacterium tuberculosis, M. bovis BCG and M. smegmatis. *Microbiology, 148*, 3007–3017.

Bardarov, S., Kriakov, J., Carriere, C., Yu, S., Vaamonde, C., McAdam, R. A., et al. (1997). Conditionally replicating mycobacteriophages: a system for transposon delivery to Mycobacterium tuberculosis. *Proceedings of the National Academy of Sciences of the United States of America, 94*, 10961–10966.

Beichner, R., Bernold, L., Burniston, E., Dail, P., Felder, R., Gastineau, J.G., et al. (1999). Case studies of the physics component of an integrated curriculum. *Physics Education Research, 67*, 16–24.

Brown, J., Collins, A., & Duguid, P. (1989). Situated cognition and the culture of learning. *Educational Researcher, 18*(1), 32–42.

Bryce, T., McCall, J., MacGregor, J., Robertson, I., & Weston, R. (1983). *Techniques for the Assessment of Practical Skills in Foundation Science.* London: Heinemann.

Call, G. B., Olson, J. M., Chen, J., Villarasa, N., Ngo, K. T., Yabroff, A. M., et al. (2007). Genomewide clonal analysis of lethal mutations in the Drosophila melanogaster eye: comparison of the X chromosome and autosomes. *Genetics, 177*, 689–697.

Chen, J., Call, G. B., Beyer, E., Bui, C., Cespedes, A., et al. (2005). Discovery-based science education: functional genomic dissection in Drosophila by undergraduate researchers. *PLoS Bio, 3*, e59.

Chinn, C. A., & Malhorta, B. (2002). Epistemologically authentic inquiry in schools: A theoretical framework for evaluating inquiry tasks. *Science Education, 86*(2), 175–218.

Cumming, J., & Maxwell, G. (1999). Contextualizing authentic assessment. *Assessment in Education, 6*(2), 177–194.

Darling-Hammond, L., & Falk, B. (1997). Using standards and assessments to support student learning. *Phi Delta Kappan, 79*, 190–199.

Davis, B. (1989). *GASP: Graded Assessment in Science Project.* London: Hutchinson.

Doran, R., Chan, F., Tamir, P., & Lenhardt, C. (2002). *Science Educator's Guide to Laboratory Assessment.* Arlington: National Science Teachers Association Press.

Ebert-May, D., Batzli, J., & Lim, H. (2003). Disciplinary research strategies for assessment of learning. *BioScience, 53*, 1221–1228.

Firestone, W., Mayrowetz, D., & Fairman, J. (1998). Performance-based assessment and instructional change: The effects of testing in Maine and Maryland. *Educational Evaluation and Policy Analysis, 20*, 95–113.

Gandhi, N. R., Pawinski, R., Govender, T., Lalloo, U., Zeller, K., Andrews, J., et al. (2006). Extensively drug-resistant tuberculosis as a cause of death in patients co-infected with tuberculosis and HIV in a rural area of South Africa. *Lancet, 368*, 1575–1580.

Germann, P., Haskins, S., & Auls, S. (1996). Analysis of nine high school biology laboratory manuals: Promoting scientific inquiry. *Journal of Research in Science Teaching, 33*(5), 475–499.

Gott, R., & Duggan, S. (2002). problems with the assessment of performance in practical science; Which way now? *Cambridge Journal of Education, 32*(2), 183–201.

Gulikers, J. T. (2006). *Authenticity is in the Eye of the Beholder: Belief and Perceptions of Authentic Assessment and the Influence on Student Learning (Doctoral Dissertation, Open University of Nederland, 2006).* Retrieved January 17, 2008, from http://hdl.handle.net/1820/1043

Hake, R.R. (1998). Interactive-engagement versus traditional methods: A six-thousand-student survey of mechanics test data for introductory physics courses. *American Journal of Physics, 66*(1), 64–74.

Hanauer, D. I., Jacobs-Sera, D., Pedulla, M.C., Hendrix, R., & Hatfull, G. (2006). Teaching Scientific Inquiry. *Science, 314*(5807), 1880–1881.

Hanauer, D. (2006). *Scientific Discourse: Multiliteracy in the Classroom.* London: Continuum.

Hanauer, D. (2007). *Undergraduate Assessment: A Genre Analysis of Microbiological Laboratory Literacy.* Bacteriophage Institute of Pittsburgh, Hatfull Laboratory, University of Pittsburgh, Pittsburgh.

Handelsman, J., Ebert-May, D., Beichner, R., Bruns, P., Chang, A., DeHaan, R., et al. (2004). Scientific Teaching. *Science, 304*, 521–522.

Handelsman, J., Miller, S., & Pfund, C. (2007). *Scientific Teaching.* New York: W.H. Freeman and Company.

Hargrove, T. Y., & Nesbit, C. (2003). *Science Notebooks: Tools for Increasing Achievement Across the Curriculum* (ERIC Digest ED482720). ERIC Clearinghouse for Science Mathematics and Environmental Education.

Handelsman, J., Pfund, C., Miller Lauffer, S., & Maidl, C. (2005). Entering Mentoring: A Seminar to Train a New Generation of Scientists. Wisconsin: University of Wisconsin Press.

Hatfull, G. F. (1994). Mycobacteriophage L5: A toolbox for tuberculosis. *ASM News, 60*, 255–260.

Hatfull, G. F. (2004). Mycobacteriophages and tuberculosis. In K. Eisenach, S. T. Cole, J. W. R. Jacobs, & D. McMurray (Eds.), *Tuberculosis* (pp. 203–218). Washington, DC: ASM Press.

Hatfull, G. F., Pedulla, M. L., Jacobs-Sera, D., Cichon, P. M., Foley, A., Ford, M. E., et al. (2006). Exploring the mycobacteriophage metaproteome: phage genomics as an educational platform. *PLoS Genetics, 2*, e92.

Hendrix, R. W. (2002). Bacteriophages: evolution of the majority. *Theor Popul Bio, 161*, 471–480.

Hennes, K. P., & Suttle, C. A. (1995). Direct counts of viruses in natural waters and laboratory cultures by epifluorescence microscopy. *Limnol Oceanogr, 40*, 1050–1055.

Herrington, J., & Herrington, A. (2006). *Authentic conditions for authentic assessment: Aligning task and assessment.* Retrieved May 17, 2007, from HERDSA: http//edserver2.uow.edu.au/~janh/assessment/authentic%20assessment_files/HERDSAHerringtonFinal.doc

Herrington, J., & Herrington, A. (1998). Authentic assessment and multimedia: How university students respond to a model of authentic assessment. *Higher Educational Research and Development, 17*(3), 305–322.

Herron, M. D. (1971). The nature of scientific enquiry. *School Review, 79*(2), 171–212.

Herron, J. (1995). The nature of scientific inquiry. *School Review, 79*(2), 557–560.

Hodson, D. (1996). Laboratory work as scientific method: Three decades of confusion and distortion. *Journal of Curriculum Studies, 28*(2), 115–135.

Hofstein, A., & Lunetta, V. N. (2003). The laboratory in science education: Foundations for the twenty-first century. *Science Education, 88*(1), 28–54.

Inhelder, B., & Piaget, J. (1958). *The Growth of Logical Thinking from Childhood to Adolescence.* New York: Basic Books.

Jacobs, W. R., Jr., Barletta, R. G., Udani, R., Chan, J., Kalkut, G., Sosne, G., et al. (1993). Rapid assessment of drug susceptibilities of Mycobacterium tuberculosis by means of luciferase reporter phages. *Science*, *260*, 819–822.

Knight, J., & Wood, W. (2005). Teaching more by lecturing less. *Cell Biology Education*, *4*, 298–310.

Latour, B., & Woolgar, S. (1986). *Laboratory Life: The Construction of Scientific Facts*. Princeton: Princeton University Press.

Lave, J., & Wenger, E. (1991). *Situated Learning: Legitimate Peripheral Participation*. Cambridge: Cambridge University Press.

Lawrence, J. G., Hatfull, G. F., & Hendrix, R. W. (2002). Imbroglios of viral taxonomy: genetic exchange and failings of phenetic approaches. *Journal of Bacteriology*, *184*, 4891–4905.

Lee, H. S., & Songer, N. (2003). Making authentic science accessible to students. *International Journal of Science Education*, *25*(8), 923–948.

Linn, R. L., Baker, E., & Dunbar, S. (1991). Complex performance based assessment. *Educational Researcher*, *20*(8), 15–21.

Lopatto, D. (2004). Survey of Undergraduate Research Experiences (SURE): first findings. *Cell Biology Education*, *3*, 270–277.

Lopatto, D. (2007). Undergraduate research experiences support science career decisions and active learning. *CBE Life Science Education*, *6*, 297–306.

Lunetta, V., & Tamir, P. (1979). Matching lab activities with teaching goals. *The Science Teacher*, *46*, 22–24.

Lunsford, E., & Melear, C. T. (2004). Using scoring rubrics to evaluate inquiry. *Journal of College Science Teaching*, *34*(1), 34–38.

McDowell, L. (1995). The impact of innovative assessment on student learning. *Innovations in Education and Training International*, *32*, 302–313.

Messick, S. (1994). The interplay of evidence and consequences in the validation of performance assessments. *Educational Researcher*, *23*(2), 13–23.

Meyer, C. (1992). What's the difference between authentic and performance assessment? *Educational Leadership*, *49*(8), 39–40.

Millar, R. (1998). 'Rhetoric and reality: What practical work in science education is really for'. In J. Wellington (Ed.), *Practical Work in School Science: Which Way Now?* London: Routledge.

National Research Council. (2003). *Bio2010:Transforming unndergraduate education for future research biologists. Committtee on Undergraduate Biology Education to Prepare Research Scientists for the 21st Century.* Board on Life Sciences, Division on Earth and Life Sciences. Washington, DC: National Academy Press.

National Research Council. (2001). *Classroom Assessment and the National Science Education Standards*. In J. Myron Atkin, P. Black, & J. Coffey (Eds.). Washignton, DC: The National Academies Press.

National Research Council. (1996). *National Science Education Standards*. Washington DC: US Government Printing Office.

Newman, F., & Archbald, D. (1992). The nature of authentic academic achievement. In H. Berlak, E. Newman F.M. Adams, D. Archbald, T. Burgess, J. Raven, & T. Romberg (Eds.), *Towards a New Science of Educational Testing and Assessment* (pp. 71–84). Albany: State University of New York Press.

Newman, F., & Wehlage, G. (1993). Five standards of authentic instruction. *Educational Leadership*, *50*(7), 8–12.

Nott, M., & Smith, R. (1995). "Talking your way out of it", "rigging" and "conjuring": What science teachers do when practicals go wrong. *International Journal of Science Education*, *17*(3), 399–410.

Pedulla, M. L., Ford, M. E., Houtz, J. M., Karthikeyan, T., Wadsworth, C., Lewis, J. A., et al. (2003). Origins of highly mosaic mycobacteriophage genomes. *Cell*, *113*, 171–182.

Polman, J. (1999). *Designing Project-Based Science: Connecting Learners through Guided Inquiry.* New York: Teachers College Press.

Raviglione, M. C. (2003). The TB epidemic from 1992 to 2002. *Tuberculosis (Edinb)*, *83*, 4–14.

Reeves, T. (2000). Alternative assessment approaches for online learning environments in higher education. *Journal of Educational Computing Research*, *23*(1), 101–111.

Reeves, T., & Okey, J. (1996). Alternative assessment for constructivist learning environments. In B. Wilson (Ed.), *Constructivist Learning Environments: Case Studies in Instructional Design* (pp. 191–202). Englewood Cliffs: Educational Technology Publications.

Roberts, R., & Gott, R. (2003). Assessment of biology investigations. *Journal of Biological Education*, *37*(3), 114–121.

Roberts, R., & Richard, G. (2003). Assessment of biology investigations. *Journal of Biological Education*, *37*(3), 114–121.

Roth, W. (1995). *Authentic Science: Knowing and Learning in Open Inquiry Science Laboratories.* Dordrecht: Kluwer.

Ruiz-Primo, M. A., Li, M., & Shavelson, R. J. (2002). Looking into students' science notebooks: What do teachers do with them? (CSE Technical Report 562). Los Angeles, CA: Center for the Study of Evaluation, National Center for Research on Evaluation, Standards, and Student Testing, University of California, Los Angeles.

Sambell, K., McDowell, L., & Brown, S. (1997). But is it fair? An exploratory study of student perceptions of the consequential validity of assessment. *Studies in Educational Evaluation*, *23*, 349–371.

Shavelson, R., Baxter, G., & Pine, J. (1992). Performance assessments: Political rhetoric and measurement reality. *Educational Researcher*, *21*(4), 22–27.

Shavelson, R., Solano-Flores, G., & Araceli Ruiz-Primo, M. (1998). Toward a science performance assessment technology. *Evaluation and Programming Planning*, *21*, 171–184.

Shymansky, J., Chidsey, J., Henriquez, L., Enger, S., Yore, L., Wolfe, E., et al. (1997). Performance assessment in science as a tool to enhance the picture of student learning. *School Science and Mathematics*, *97*, 172–183.

Solano-Flores, G., & Shavelson, R. J. (1997). Development of performance assessments in science: Conceptual, practical and logistical issues. *Educational Measurement: Issues and Practice*, *16*(3), 16–25.

Solano-Flores, G., Jovanovic, J., Shavelson, R., & Bachman, M. (1999). On the development of a shell for generating science performance assessments. *International Journal of Science Education*, *21*(3), 293–315.

Stenmark, J. (1991). *Mathematics Assessment: Myths, Models, Good Questions and Practical Suggestions.* Reston, VA: National Council of Teachers of Mathematics.

Strobel, S. A., & Strobel, G. A. (2007). Plant endophytes as a platform for discovery-based undergraduate science education. *Nature Chem. Biol.*, *3*, 356–359.

Tamir, P., & Lunetta, V. N. (1978). Analysis of the laboratoryinquiries in the third edition of the BSCS yellow version. *American Biology Teacher*, *40*(6), 353–357.

Tamir, P., & Lunetta, V. N. (1981). Inquiry related tasks in high school science laboratory handbooks. *Science Education*, *65*(5), 477–484.

Torrance, H. (1995). Introduction. In H. Torrance (Ed.), *Evaluating Authentic Assessment: Problems and Possibilities in New Approaches to Assessment* (pp. 1–8). Buckingham: Open University Press.

Udovic, D., Morris, D., Dickman, A., Postlethwait, J., & Wetherwax, P. (2002). Workshop biology: Demonstrating the effectiveness of active learning in an introductory biology course. *BioScience*, *52*, 272–281.

Welford, G., Harlen, W., & Schofield, B. (1985). *Practical Testing at Ages 11, 13 and 15.* London: Department of Education and Science.

Wenger, E. (1998). *Communities of Practice: Learning, Meaning and Identity.* New York: Cambridge University Press.

Wenning, C. (2007). Assessing inquiry skills as a component of scientific literacy. *Journal of Physics Education Online*, *4*(2), 21–24.

Wenning, C. (2005). Levels of inquiry: Hierarchies of pedagogical practices and inquiry processes. *Journal of Physics Teacher Education Online*, *2*(3), 3–11.
White, R., & Gunstone, R. (1992). *Probing Understanding.* London: Falmer Press.
Whitman, W. B., Coleman, D. C., & Wiebe, W. J. (1998). Prokaryotes: the unseen majority. *Proceedings of the National Academy of Sciences of the United States of America*, *95*, 6578–6583.
Wiggins, G. (1993). *Assessing Student Performance.* San Francisco: Jossey-Bass.
Wiggins, G. (1990). *The Case for Authentic Assessment.* Washington, DC.: Eric Clearing House.
Williams, S., & Hmelo, C. (1998). Guest editors' intorduction. *The Journal of Learning Sciences*, *7*, 265–270.
Wommack, K. E., & Colwell, R. R. (2000). Virioplankton: viruses in aquatic ecosystems. *Microbiology and Molecular Biology Reviews*, *64*, 69–114.
Young, M. (1995). Assessment of situated learning using computer environments. *Journal of Science Education and Technology*, *4*(1), 89–96.
Zachos, P. (2004). Pendulum phenomena and the assessment of scientific inquiry capabilities. *Science and Education*, *13*, 743–756.
Zachos, P., Hick, T. L., Doanne, W. E., & Sargent, C. (2000). Setting theoretical and empirical foundations for assessing scientific inquiry and discovery in educational programs. *Journal of Research in Science Teaching*, *37*(9), 938–962.

Index

Note: The locators with the letters '*f*' and '*t*' refers to figures and tables respectively

I

K

L

M

N

P

Color Plates

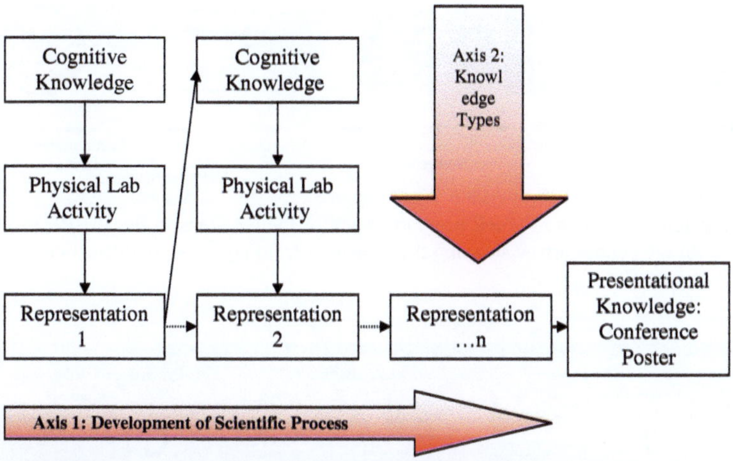

Fig. 2.2 A Schematic Representation of the Scientific Inquiry Process

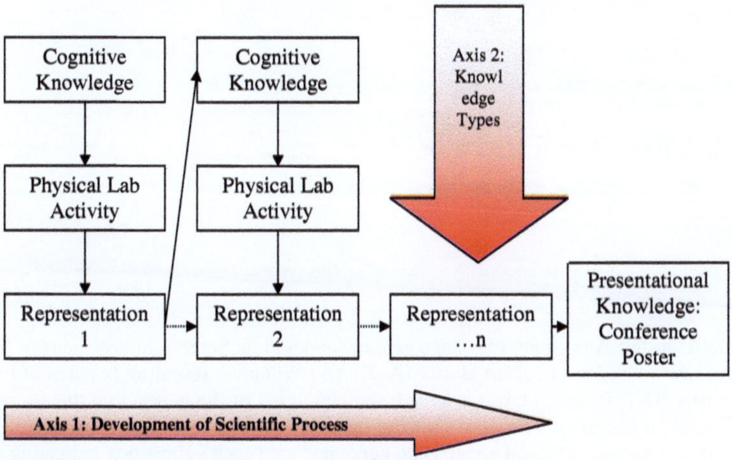

Fig. 5.2 A schematic representation of the scientific inquiry process

Color Plates

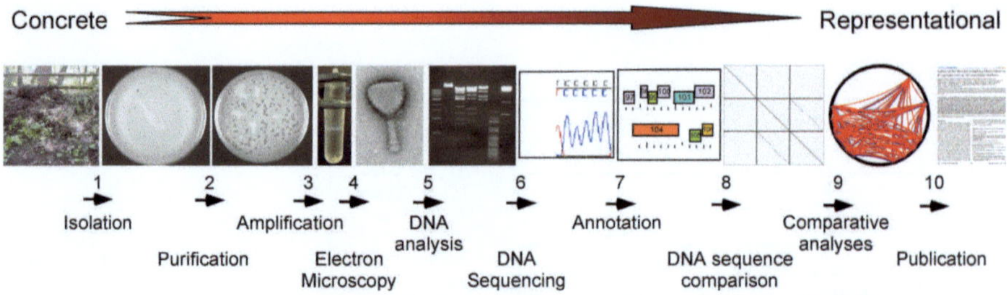

Fig. 6.3 The ten steps of the PHIRE program. Each of the ten steps in the PHIRE program are illustrated with the central arrow showing the transition from concrete to abstract comprehension from step 1 to step 10

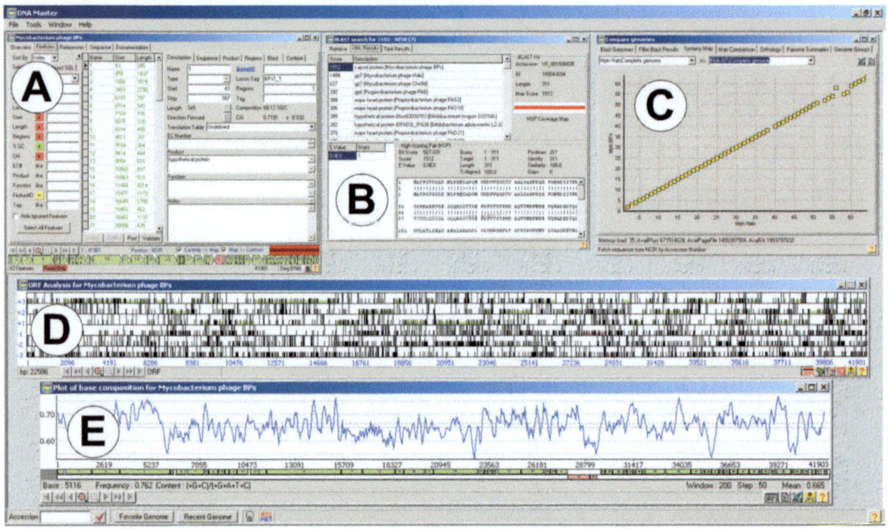

Fig. 6.6 DNAMaster: A program for phage genome annotation. Screen shots are shown from several representative windows of DNAMaster (**A–E**). (**A**) Window presenting features of mycobacteriophage BPs. The "Feature" tab is selected, showing a list of the genes with their coordinates. (**B**) The "Compare Genomes" window showing the results of a BlastP search of phage BPs gp7. (**C**) Comparison of phage BPs and phage Halo genomes, with each yellow box indicating the position of genes that are shared between the two genomes. (**D**) The "Frames" window showing the positions of stop and start codons in all six reading frames. The positions of identified opening reading frames are colored either *green* (forward direction) or *red* (reverse direction). (**E**) Plot of base composition showing the average GC% content across the BPs genome. These represent just a small subset of the available functions with DNAMaster (available as a free download from http://cobamide2.bio.pitt.edu)

Color Plates

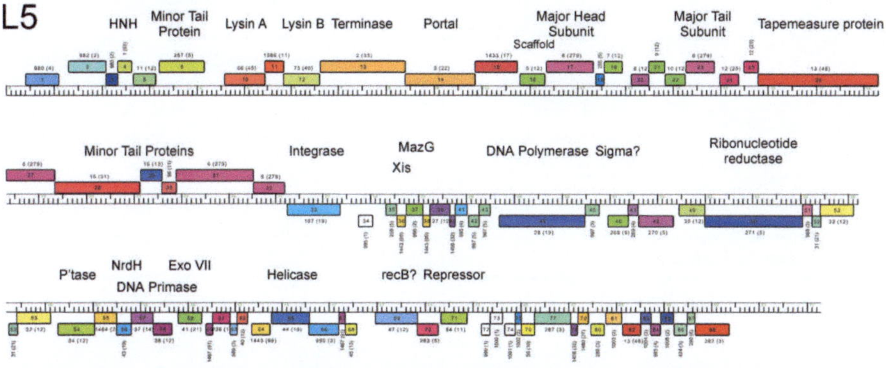

Fig. 6.8 Genome map of mycobacteriophage L5. The L5 genome is represented as a *horizontal bar* with markers spaced at 1 kbp intervals. Each of the predicted genes is shown as a colored box either above or below the genome; those above are transcribed rightward, and those below are transcribed leftward. The map was generated by the program Phamerator, which sorts the predicted genes into phamilies (Phams) as functions of their predicted amino acid sequence relatedness. The Pham number is shown above each gene with the number of Pham members in parentheses, and each gene is colored according to its Pham. Some of the predict gene functions are noted

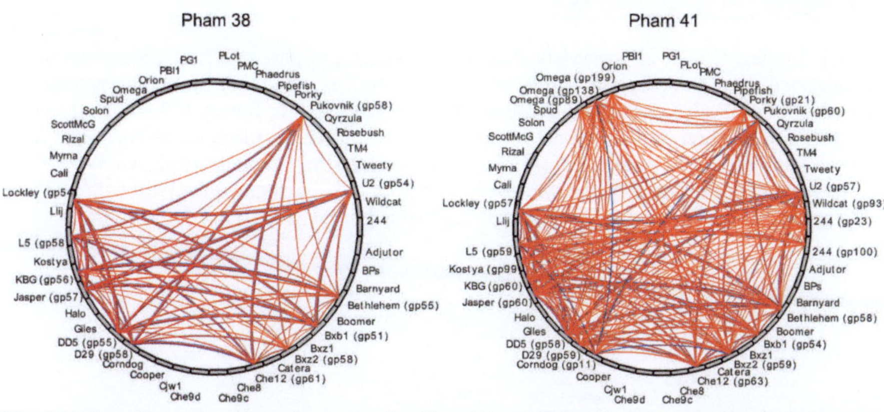

Fig. 6.9 Phamily circles. Phamily circles for Pham38 and Pham41 are shown. In the L5 genome (see Fig. 6.8), genes 58 and 59 are members of these two Phams, respectively, and the phamily circles suggest that they have distinct and different evolutionary histories. Each of the phages is listed around the circumference of each circle and an arc is drawn between members of each phamily with line thickness corresponding to strength of the relationship

Color Plates

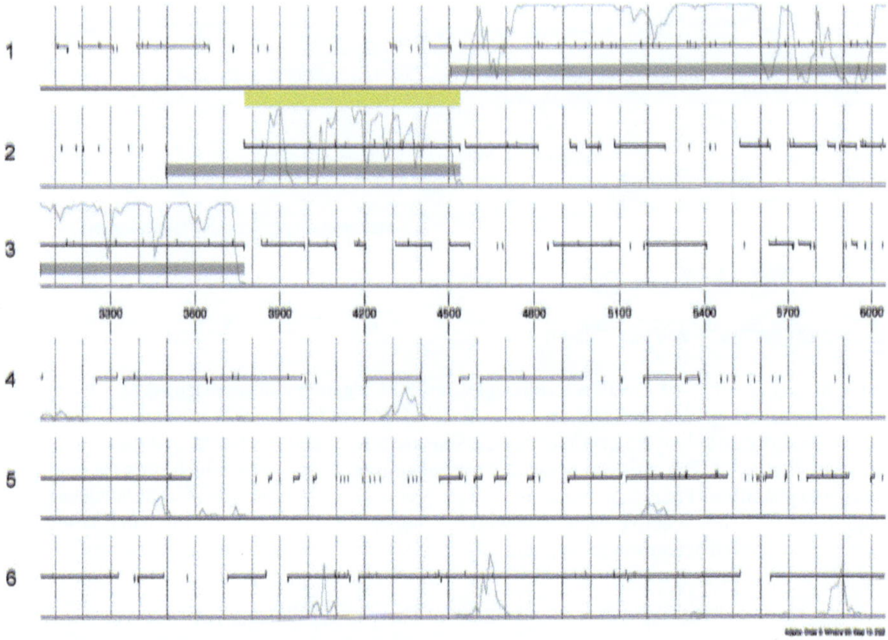

Fig. 7.1 Graphic Output of GeneMark Program. A segment of phage Adjutor genome sequence was analyzed using the program GeneMark, which generates a graph of the coding potential in each of the six possible open reading frames (ORFs) (labeled 1–6; frames 1–3 are expressed in the rightward direction, and 4–6 in the reverse direction). ORFs are identified as *horizontal lines* between translation stop codons (*down ticks*), and potential start codons are shown as *up ticks*. Coding potential is indicated by the line graph. The thick horizontal gray lines (still italicized) are considered areas of interest. One such gene is highlighted in *green*

Color Plates

Microbial Genomes

```
GLIMMER (ver. 3.02; iterated) predictions:
 orfID          start       end  frame   score
--------        -----     -----   --     -----
>Adjutor
orf00001           43       309   +1      5.50
orf00002          421      1524   +1     11.60
orf00003         1568      1762   +2      7.44
orf00004         1772      1936   +2     19.55
orf00005         1946      2125   +2      2.27
orf00006         2136      3776   +3      9.08
orf00008         3773      4543   +2      7.48
orf00010         4540      6306   +1     13.68
orf00011         6328      7914   +1     15.10
orf00012         7925      8137   +2      8.51
orf00013         8134      8586   +1      6.27
orf00014         8555      8734   +2      9.56
orf00015         8822      9067   +2      1.62
orf00016         9235      9636   +1      6.98
orf00017         9669     10376   +3     10.88
orf00019        10392     10811   +3     10.24
orf00020        10848     12032   +3     12.62
orf00022        12029     12397   +2     12.81
orf00023        12400     12732   +1      7.05
orf00024        12729     13136   +3      7.45
orf00025        13129     13491   +1      8.23
orf00026        13488     13907   +3      5.12
orf00027        13944     14300   +3      8.89
orf00028        14312     14512   +2      4.14
orf00029        14541     15344   +3      9.78
orf00030        15426     16079   +3     10.30
orf00032        16102     16320   +1      8.00
orf00034        16322     21094   +2     10.80
orf00036        21084     22604   +3     14.22
orf00038        22601     24256   +2     12.44
orf00039        24256     26526   +1     13.24
orf00040        26526     28574   +3     11.64
orf00043        28574     29440   +2      4.49
orf00044        29450     29770   +2     11.76
orf00046        29773     30201   +1      4.90
orf00048        30210     31193   +3     10.50
orf00049        31190     31444   +2      7.17
orf00051        31715     32254   +2      2.39
orf00053        32238     32693   +3      6.68
```

Fig. 7.2 Glimmer Program Output. A segment of the phage Adjutor genome sequence was analyzed by Glimmer generating a list of potential ORFs, their start and stop codons, reading frame, and evaluative score. The *red box* designates one specific candidate gene

Color Plates

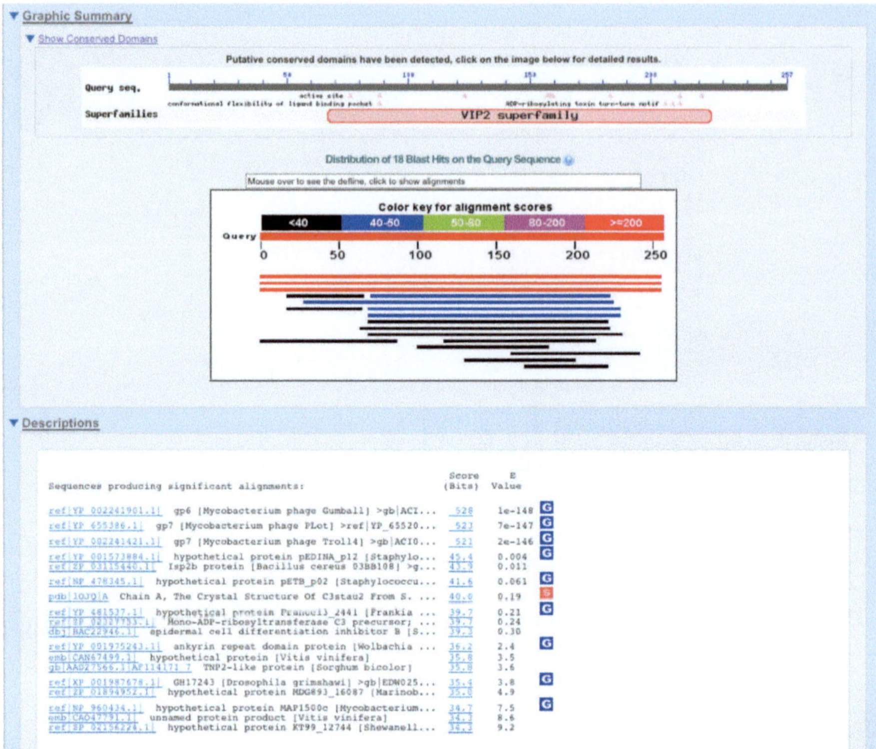

Fig. 7.3 Output of a BLASTP search using the BLAST server at NCBI. The amino acid sequence of a predicted phage protein was submitted as a search query to the server, which returned a summary of the search results; a screen shot of the results window is shown. At the *top*, a diagram shows the correspondence of a putative conserved domain identified in the search with a linear representation of the query sequence. Below that is a diagram of related sequences identified in the search, with the closest matches shown in *red*. The identities of the specific matches and their scores are shown in the *bottom panel*

Color Plates

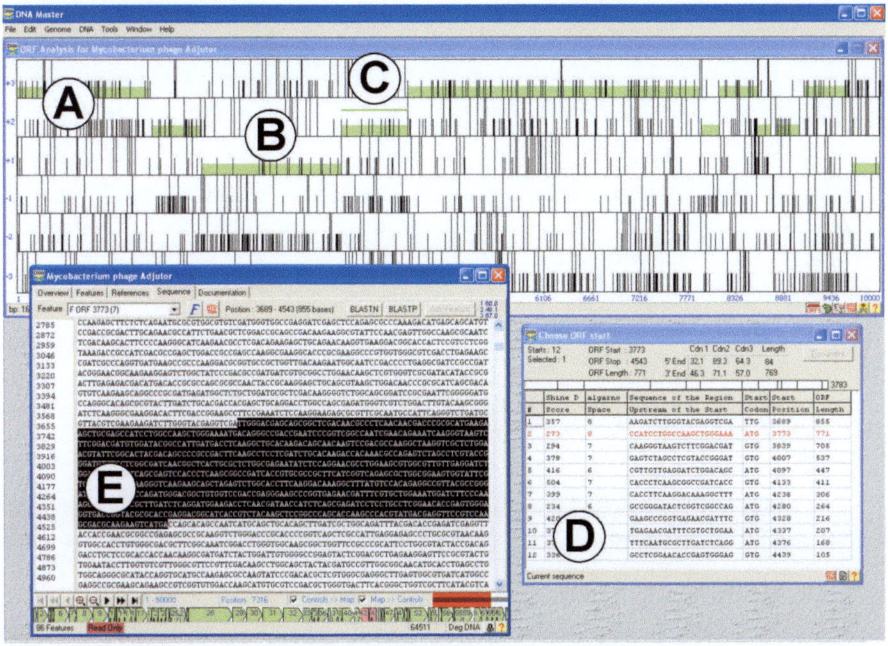

Fig. 7.4 Representations of genome analyses using DNA Master. (**A**) The output from the "Frames" routine in DNA Master showing six reading frames, with start (*short vertical lines*) and stop codons (*full height lines*) indicated. (**B**) ORFs with strong prediction for coding potential predicted by GenMark and Glimmer are designated by a *thick green horizontal line*. (**C**) Clicking on a segment of a frame of interest produces a *thin green* line and also links to the "choose start" routine shown in (**D**) the ORF and start codon corresponding to the frame segment in (**C**) is in *red*. (4). (**E**) The genome segment highlighted in (**C**) is revealed as a selected segment (black background) in the "Sequence" panel of DNA Master, and can be added to the annotation or copied as either a nucleotide or a translated amino acid sequence for BLAST analyses

Color Plates

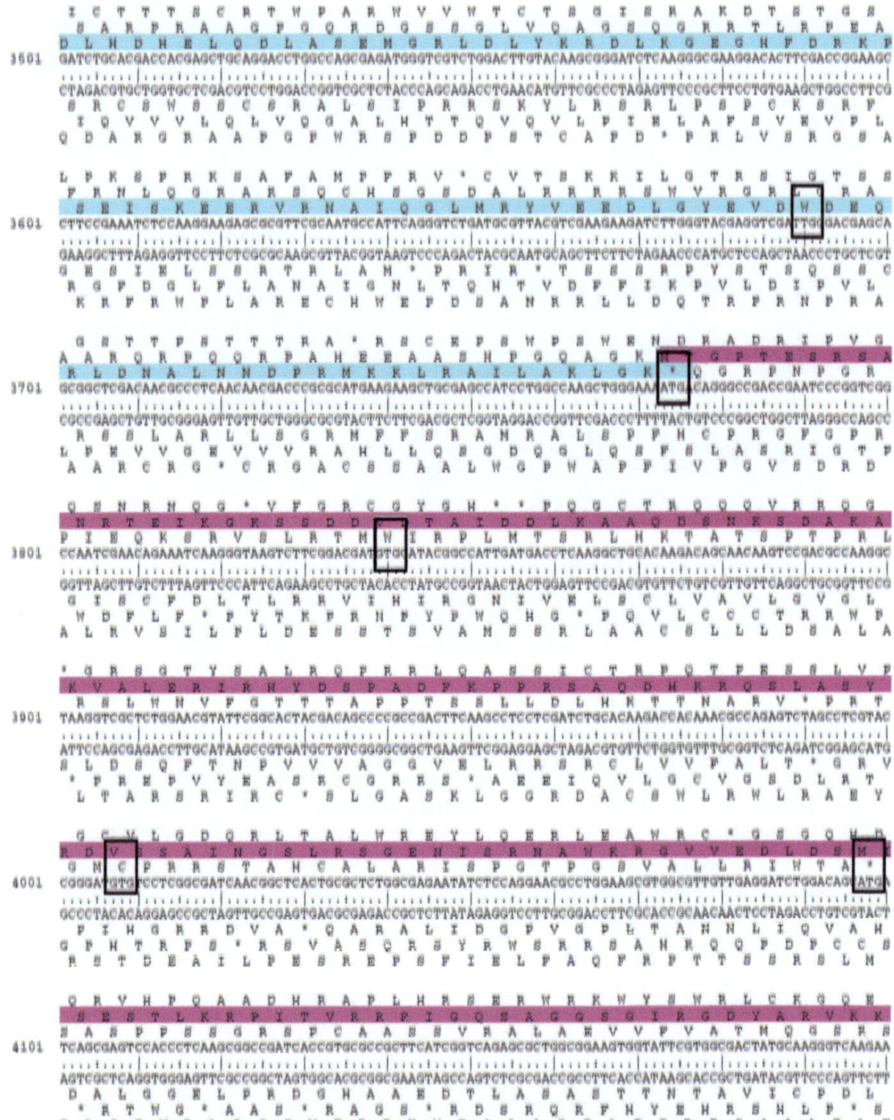

Fig. 7.5 Six-frame translation of a phage genome segment. DNAMaster provides an output showing the DNA sequence of both strands as well the amino acid sequences in each of the potential six reading frames. The amino acid sequences of the potential ORFs predicted by Glimmer and GenMark are colored. Each of the potential start codons shown in Fig. 7.4E (and within this DNA segment) are shown *boxed*

MIX
Papier aus verantwortungsvollen Quellen
Paper from responsible sources
FSC® C105338

If you have any concerns about our products,
you can contact us on
ProductSafety@springernature.com

In case Publisher is established outside the EU,
the EU authorized representative is:
Springer Nature Customer Service Center GmbH
Europaplatz 3, 69115 Heidelberg, Germany

Printed by Libri Plureos GmbH
in Hamburg, Germany